Staying Well in a Toxic World

Staying Well in a Toxic World

Understanding Environmental Illness, Multiple Chemical Sensitivities, Chemical Injuries, and Sick Building Syndrome

Lynn Lawson

Foreword by Theron G. Randolph, MD

The Noble Press, Inc.

CHICAGO

Library of Congress Cataloguing-in-Publication Data

Lawson, Lynn, 1925–
    Staying well in a toxic world : understanding environmental illness,
    multiple chemical sensitivities, chemical injuries, and sick building
    syndrome / Lynn Lawson : foreword by Theron G. Randolph, MD.
    488 p. cm.
    Includes bibliographical references and index.
    ISBN 1-879360-33-0 : $15.95
    1. Environmentally induced diseases.   2. Sick building syndrome.
    3. Chemicals—Health aspects.   4. Environmental health.   I. Title.
    RB152.L385 1994 1993
    616.9'8—dc20   94-13962
                                                    CIP

Noble Press books are available in bulk at discount prices. Single copies are
available prepaid direct from the publisher.

The Noble Press, Inc.
213 W. Institute Place, Suite 508
Chicago, Illinois 60610
(312) 642-1168

The material in this book is for information only and is not to be construed as medical advice, which should be obtained from your licensed medical practitioner.
Companies and products are listed for information only and not as recommendation.
Names of persons interviewed have been changed or deleted. Additional documentation is available on request.

To all who are as sick as I was without
knowing the cause.

Contents

Foreword by Theron G. Randolph, MD 9

Acknowledgments 13

Introduction: Notes from a Human Canary 15

Chapter 1: Your Allergies, My Headaches, Our Problem 31

Chapter 2: Breathing Easier? 59

Chapter 3: Warning: Your Job May Be Hazardous 99
to Your Health

Chapter 4: Warning: Your Home May Be Hazardous 133
to Your Health

Chapter 5: In and Under the Rug 167

Chapter 6: Why We Are So Well Preserved 187

Chapter 7: Which Pesticides Are Safe: 205
Fighting the Deadly Dandelion

Chapter 8: Factory Food 241

Chapter 9: Skunk Mail and Other Invasions 277
of Personal Airspace

Chapter 10: Who Is Most at Risk 299

Chapter 11: Recourse 323

Chapter 12: Shooting Arrows at the Storm: 357
What Is Wrong with Modern Medicine

Chapter 13: How Good Is Green: 393
We the Endangered Species

Chapter 14: Riders on the Earth Together 415

Afterword: Who Is Most to Blame 431

Appendix: An EPA Epiphany 435

Glossary: The Players: Who's Who and What's What 439

Notes 443

Index 481

Foreword

WHEN LYNN LAWSON walked into my clinic in 1986, I had no idea that seven years later she would know more about the illness now called environmental illness/multiple chemical sensitivities (EI/MCS) than any other nonmedical person I know. In those years she has not only improved her own health drastically, but has educated herself about the health effects of the derivatives of gas, oil, and coal to an extent that enabled her to complete the best-written and best-documented book on EI/MCS done so far for the lay reader.

Though her book is as up-to-the-minute as possible, much remains to be learned about this illness and its causes. We don't know, for instance, why the man who works in a filling station and the woman who sprays synthetic perfume on herself every day don't seem bothered by their chemical exposures. We don't know why some workers can clean out tank cars seemingly without ill effect, while others doing the same thing can, ever afterwards, have a serious problem with chemicals. The difference may be genetic, but if so, we don't know the modus operandi.

We do know that EI/MCS is mediated by nonimmunologic mechanisms (antigens or antibodies are not commonly involved), but we don't know which mechanisms to blame. To the best of my knowledge, there have been no scientifically oriented investigative efforts to find out. We do know, also, that the degree of exposure is important. Exposure at a given level will hit one person out of ten,

but not nine out of ten. Exposure at a threefold increase will probably hit three out of ten instead of one out of ten. Exposure is a dose-
related curve. Though we don't have hard evidence of this, our
experience with thousands of patients makes this relationship clear.
With this illness, "hard" evidence is hard to come by. There are too
many chemicals, too many exposures, too many environmental factors, and too many individual differences for the customary randomized, double-blind, controlled tests (of usually only one
variable) to be conclusive. Instead, clinical evidence has to be the
touchstone. This book presents dozens of personal stories typical of
the clinical evidence that environmental physicians are all too familiar with.

Despite the paucity of controlled, double-blind studies of
EI/MCS, what is becoming clear is that millions of the residents of
the world are in jeopardy as far as their health is concerned. The
more developed the country, the greater the jeopardy. So our jeopardy in the U.S. is greater than that of someone living in Peru, for
instance, where the population density is much less, the pollution is
less, and the cleansing winds from the Pacific are prevalent. In the
developed countries, millions of people are chronically ill from
chemicals in the environment and don't know why, and the medical
profession is still not recognizing the connection with any degree of
accuracy.

In fact, if technology continues racing ahead as it has been, it is
conceivable that everyone will eventually develop this illness to
some degree. We need to slow this process, or the human race is
going to be impaired to the point where it will not be productive, or
as productive as if we had not had these exposures. We're bringing
up a younger generation in the public schools who are chemically
sensitive before they get out of school. Some children have so much
sensitivity that they are not educable; other children become sensitized before they even get to school.

That's why this book is so important. It tells the reader how we
got where we are today, environmentally and medically. It tells
what our government is doing and not doing to protect our health.
Urgent and compelling, it will stir up action at the patient level. The
chronically ill who read it will bug their doctors; and if the doctors
don't listen, the patients will change doctors. Already millions of

Americans, impatient with their traditional doctors' lack of success with the chronic diseases so common today, are turning to better nutrition and alternative practitioners. Medical school teaching is slowly being passed by, and doctors are beginning to realize the need to take the environment into their thinking. This change can come none too soon.

Theron G. Randolph, MD
President, Human Ecology Research Foundation
700 West Fabyan Parkway #1103-F
Batavia, Illinois 60510

Acknowledgments

THIS BOOK WOULD NOT have been written, nor would I have gotten better, without the help of Court, my husband of thirty-five years. Unfailingly he accepted my illness and believed that it really existed—the single most important thing that anyone can do for the chemically injured. When I felt most miserable, he held my hand, filled ice bags for me, and stood by while I dunked my head in ice water. After I got better and began writing this book, he ran countless errands to free up my time, made photocopies, brought home books from the library, and read many articles on EI/MCS. He also read (and painstakingly edited) every chapter and every footnote.

My gratitude also goes to Steve Bates, who encouraged me at every step and who did a thorough and thoughtful editing of several chapters. Both Steve and Court graciously allowed me to talk endlessly on this most absorbing (to me) subject. Others who read chapters and commented helpfully on them were Julie Accola, Marjorie Fisher, Beatrice Trum Hunter, Judy Juers, Bill Kaplan, Jim Kepler, and my cousin Lee Valentine. Andy Fisher and Nancy Liskar provided invaluable help at crucial moments. I am grateful to my friends at the Noble Press—David Driver, Doug Seibold, Mary Jean Jones, Denise Lewis, Kristin Field, and especially my skillful and tactful editor, Julia Bogardus. Thanks to Kathleen Flaherty, Phil Franchine, and Kay McCarty for their moral support. I also offer my love and gratitude to the other members of my EI/MCS support group, who, like me, have suffered not only from the illness itself but from others' disbelief and denial. It was the thought of our shared suffering and our mutual need to make our stories known that kept me going to the final sentence.

Introduction:
Notes from a Human Canary

IN SEPTEMBER 1987 a group of us were sitting in saunas in a Los Angeles detoxification clinic to try to rid our bodies of unwanted toxic chemicals. We came from many places and varied backgrounds. We had all been poisoned. Each of us carried a toxic load from the thousands of synthetic chemical compounds introduced into our environment since World War II. Most of these compounds have been derived from petrochemicals or coal tar. The large majority are untested for chronic human health effects. New synthetic chemical compounds continue to be added to this arsenal at the rate of over one thousand every year.

Several men in the group were firefighters suffering from an acute exposure to polychlorinated biphenyls (PCBs) while fighting a hospital fire. One woman (I'll call her Annemarie), from a small city ringed by mountains, had had multiple exposures to pesticides and more recent exposures to paint and other pollutants at her workplace. Tom, a young, lean, muscular professional golfer, had been incapacitated by pesticides on golf courses. Julia had been poisoned by formaldehyde in her house. Ironically, her husband is a building contractor. Valerie, exquisitely sensitive to chemicals, often sat in the sauna holding an ice pack to her jaw to relieve the intense pain. Her problem was thought to be caused in part by old silver/mercury amalgam fillings, removed but, unfortunately, replaced with other toxic substances that her dentist had not adequately tested for compatibility before placing in her mouth. Roger, a tall, tanned, handsome actor and former television star, had become chemically sensitive from pesticide spraying in his apartment building. The pesticide company, we heard, was paying for his detoxification.

Carl, another young, good-looking actor, sat in the sauna reading books on acting, saying nothing about his symptoms or their cause. George, a youthful executive, was equally mysterious. His company's defense contracts seemed implicated in his condition. Linda, a grade-school teacher, was apparently made ill by her school's heating system, and Anne, another teacher, was disabled by her school's use of a pesticide containing dioxin. Al, a Vietnam veteran, was thought to be suffering from dioxin exposure. Juanita had been exposed to sprayed produce during a stay in Italy, though her primary problem, candidiasis (an overgrowth of the yeast *Candida albicans* that we all carry in our bodies), had weakened her to the extent that she would be unable to continue the detoxification. Mollie, a social worker, was so chemically sensitive that in her parents' house she could sit on only one chair—an untreated wooden one. She reacted to the paints, stains, and fabrics on the other chairs. Don, a housepainter, could no longer work with paint. Several other people—a teenaged girl, her mother, two chiropractors and the girl friend of one—completed the group during my stay. Most were young; the oldest were in their sixties. Except for Juanita, we all looked healthy.

What is this program that attempts to lessen the body's burden of its bioaccumulation of toxic materials? Begun in the late 1970s, it was originally developed to help people damaged by so-called recreational drug use. By the mid-1980s the program had been expanded to include the chemically sensitive—those diagnosed with multiple chemical sensitivities, also known as environmental or ecological illness, twentieth-century disease, or chemical injury.

Megan Shields, MD, a family physician with a large Los Angeles practice, medically supervised the clinic, called HealthMed, then located in a converted health club. R. Michael Wisner, a largely self-educated toxicologist, managed HealthMed's day-to-day operation and the staff, which consisted of a nurse, nurse's aides, and patient supervisors specially trained in the detoxification program.

During our stays at HealthMed, which could last from two to

eight weeks of usually consecutive days at the facility, we were given extensive tests by the staff—physicals, blood and hair analyses for the presence of toxins, fat biopsies, eye tests, intelligence tests (to measure any changes), and so on. For us patients, each day began with an interview by a supervisor, who took our pulse and blood pressure and questioned us about how we had fared over the evening. The supervisor decided whether or not to increase our dose of niacin (one of the B vitamins), which we then took before heading off for a brisk half-hour walk or jog on Los Angeles sidewalks. The niacin "mobilizes" some of the toxins stored in the body fat and releases them into the blood stream. The exercise stimulates the body to excrete the toxins through the sweat glands and the gut, and that is how the program works.

Once back in the building, we immediately changed into swim suits, weighed ourselves, showered, and began our first sauna of the day. Each of us entered one of the building's three saunas carrying towels and balancing on our clipboards a carefully measured glass of filtered water and an estimated quantity of sodium and potassium pills to replenish our bodies' supplies of these nutrients. After up to thirty minutes in the sauna, spent talking, reading, filling in the elaborate daily records we kept on our clipboards, or playing cards in sometimes desperate attempts to pass the time, we again showered and spent a few minutes on cedar benches in the cool-down area. Then into the sauna again, for a daily total of as much as 180 sauna-minutes. Though the staff sometimes provided platters of colorful, crunchy vegetables, we were expected to bring our own lunches and to keep to our own usual diets.

At the end of each sauna day, we again weighed ourselves and saw our supervisor—for pulse and blood pressure, a measured dose of oil to replace the fat lost by the body during the day, and our vitamin and mineral supplements for the evening. With the supervisor we discussed our daily record of any adverse reactions to food or saunas, any changes in sleep patterns, and any external or psychological pressures that might be interfering with the treatment. We especially mentioned any symptoms—known in HealthMed talk as "manifestations"—occurring during or after the saunas. Manifestations were important, for they meant that the toxins, back in the bloodstream from their resting place in our body fat, were once again making us sick. As one thing that could add to our total body burden was synthetic scents of any kind, scented products were banned at the clinic. If a person wearing a scented product happened to enter the building, the staff diplomatically handled the offender.

Though well supervised, the program was stressful for most patients—away from home, family, and friends, living in musty, heavily scented motel rooms on a busy, four-lane street. Some of us suffered severe manifestations, such as a full-day's diarrhea or an eight-hour headache. During my thirty-one consecutive days in the saunas I suffered six ghastly headaches, which began toward the end of my daily saunas, leaving me unable to eat, read, talk, or even watch television, barely able to get to the motel's ice machine to fill my ice bag. By morning they were gone, mercifully. At first the staff wanted me to go back in the sauna after the headache started, so that I could continue sweating out the toxins. Later, after they saw that doing so only aggravated my misery, they concluded that I was one of a few patients who "did not fit the pattern," and they recommended that I not stay in the sauna for the full thirty minutes, but leave at the first hint of head pain. Thus I logged in less sauna time than most, but still felt certain that I was getting rid of some toxins down the clinic's drains.

Not all was grim at the clinic, however. Friendships and camaraderie developed easily among people who had experienced similar ordeals—years of pain, bewilderment, and misdiagnosis by doctors who had never been trained to search for the ultimate causes of our illness. Instead, we had been poked, prodded, and bled, given expensive and sophisticated tests and a variety of symptom-masking drugs, many doing more harm than good. Illnesses like ours often involve several organ systems, can produce a variety of symptoms, and seldom show up on conventional medical tests. Many of us had been told "it's all in your mind" and referred to psychotherapy; those who took this advice usually found they remained just as sick. Though the staff discouraged us from talking about our illnesses because they thought it might depress us, we nevertheless did a lot of therapeutic sharing. Jokes and funny stories abounded. We were travelers together.

The Chemical Buildup

How did I become chemically sensitive? I am now in my sixties. My first seventeen years were spent in a tiny farming town in southern Wisconsin, at a time when farmers fertilized fields with manure, not chemicals. There were no petroleum-based pesticides: flyswatters or sticky pest strips caught flies. Housewives washed clothes with soap, not detergents. Synthetic fabrics, except for rayon, did not exist; there was no "need" for fabric softeners. Women wore cotton or, rarely, silk stockings. Perfumes were made from flowers, medications mostly from plants. My teeth were poor; a local dentist put in the first of many fillings, probably silver/mercury amalgams. I remember playing, fascinated, with the mercury from a broken thermometer. At twelve I had my first classical migraine (headache preceded by a visual disturbance called an "aura"—in my case flashing zigzag lights lasting up to a half hour and gradually filling half of my vision). Except for the usual childhood diseases and an occasional headache of this type, I was reasonably healthy and remained so through four years of college in a small Wisconsin industrial city, where I was a chemistry major at the beginning of the chemical revolution.

In 1946 I moved to Hyde Park, on Chicago's South Side. There I spent many hours on the 55th Street promontory, excited by the dramatic contrast between the Loop skyscrapers on my left, the scrubber-less smokestacks of Gary and Hammond on my right, and ever-changing Lake Michigan in front of me. This was surely the best of both worlds, I thought—manmade and natural. Later, after I bought my first car, in 1953, driving with open windows through Gary and Hammond also excited me. Clichés flowed through my manipulated mind like pollutants through the Little Calumet River: "America's industrial might," "the industrial heartland," "city of the big shoulders." Though I hadn't yet heard of Ayn Rand, I was thinking like her. She is the conservative author who said, during the environmental movement of the late 1960s, that we should go down on our knees daily and thank God for belching smokestacks. Years later, I would remember that one of the smelly, belching smokestacks I passed on my way to work belonged to Argo, a major corn product company.

In the fall of 1947 I worked briefly for Marshall Field's department store in Chicago's Loop. As Christmas approached, I became very aware of the pungent odor from the store's elaborate Christmas decorations—probably fireproofing of some sort. From 1948 to 1954 I worked in an office surrounded by chemistry laboratories, where negative air pressure was carefully maintained in order to prevent radioactive and other substances from escaping. My teeth required more dental work—bridges, root canal work, and more "silver" fillings. My classical migraines recurred; since then I have had perhaps one a year. In addition, however, I began to have fairly severe aura-less headaches, about one or two a month.

From 1955 to 1956 I worked at the Art Institute of Chicago, where walls were usually painted before each new exhibit. The following year I moved to a suburb, where I have lived ever since. Just before and after my marriage in 1959, I painted, stained, or refinished over sixty pieces of furniture, often working in cramped, inadequately ventilated areas. (Who takes those label warnings seriously!) For a year and a half I worked for a major pharmaceutical company, where I walked from the train stop to my office building amid clouds of chemicals. The building was old and had windows that opened, letting in the fumes; my non-aura headaches worsened. Once, miserable with pain and nausea and thinking my condition caused by stress, I drank a beer "to relax," and felt much worse. Another time, after taking a mild tranquilizer "to relax," I drank a martini . . . and discovered that alcohol and tranquilizers don't mix. Together they were poisonous.

In the summer of 1961 my husband and I bought our present home at a time when the spraying of elm trees with pesticides (to curb Dutch elm disease) was in full swing. The spraying was not always successful, and we often awoke to the sound of saws. That summer I found several dying robins in our yard. I brought one into our house, hoping to revive it, to no avail; the next year, after reading Rachel Carson's *Silent Spring,* I began to realize what had killed them. That same year I stopped smoking; I had been a pack-a-day smoker for sixteen years.

The sixties moved on. My own awareness of environmental issues was slowly awakening; not so my awareness of toxicity in humans, or of how potentially hazardous were even my own personal routines. Almost daily, I treated my continuing headaches with Fiorinal, a potent prescription drug containing phenacetin (now suspected of causing kidney damage). My then-internist also recommended buffered (aluminum-containing) aspirin, which I bought in bottles of five hundred. Though I switched to hypoallergenic cosmetics (I had discovered a severe allergy to orrisroot, a common ingredient in cosmetics and potpourri), I continued to use perfume: after all, one is not completely dressed without a squirt of some highly touted scent. I welcomed the new synthetic fabrics that soon dominated the market: cotton/polyester sheets and easy-care, no-iron clothes washed in miracle-white detergents and no-cling fabric softeners all seemed the housewife's best friend. The miracle of modern chemistry had arrived.

In 1970, having become an ardent environmentalist, I felt fortunate to be able to teach several sections of a special freshman composition course on environment and population at a local university. My enthusiastic students wrote term papers on subjects ranging from the U.S. Bureau of Land Reclamation's depredations to the dangers from auto pollution to the harmful effects of pesticides. Yet I failed to connect my headaches with these issues. In the mid-1970s our house received its only (to our knowledge) indoor spraying of pesticides; in the mid-1980s we had several trees sprayed for cottony maple disease.

After I began full-time work in offices housed in new, tightly constructed buildings, with nearby copy machines, wall-to-wall carpeting, and sealed windows, my headaches worsened. Danger had moved indoors. Finally I went to a well-publicized Chicago headache clinic, where extensive testing failed to reveal anything organically wrong. There, with visits every three months, I was treated with a succession of prescription drugs, including Cafergot, Periactin, Migral, Midrin, Darvocet, Inderal, Decadron, and Miltown. None helped very much. Each time I went to the headache clinic, which was usually packed with sufferers, a nurse ushered me into an examining room, took my blood pressure, and asked a few questions. When the doctor finally came in, he would smile, shake my hand perfunctorily, look at what the nurse had written, and ask, "I've helped you, haven't I?" Foolishly, always the obedient patient,

I would reply "Yes." Whereupon he would continue or change the prescription, smile again, and leave the room.

After seven years of this, I asked my present internist, Dr. William D. Kerr, Jr., if he would try to help me with my headaches. He prescribed Verapamil, a calcium channel blocker. It helped for a while, but had bad side effects. Finally, it stopped helping, my body apparently having developed a tolerance for it.

At last, working in an office with windows that opened, I was happier. However, I was increasingly bothered by odors of newsprint and cleaning solutions, and by other people's tobacco smoke, perfumes, shampoos, deodorants, and other cosmetic products. The office copier was in a small, unventilated room, and for a while the old stove in the building basement leaked carbon monoxide. I stopped walking down supermarket detergent aisles, because the smells had become obnoxious. I was becoming desperate, awakening early two or three days a week with a headache, nausea, and stiff neck. "Headache" is inadequate to describe my condition: it would be more accurate to call it a "sick-all-over-all-day-misery."

Most days I disciplined myself to get through the office routine somehow, but some days I would have to go home early, able to tell my supervisor only "I'm so sick." When the "headaches" were at their worst, I could not read, sleep, watch television, talk, or think. I was only able to lie motionless on a sofa with an icebag on my forehead. Many nights I tied the icebag to my head to help myself get to sleep. My husband would fill the icebag for me, even in the middle of the night.

I continued to take aspirin in large quantities. Sometimes, in desperation, I would take any other prescription or over-the-counter drug in our medicine cabinet that I thought might possibly help— tranquilizers or antihistamines or diuretics. For the nausea, I tried Coca-Cola syrup, purchased from a local pharmacist, and Emetrol, a nonprescription anti-nausea drug recommended by another pharmacist. Nothing helped very much.

Years of psychotherapy had given me valuable insights into my emotions, but did nothing for my "headaches." Biofeedback and relaxation techniques, learned at the headache clinic and probably the only truly safe treatment the clinic offered me, nonetheless rarely had any effect. Two sessions with a hypnotist did not help. Fish oil supplements, thought to help migraine sufferers, appeared to have little effect. Plunging my head into ice-cold water and keeping it there until I could no longer stand *that* pain offered five minutes of relief. After reading that the plant feverfew had helped migraine sufferers in England, I planted some seedlings in our garden. Finally, unable to tolerate feeling so ill at work, I "retired" from a job that I had enjoyed. I thought that perhaps being away from professional stress would relieve my condition.

It didn't. Finally, in 1986, I went to Dr. Kerr and pleaded, in tears, "I'm desperate. Tell me again about your Dr. Randolph." Fifteen years before, he had told me about an allergist, Theron G. Randolph, MD, who hospitalized people with "unmanaged" chronic illnesses in special "safe" environmental units, fasted them for four to five days, and then tested them for food and chemical sensitivities. With horror I had rejected the suggestion, for I knew that missing or delaying even one meal had given me excruciating headaches in the past. Would that I had taken that suggestion then! I could have saved myself fifteen years of pain.

Readiness Is All

This time I made an appointment with Dr. Randolph right away. I was ready. By then he no longer had an environmental unit, but his clinic sent an extensive questionnaire, covering my lifestyle as it related to foods and chemicals: What foods do you eat three or more times a week? Do you like/dislike the smell of gasoline and road-tarring compound? What medications have given you adverse side effects? Do you dislike perfumes? If so, which ones? And so on. At my first appointment, one of his nurse assistants took the most extensive medical history anyone had ever taken. Were you breast-fed? Where have you worked? Do you feel better when you travel? Do you feel better indoors or outdoors? The history took three hours and produced seven single-spaced pages. By then, I was beginning to think of possible connections between my health and my exposures, such as the corn product and pill-factory fumes of long ago. Dr. Randolph looked over the history and decided what I should be tested for.

The tests, sublingual and intradermal, given blind (I did not know what I was getting), revealed subtle but unmistakable reactions to several common foods, primarily corn and milk; several common chemicals, primarily phenol, formaldehyde, and ethanol; and several common mixtures of chemicals, primarily auto exhaust and tobacco smoke. The tobacco smoke extract produced so much choking that the nurses gave me oxygen.

During my six days in the testing room, I heard others' stories and saw others' reactions. I saw a six-year-old girl become agitated and hyperactive after receiving a food or chemical and calm down after receiving a "neutralizing" dose. I heard a patient describe her uncontrollable tears while buying lunch in the building's grocery— tears that stopped as soon as she returned to the clinic's environmentally "safe" surroundings and filtered air. As I read materials in the testing room, especially Dr. Randolph's book *An Alternative Approach to Allergies: The New Field of Clinical Ecology Unravels the Environmental Causes of Mental and Physical Ills*, I began to think that the mystery of my illness might now be solved . . . at last.

In the post-testing interview with Dr. Randolph, who had just turned eighty, he kindly but firmly warned me: "Your health is deteriorating and will continue to deteriorate until you find out what is causing this and do something about it." He knew what I had reacted to in the testing, but it was now up to me to find out what in my foods and surroundings I needed to avoid. Avoidance, he told me, is the "cure," not medications that only mask the symptoms. And though informally this condition is known as environmental illness, on the insurance form Dr. Randolph listed my major symptoms: migraine, rhinitis, gastroenteropathy, and chronic fatigue. Doctors and insurance companies tend not to accept the term "environmental illness," though "multiple chemical sensitivities" is gaining broader acceptance.

The clinic sent me home with a prescription for aspirin in capsule form, without cornstarch, and elaborate instructions for starting the four-day rotation diet known as the "rotary diversified diet." Based on the biological food families, this diet forbids the person with suspected food allergies from repeating any food until three days have elapsed; one day if the foods are in the same biological family. For example, broccoli and cabbage are in the same family. If you have broccoli on Monday, you should not have it again until at least Friday, though you could have cabbage on Wednesday. This applies to every single food you eat. It is intended to keep you from developing new food allergies or reactivating old ones.

Sound bizarre? Probably, if you have never heard of it before. That night, determined to get better, I drew up a two-week schedule on a sheet of typing paper and tried to plan this weird diet with whatever foods I had on hand or could buy. The next day I started it, avoiding mainly milk and corn, plus other members of the grain family like wheat, rye, oats, barley, rice, and millet. What on earth does one eat for breakfast on this diet? Somehow I found enough to survive, though I had an extremely severe "headache" for two days, just as if I had been in the hospital environmental unit that I had declined to enter fifteen years earlier. My worst fears were realized, but I now knew that this reaction merely proved the point. As I knew by then from my reading, I was experiencing the symptoms of withdrawal from the foods to which I had become addicted. From that moment on, unbelievable though it may seem, I have never once awakened early with a stiff neck and a headache, my common pattern: because those headaches ended so abruptly with my change of diet, I knew that they had been food-induced. Before I was properly diagnosed by Dr. Randolph, I used to have a glass of milk by my bed every night, for taking aspirin in the middle of the night. Those middle-of-the-night headaches, I now realized, occurred because of the long time lapse between dinner and breakfast: by five a.m. my body missed its "food fix." The sip of milk came too late.

The Detective Work

After those first two days were over, I began feeling better than I had for years. When I tested myself for corn, however, by eating a bowl of corn meal mush doused with corn syrup, several hours later I developed an excruciating two-day "headache" that confirmed for me my worst food allergy. I knew I had to avoid corn in all forms. Corn is the most common food allergy, possibly because, as corn syrup, corn starch, corn oil, and other less obvious names, it is present in almost all processed foods and many medicines (just read the labels). Food allergies, according to Dr. Randolph and the many environmental physicians he has trained, are closely related to addictions. When we first react with dislike to a new food, we may still go on eating it for a variety of reasons, one being difficulty in avoiding it. After a while, we may become addicted to it and find it hard to give up. Tobacco is a good example of this phenomenon; those who choke on cigarettes at first try may eventually find themselves addicted.

During the first three weeks I was on the rotation diet, I lost eighteen previously hard-to-lose pounds. My meals consisted of only two or three foods each—dinner, for example, might consist entirely of turkey, sweet potato (without butter), and peas; lunch of almonds and cherries. Because at first I had a hard time finding enough "safe" foods to eat, the pounds melted off. They never have returned; now that I am no longer addicted to any food, it is easy to maintain my desired weight.

Actually, I got better in two stages—first from rotating my foods and avoiding those I was allergic to, second from avoiding chemicals. During the first year after I was diagnosed I continued to have headaches that usually came on during the day. As I became more sophisticated about chemicals, I could usually tell what exposure was causing the headache, though as a "delayed reactor"—one who does not react immediately to an exposure—I found the detective work somewhat tricky.

One night about a month after I was diagnosed, I smelled formaldehyde on my pillowcase. Formaldehyde, a suspected carcinogen, is in many, many products, including synthetic fabrics such as cotton/polyester sheets. I immediately put some old cotton sheets and pillowcases on my bed. A few days later, I detected the same smell in soap from a filling station dispenser. Now I avoid using public soap dispensers and try to carry my own soap. And once again I hang my all-cotton sheets on lines in our basement after they have been washed in our washing machine with a plant-based liquid soap without fabric softeners. Fabric softeners from neighbors' dryers and others' clothes now smell nauseating to me.

One's sense of smell is invaluable in detecting possible chemical injury from modern synthetic products. As my husband and I gradually removed all or most smelly, suspect, petrochemically based products from our home, we both began to be aware when someone who had used or was wearing such products entered our house or car. At first, such exposures were likely to bring on a headache the next day (now not so likely). Because of my sensitivity (my husband is aware of the smells but does not apparently react), I became homebound for a time. We stopped going out to public places and to restaurants, where there was no way I could stick to my rotation diet. Dr. Randolph had advised me to stay on the diet the rest of my life. I did observe it rigidly for about a year; now I follow a modified rotation, eating mostly organic (chemically less contaminated), whole, fresh, unprocessed foods. To my surprise, I really like the diet.

Cleaning Up

The greatest shock came shortly after I was diagnosed, when I got the results of a blood test that Dr. Randolph had prescribed. I was in high percentiles for two chemical solvents (toluene and tetra-chloroethylene) and five pesticides, including a metabolite of DDT (DDE), heptachlor, and dieldrin—the latter three restricted by the EPA since the early 1970s as carcinogenic. I had not known that I had these toxic chemicals in my body. I did not want them in my body. No one had asked for my consent to put them in my body. I had never worked for an exterminator. Our house had only been sprayed once. Where had they come from? Apparently the pesticides were from food and other common exposures, the toluene possibly from printer's ink and self-service gasoline, the tetrachloroethylene from dry-cleaned clothes left in their bags in my closet and from spending hours at a do-it-yourself dry cleaner in order to save money. I was not alone, I discovered: the EPA's ongoing National Human Adipose Tissue Survey (see Chapter 2) tells us that most Americans have modern toxic chemicals in their body fat and in their bloodstreams.

This knowledge hit home when I found myself having severe headaches after I finished each aerobic class at the local YMCA—a post-retirement attempt to achieve some long-overdue physical fitness. What was causing these headaches? Probably the scented soap handed out by the Y, others' shampoos, the pesticides sprayed monthly throughout the building—and, though I didn't realize it then, the sweating that was mobilizing the toxins in my body fat into my bloodstream, causing my typical symptoms. It was at this point that Dr. Randolph suggested I try detoxification at HealthMed.

First, however, I wanted to clean up my house and lifestyle. I tried almost everything I read or heard about concerning health and the environment. My husband and I had our unvented gas kitchen stove removed and an electric one installed. We bought air filters that removed chemicals, one for our living room, one for our bedroom, and one for our car. We started driving our car with windows closed, the filter going, and the ventilating system on "recirculate." We try to leave ample space between our car and other cars' exhaust pipes. My husband reads our daily paper first, then puts it in a zippered nylon mesh bag and "bakes" it for forty minutes in our electric dryer vented to the outside, which outgases chemicals in the paper and ink so that I can read it. (Heat activates molecules.) We gave away most of our synthetic clothes and bought only natural fabrics. We have clothes dry-cleaned as little as possible; when we do, we take them out of the bag immediately and air them out in our basement for months before wearing them. I threw out all aerosol spray cans and other petroleum-based products (wishing that our community had a hazardous waste disposal system). We switched to plant-based toothpaste, shampoos, deodorants, soaps, detergents, and other cleaning products. I put away my electric blanket (the heated wires give off fumes) and sleep under down, wool, or cotton, as pure as possible. Essentially, it was back to the thirties— to the products that I remember my mother using.

Plus a few new products. After reading about them, I bought a negative-ion generator (positive ions are found in polluted areas, negative ions on unpolluted mountains and beaches), full-spectrum fluorescent tubes for our kitchen, and full-spectrum sun glasses (full-spectrum products maintain the natural balance of sunlight). I tried acupuncture, took vitamin and mineral supplements. (I rarely need prescription drugs and have not had colds or flu since returning from HealthMed, a welcome change from previous years.) In 1991 a dentist well-versed in nontoxic dentistry replaced my mercury amalgams with a composite to which I tested nonreactive. The only major thing not done is to change our gas forced-air heating system to electric in order to avoid exposure to combustion products (too expensive).

A Runaway Chemical Technology

By a year after my diagnosis, I was feeling much better. My headaches stopped almost completely, occurring only after unavoidable exposures. Which of these measures helped? I did not know—perhaps all of them. I did know, finally, what had been causing my headaches: for forty years I had been slowly poisoned. I also knew that for the first time in years, I felt the way most fairly healthy people must feel, the way the average healthy person daily takes for granted. I no longer suffered from recurrent severe pain and the ever-present fear of having to force myself through work or a social situation while feeling extremely sick. I began to consider myself 80 to 90 percent "cured," but my now-infrequent, less-severe headaches could still be unpleasant. Also, maintaining my health still required considerable avoidance of certain places and situations, and I knew that I could not go back to work in an office. It also required certain precautions, such as using a mask in theaters and traveling with my own bedding. It was then that I decided to try HealthMed.

Getting better when you are chemically injured—and millions of people are without knowing it—is obviously not a quick fix, like getting a prescription from your doctor. It may also be impossible to get completely well as long as the world is as contaminated as it is. The chemical revolution that I did not even dream of in my college chemistry lab has now taken place, and I will probably have to be careful the rest of my life.

Samuel S. Epstein, MD, professor of occupational and environmental medicine at the University of Illinois Medical Center in Chicago, has written of a "runaway chemical technology": "With the dawn of the petrochemical era in the early 1950s, annual U.S. production of synthetic organic chemicals was about one billion pounds. . . . By the 1980s [it was] over four hundred billion pounds. The overwhelming majority of these industrial chemicals has never been adequately, if at all, tested for long-term toxic, carcinogenic, mutagenic, and teratogenic effects."

Actually, of course, it is we who are doing the testing. All of us, but especially those with environmental illness/multiple chemical sensitivities. We are the canaries in the modern chemical mines, the living environmental-impact statements, the not-so-distant early warning systems. Rachel Carson wrote, more than thirty years ago (a time when "he" was commonly assumed to mean both "he" and "she"), "The contamination of our world is not alone a matter of mass spraying. Indeed, for most of us this is of less importance than the innumerable small-scale exposures to which we are subjected day by day, year after year. Like the constant dripping of water that in turn wears away the hardest stone, this birth-to-death contact with dangerous chemicals may in the end prove disastrous. Each of these recurrent exposures, no matter how slight, contributes to the progressive buildup of chemicals in our bodies and so to cumulative poisoning. . . . Lulled by the soft sell and the hidden persuader, the average citizen is seldom aware of the deadly materials with which he is surrounding himself; indeed, he may not realize he is using them at all."

1

Your Allergies, My Headaches, Our Problem

O N   A N   U N S E A S O N A B L Y   W A R M   February afternoon, I waited for my friend John in a popular smoke-free, vegetarian, health-food restaurant in a suburb of a large midwestern city, looking forward to a leisurely conversation over a raisin bran muffin, carob tofu cheesecake, or oatmeal peach pie. After we were seated, John ordered his usual: mineral water. But instead of lingering, we soon left, aware of the smell of new carpeting. Outside I said to John, "I'm going back to speak to the manager." When I told the manager that we were leaving because we both react to chemicals like those in the carpeting, she said that she that some of her employees were also reacting to the carpeting . . . but "you have allergies; I have headaches."

Outside again, in purer air, I remarked to John, "That says it all." She thinks that we are "allergic," while she has only headaches. What she doesn't realize is that all three of us are feeling the effects of the twentieth century. Especially since World War II, thousands upon thousands of new chemicals have poured into our environment. Most have been derived from petroleum or coal tar. Governmental agencies do some testing and regulating, but they cannot begin to keep up with the more than one thousand new chemicals that chemists synthesize each year for commercial use. Often the only testing is that done on animals by the manufacturer that markets the products incorporating these chemicals. Most are untested for human health effects.

More and more people are becoming ill from these chemicals and the products—from synthetic carpeting to oven cleaner—that contain them, often without realizing the source of their chronic symptoms. In 1987 a workshop of experts convened by the Board on Environmental Studies and Toxicology of the National Academy of Sciences, the nation's most prestigious scientific organization, estimated that approximately 15 percent of the U.S. population experiences sensitivity to chemicals found in common household products.

Two 1993 studies reinforced that estimate. Fifteen percent of 643 presumably healthy young adult college students reported feeling ill from smelling one or more of the chemicals in pesticides, auto exhaust, paint, new carpet, and perfume. Seventeen percent of 263 adults aged sixty to ninety felt ill after low-level exposures to at least four out of five of the same substances.

That's right—you may be one of those reacting to pesticides, perfumes, carpets, cleansers, waxes, polishes, paints, detergents, fabric softeners, air "fresheners," deodorant soaps, glues, and a number of other products that you may be exposed to daily. And you may not be connecting these products with your headaches, coughing, dizziness, nausea, joint pains, fatigue, dizziness, or feelings of depression or "spaciness." With all the media emphasis on stress, you probably blame stress for your symptoms. Certainly we are all somewhat stressed out by our fast-moving modern world, but stress is by no means the only culprit.

Naming the Illness

For forty years I thought I had an incurable disease called "migraines." Now I know that what I had was neither incurable nor a disease. It was a symptom. I suffered from both the so-called "classical" migraines—those with visual auras—and the so-called "common" migraines. Both, I finally learned, were caused by either the foods I was allergic to or the petroleum-derived chemicals in my environment. Once I was properly diagnosed and began to see the cause-and-effect connection between exposure and symptom, I cleaned up my diet and home (got rid of toxic products). My headaches virtually ceased—to my intense relief. The process of getting well took much effort and the better part of a year—and is still going on—but it is definitely worth it.

John's story is different. In 1982, previously very healthy, he fell ill with flu-like aches and pains and fatigue that did not go away. Then he developed symptoms like trouble concentrating and unusual mood swings, making it hard for him to think and work. Though he began to feel better after he cleaned up his apartment and his diet, his fatigue and flu-like symptoms have persisted. He seems to have been hit by a triple whammy—chemical sensitivity; chronic fatigue syndrome (CFS), also known as chronic fatigue immune deficiency syndrome (CFIDS); and candida-related complex, also known as candidiasis. *Candida albicans* is a yeast that occurs naturally in our intestines; the overuse of antibiotics, birth-control pills, and immunosuppressive drugs like steroids and hormones can cause an overgrowth of candida, producing a variety of symptoms. Treatment consists of antifungal medications and avoidance of foods, such as sugar, that the yeast feeds on. Hence John ordered only mineral water in the health-food restaurant.

As you can see, the condition is complex, and the names for it are confusing. One name is *total allergy syndrome*—but are these reactions really allergies? The definition of allergy used in the early 1900s was "altered reactivity," meaning that I react to something that you don't react to. In that sense, John, the restaurant manager, and I all have allergies. After all, many people live with new carpeting, pump gas, drive with car windows open, refinish furniture, have gas stoves, wear perfumes, and use supermarket detergents without apparent ill effects. By this definition, these fortunates are not allergic—and we three are. But by the definition of allergy that evolved in the 1920s—one involving reactions between antigens and antibodies in the body—we three do not have allergies. Our bodies do not produce the antibody immunoglobulin E (IgE) in response to chemical exposures in the way that the bodies of those with hay fever produce IgE in response to ragweed. Therefore our reactions, say the traditional (post-1925) allergists, are not "IgE-mediated"; and John, the restaurant manager, and I do not have allergies.

So where does this leave us? In their 1991 book *Chemical Exposures: Low Levels and High Stakes*, Nicholas Ashford, a lawyer and

MIT scientist, and Claudia Miller, a physician, distinguish three types of sensitivity: classical toxicity, or poisoning, as with well-documented reactions to lead or benzene; IgE-mediated allergy, as with the well-known reactions to ragweed or bee venom; and multiple chemical sensitivities (MCS), the less well-known and less understood phenomenon of persons reacting with multiple symptoms to multiple chemicals. Sometimes such persons acquire MCS after an acute or traumatic exposure to one or two chemicals. After that transforming experience, they find that they have become acutely "sensitized" to very low levels of many chemicals, perhaps permanently. The former head of the Art Institute of Chicago, Welshman Tony Jones, is an example of this kind of "sensitizing." Once a sculptor creating large outdoor pieces from fiberglass and synthetic resin, Jones lost consciousness one day from breathing the toxic resin fumes, even though he was wearing a double-nozzled gas mask; luckily, he was found by students sharing his studio. Now extremely sensitive to all plastics, he has exchanged sculpting for administering.

Thus "sensitivity" means quite different things to toxicologists, to allergists, and to environmental physicians, the practitioners of the specialty known as environmental medicine. Environmental physicians say that John, the restaurant manager, and I have *environmental* or *environmentally-induced illness* (EI), also known as *ecological illness* and MCS. For insurance purposes, they may simply describe the illness by its symptoms, such as migraines or gastroenteritis or seizures or fibromyalgia. Environmental physician Grace Ziem has proposed a working definition: "Multiple chemical sensitivity (MCS) is defined as illness reactions associated with exposure to more than one chemical, at significantly lower exposure levels than would cause noticeable illness in the general population, not mediated solely by known immune mechanisms, often accompanied by unusual fatigue, involving symptoms in multiple organ systems, and usually including symptoms of the central nervous system." A less technical definition comes from chemically sensitive Adie Zuckerman: "It's a rain barrel effect. Your life, drop by drop, is being filled up with exposure that causes your body to react. It may just take that last drop of water to make your rain barrel overflow."

Some environmental physicians refer to EI/MCS as *immune system dysfunction*, because our immune systems do not seem to be able to handle, or adapt to, modern chemicals without either malfunctioning or over-functioning. But no one seems to know why I am chemically sensitive and the person working the gas pumps at the local filling station is not, or why my husband has hay fever and I do not, or why John has flu-like symptoms and I have headaches, or why some of the health-food restaurant's workers react to the new carpeting and some do not. Genes? An inherited susceptibility? One's total body burden of "xenobiotics" (substances foreign to the body)? Chemically sensitive Judy Polkow suggests still another name, *xenobiotic response syndrome*, for what she calls "a major epidemic of monstrous proportions." An acquired deficiency in one's immune system? Only time and much research will tell. Fortunately, a few scientists are now beginning to look into multiple chemical sensitivities.

Even the word "sensitivity," however, does not sit well with some people. In Colorado, Ed and Suzanne Randegger publish a newsletter, *The Wary Canary*, so named because people with EI/MCS see themselves as canaries in the coal mine, warning others of dangerous fumes. A reader suffering from exposure to the pesticide chlordane and the wood preservative pentacresol wrote the Randeggers: "Lay off that 'sensitive' crap! If your kid plays in the street and is run over by a truck, do you say, 'Poor thing, he's sensitive to Fords'? We're basically dealing with poisons, not frail health."

Because this type of acute reactivity is relatively new, it has spawned another name—*twentieth-century disease*. As San Francisco allergist/immunologist Alan S. Levin has written: "Over many centuries, our bodies have miraculously evolved to tolerate or require most of the naturally occurring substances that surround us. Yet there are many synthetic substances in our environment to which our bodies have not had sufficient time to adapt. At the present moment we're being exposed to concentrations of these chemicals that . . . tax our adaptive mechanisms to their maximum." Levin says that today's chemical pollutants are like "germs" a hundred years ago, germs being those microorganisms that cause infectious diseases, a relationship discovered by Louis Pasteur. Both chemical pollutants and germs are invisible; both have caused controversy.

In his practice, Levin distinguishes between the more-familiar "Type 1" allergy, producing symptoms such as rhinitis, hay fever, asthma, skin disorders, and gastrointestinal problems; and the less-recognized "Type 2" allergy, producing symptoms such as headaches, mood and behavior changes, heart palpitations, blurred vision, fatigue, numbness, muscle and joint aches, and skin and gastrointestinal disorders. Type 2 symptoms, which to him can also include arthritis, epilepsy, depression, multiple sclerosis, and some forms of cancer, are, he believes, produced by modern synthetic chemicals and other environmental pollutants. Hence the informal, commonly used name for this condition—*environmental illness*. John, the restaurant manager, and I all have EI in varying degrees. Yet everything is in some sense "environment"; and everything in the world, including our bodies and our personal environments, is composed of chemicals. Most of these chemicals are essential or obviously benign; we could not exist if they were not. The primary cause of EI/MCS is the new chemicals that have been synthesized in this century. Before World War II, most common products, such as soap, were derived from plants or animals, natural substances that our bodies have adapted to over thousands of years. Since World War II, many of these same products, such as detergents, have come to contain synthetic chemicals, usually derived from petroleum or coal tar; these new chemicals are foreign to our bodies.

Psychiatrist Thomas Stone, now practicing environmental medicine, believes that many people are adapting to these chemicals, but, he warns, "the price we pay for chronic adaptation is chronic illness." Another environmental physician, Dr. William J. Rea, says that "in my opinion, it's not *why* one gets sick [from a toxic environment] and one doesn't, it's *when* one gets sick. If you're one of those who can adapt real fast you won't perceive damage until it's too late. The people who seem to adapt may come down with cancer or heart disease or liver failure thirty years later." Scientists now finding objective biological markers in people with chemically induced illness are calling it by what is probably its most accurate name: *chemical injury*. It is important, however, not to wait for the perfect name before taking steps to prevent this most difficult of all illnesses.

Black Gold?

Nineteenth-century coal miners knew that the gases in mine tunnels were lethal. That is why they took canaries into the mines with them; when the canaries stopped singing or died, the miners knew that they, too, were in danger.

In this century, television pictures from Alaska's Prince William Sound, California's Huntingdon Beach, and the Persian Gulf have shown us new "canaries": otters, seals, cormorants, and creatures across numerous species struggling to survive while coated with gooey, toxic oil. These victims symbolize for us the dangers of a new contaminant, petroleum. The effects of the Alaska spill may be permanent: scientists have found possible genetic defects in salmon returning to Prince William Sound, as well as declines in the numbers of several bird species. The effects of petroleum and its byproducts on us are as yet uncalculated.

Some of the chemicals derived from petroleum seem to have retained the poisonous properties of their source. Crude oil itself contains benzene, toluene, and xylene, as does coal tar. Benzene is known to cause cancer. One of six toxic chemicals for which the U.S. Environmental Protection Agency (EPA) requires special controls, benzene reaches us mainly in auto exhaust, industrial emissions, and tobacco smoke. In 1989, twelve years after the EPA began considering curbs on benzene, that agency finally issued tight controls on benzene releases from steel plants, service stations, and other industrial sources—but not from automobiles. Also in 1989, southern California's South Coast Air Quality Management District found that commuters on that area's expressways, typically either congested or in gridlock, are exposed to four times as many pollutants inside as outside their cars, especially at slow speeds; and the levels of benzene were higher than those of other pollutants. The 1990 Clean Air Act should reduce auto emissions somewhat, but major improvement is still a long way off.

Benzene also made news when Perrier removed millions of bottles of its water from the market in 1990 because a faulty filter had allowed benzene into some bottles. The Perrier flap was a tempest in a tankard, however; Action on Smoking and Health, a leading anti-smoking organization, estimated that nonsmokers sitting in a bar for one hour drinking a contaminated bottle of Perrier will suffer a cancer risk at least ten thousand times higher from breathing other people's tobacco smoke than they will from their drink.

Toluene, found in cleaning compounds, cosmetics, printers' ink, and many other products, can damage the kidneys, liver, and central nervous system and can cause dizziness, headaches, fainting, muscle fatigue, confusion, and weakness. Kids on inner-city streets know the intoxicating effects of toluene; to get a high, they buy and sniff products from their local hardware store containing "tolly."

Xylene, found in, among other things, marking pens, caulking compounds, and air fresheners, can damage the central nervous system, gastrointestinal tract, liver, kidneys, eyes, and skin. Symptoms of xylene exposure include abdominal pain, vomiting, dizziness, incoherence, nausea, dermatitis, and, of all things, euphoria. (You might want the euphoria, but the rest?) A promotional sample of new shampoo/hair conditioner delivered to my home in 1991 contains, among eighteen other possibly toxic compounds, ammonium *xylene*sulfonate. Do I want to try this free shampoo? No way.

An EPA study of the chemicals in human body fat lets us know that most of us carry a dizzying assortment of toxic chemicals around with us. These stored chemicals plus our daily chemical exposures make up our "total body burden"; our rain barrels are filling up with toxins. A full 10 percent of the billions of barrels of crude oil we use each year goes not to auto or airplane fuel but to ordinary consumer goods—to you and me: your polyester clothes, sheets, and curtains; the pesticides you spray on your lawn; the polyvinyl chloride (PVC) pipes in your basement; the carpets and wax on your floors; your children's rubber boots, crayons, and balloons; the paint on your walls; such varied items as shoe polish, ballpoint pens, ink, toilet seats, and golf balls. Crude oil (in the form of its derivatives) is also present in things you think you need to make yourself look, smell, and feel better: aspirin, perfume, shaving cream, contact lenses, toothpaste, antihistamines, cortisone, vitamins, nail polish, and deodorant, to name a few.

Can we live without such petroleum-based products? Obviously people once did . . . and if oil industry analysts are correct, we will have to again in about forty-five years, when the earth finally runs out of oil. This estimate is based on current consumption, though world consumption levels have increased eightfold between 1950 and 1990 and world population continues to soar. In the meantime, however, plant-based substitutes are becoming more easily available. One firm, Tom's of Maine, even advertises its plant-based products on television. More and more people are becoming health-conscious consumers. They read the fine print on labels and are suspicious of the word "natural" in advertisements.

As well they might be. Dr. Samuel S. Epstein, professor of occupational and environmental medicine at the University of Illinois Medical Center in Chicago, warned in 1989 that "much cancer today reflects events and exposures in the 1950s and 1960s. Production, use, and disposal of synthetic, organic, and other industrial carcinogens were then minuscule compared with current levels, which will determine future cancer rates for younger populations now exposed. There is every reason to anticipate that the high current cancer rates will be dwarfed in coming decades." In 1960, says Epstein, cancer was striking one person in four and killing one in five; in 1990 it was striking one in three and killing one in four. He projects that it will soon be striking one in two and killing one in three.

In 1992 the American Cancer Society projected an increase in prostate cancer compared with 1991 and said that breast cancers in women have been increasing at about 3 percent per year since 1980. Yet the National Cancer Institute (NCI) spends only 10 percent of its $2 billion budget on prevention research, tending instead, after it's too late, to "blame the victim": if only he had stopped smoking! she had eaten more fiber! eaten less fat! exercised regularly! If only they had changed their lifestyle!

Actually, the NCI may have a point. Millions of new and old chemical compounds exist (indeed we are all composed of them): only about five hundred are *known* to be carcinogenic, mostly based on animal studies. Certainly, we would be wise to avoid as many of them as possible. Natural compounds in celery, figs, parsley, mushrooms, parsnips, and a few other foods are believed to cause cancer; aflatoxin, in moldy peanuts and corn, is a carcinogen.

Some scientists contend that those compounds present a greater danger than food additives and pesticide residues. Only 7 to 8 percent of cancer risk comes from food, says a Food and Drug Administration (FDA) scientist, and of that only 2 percent from additives and pesticides.

Still, because the FDA is primarily concerned with food and drugs, it tends to overlook the carcinogens we encounter every day by other means, such as auto exhaust and tobacco smoke. They all add up. Unless you have taken steps to clean up your environment, you are surrounded every day with carcinogens that you breathe, not eat. To the argument that we are in more danger from natural chemicals than synthetic ones, one can reply, "Why add toxic synthetic chemicals to our body burden of toxic natural ones?"

Residues of chemical toxins, some known to be cancer-causing in animals and many known to affect our central nervous systems, are found virtually everywhere we go: in our homes and offices, in restaurants, churches, auditoriums, and all public buildings. Synthetic chemicals, invisible though sometimes detectable by smell or by health effects, permeate our bodies, our lives, and our world. It is not hard to believe that we are all being slowly poisoned by our environment.

A Historic Discovery

One spring day in 1951, a tornado was predicted for northern Illinois. Because of the warning, all the patients of Theron G. Randolph, a young allergist/immunologist just starting his practice, had canceled their appointments—all except one, a former cosmetic saleswoman suffering from headaches, nausea, dizziness, blackouts, persistent fatigue, and nervousness. Considered a hypochondriac by previous doctors, she had been seeing Randolph for three years, during which time he had typed fifty pages of her medical history. Exasperated by his failure to make sense of her long history and determined to help her, he decided to keep the office quiet by closing the door and blocking all phone calls. He then spent three hours going over his notes with her, asking question after question. As the storm raged outside, Randolph had a sudden flash of insight: almost all of his patient's reactions were to petroleum or to its manmade products. She had been getting sick after exposures to fuel oil, auto exhaust, paint, fingernail polish, pine-scented disinfectants, and industrial emissions. Excited by his discovery, he underlined with red pencil all such substances in those fifty pages—and began the long, slow process of teaching himself how to help her (and others) avoid them. Once this was accomplished, her health improved dramatically. Medical history had been made.

Since then Randolph has diagnosed and treated more than nine thousand chemically sensitive patients and trained hundreds of physicians from a variety of specialties in the relationship of environment to health. In 1962 he published his textbook, *Human Ecology and Susceptibility to the Chemical Environment*, the medical counterpart of Rachel Carson's *Silent Spring*, also published in 1962. Giving this new specialty the name *clinical ecology*, in 1965 he and four others organized these physicians into a new group, the Society for Clinical Ecology, later changed to the American Academy of Environmental Medicine (AAEM). These environmental specialists, now numbering about five hundred, were originally trained as allergists, pediatricians, psychiatrists, otolaryngologists, and just about every sort of physician. Some were drawn into environmental medicine by their own experiences: a Washington State pathologist became ill from his frequent exposures to formaldehyde; Randolph is allergic to corn and other grains; family physician Sherry Rogers, MD, of Syracuse, New York, had both food allergies and chemical sensitivities; Dr. Rea, a Dallas chest surgeon, became chemically sensitized by operating-room anesthetics and other hospital exposures. Dr. Rea now operates the Environmental Health Center, in Dallas, Texas; in 1989 he was named the First World Professor of Environmental Medicine at the University of Surrey, in England. Like other environmental specialists, Rea looks for environmental causes rather than simply treating symptoms.

The Environmental Unit

Actually, medical awareness of the environment is not new; it's just that for generations medical training and practice have been moving away from this awareness. Hippocrates, the founder of medicine, and other physicians in ancient Greece considered air, water, and "places" to be sources of many diseases. But in the nineteenth century, with the discoveries of Pasteur, the germ theory of disease took hold. Medical science made great strides in surgical techniques and in the handling of infectious diseases. The twentieth century brought medical specialization, which meant that fewer doctors and scientists were looking at either the whole person or the environment for the causes of chronic illness. It also brought a pharmacopoeia of new ways of treating specific diseases—modern drugs, about 75 percent of which are derived from petroleum or coal tar, the rest from plants. As many of us have discovered, none of these drugs is without side effects.

All has not been lost, however. In addition to the rise of environmental medicine, other medical developments hold promise. Psychiatrist Melvyn R. Werbach, in *Third Line Medicine: Modern Treatment for Persistent Symptoms*, has recommended that medicine move away from the "doctrine of specific etiology," the one-cause-for-one-disease approach that has dominated medicine for over a century. Instead he proposes an "ecologic" model, to be achieved through what he calls "third line medicine." If you have chronic symptoms, you are likely to go first to your primary care physician—your internist or family doctor, the "first line." Referral to a specialist—the "second line"—often follows. If you don't get help there, Werbach feels, you should be seen by a "third line" physician, one who looks at the whole picture, using less orthodox but safe, immune-system-strengthening procedures to help the body resist illness. Do such doctors exist? Yes, says Werbach, but they are few, hard to find, and often self-trained. With the exception of a few continuing-education courses in environmental medicine sponsored by the AAEM and others approved by the American Medical Association (AMA), formal training for "third line" medicine does not yet exist. Nor does training in environmental toxins: a recent survey of 126 medical schools by the AMA found that only 4 required a single class in environmental medicine and toxicology.

The Institute of Medicine of the NAS agrees on the need for more training in environmental medicine, though it does not use the term "third line medicine." In its welcome 1988 report, *Role of the Primary Care Physician in Occupational and Environmental Medicine*, the authors state that "with few exceptions, physicians are in-

adequately trained in occupational and environmental medicine."
Lacking that solid foundation and inadequately trained in the related disciplines of epidemiology and toxicology, most primary care
physicians are "hard-pressed to keep up with developments in the
field." The authors' recommendations: in medical schools, more
status, more faculty, and more funding for these subjects; in doctors' practices, better, more, and more accessible information.

Despite these trends, many traditional doctors still do not believe that EI/MCS exists. It's not hard to see why. EI/MCS is a usually invisible condition caused by usually invisible substances—
many of them acting in combination with each other. Consequently, it is extremely hard to detect and diagnose. Moreover,
doctors are not trained in the relationship of environment to health,
and standard tests often fail to reveal the presence of this illness, or
even of its most common symptoms. For instance, if you have headaches, has any doctor ever given you a test that reveals the presence
of the headache or indicates the severity of the pain? Only you really
know how much it hurts. With symptoms like headaches, doctors
would do well to rely on the patient's own statements and to ask
questions about the patient's environment.

Though some researchers are finding objective evidence—biological markers—for the existence of EI/MCS (see Chapter 11), traditional medical research is no better equipped to recognize
chemical injury than are most traditional doctors. Consider the
double-blind study, an effective tool which is often considered the
standard for conclusive scientific research. Developed by pharmaceutical companies for evaluating new drugs, the double-blind
study is designed so that neither the person administering the drug
nor the person receiving it knows what it is (a third party has set up
the experiment). To further minimize the placebo effect and other
external influences, these studies include carefully selected control
groups—persons not receiving the drugs.

As yet, few controlled double-blind tests have been done on patients with suspected EI/MCS—for some fairly obvious reasons.
How is it possible to reproduce the mishmash of chemicals that im-
pinge on us every day, in order to get accurate results? What if these
chemicals have synergistic effects, as they almost certainly do, the
"whole" of their effects being greater than the sum of their "parts"?

What are the risks of exposing chemically sensitive people and their matched controls to toxic substances for purposes of such a test?

Still, one especially effective diagnostic tool exists—the controlled environmental unit. It is to these carefully monitored diagnostic environments that many EI/MCS sufferers finally turn for help.

Pioneered by Randolph, controlled environmental units are kept as free as possible of all contaminants. Ordinary ventilating systems have to be shut off or modified to keep out natural gas or heating-oil fumes. Even visitors are screened: "Do not enter this area if you are wearing perfume, hair spray, or aftershave lotion," says an entrance sign at Rea's environmental unit in Dallas. In the unit, patients are fasted for several days to help rid their bodies of food and chemical residues and then tested for their reactions to both foods and chemicals. Gradually, they are given foods thought to be safe for them. Though the process is not always pleasant, the results can be amazing.

One of Randolph's patients was virtually immobilized by rheumatoid arthritis when she entered his environmental unit in 1980. Heavily medicated, she could barely walk or use her hands and was in almost unbearable pain. After seven days of fasting, though she could drink a "compatible" water (one that she did not react to), most of her arthritic symptoms were gone. In the unit, she learned what foods and chemicals to avoid. Now on a strict diet, she is well and able to function normally in a job requiring typing! Her own study of twenty other rheumatoid arthritis patients in the unit showed that eighteen were, like her, significantly improved before their discharge from the hospital. A follow-up study of six of the eighteen found that the four who had continued to control their diet and environment were symptom-free except after unavoidable exposures. The two who had not done so were back to suffering and drugs.

For some, then, the way to good health via an environmental unit is there, but it is not easy. This route is not a quick fix. Returning to the outside world can be especially hard for those leaving the safety of the unit. When asked in 1989 about success rates, Randolph estimated that while 75 to 90 percent of all patients had been helped in the unit, approximately 20 percent of these successes cannot maintain their strict regimen upon leaving the hospital, either because of expense or for other reasons. Fortunately, add Ashford and Miller, most people can remain outpatients while they are guided through an elimination diet, avoidance of possible chemical incitants, and then a rechallenge with suspected offenders.

In any event, for researchers as well for patients, the environmental unit is an invaluable tool in cases of suspected chemical injury. To Ashford and Miller, the "environmental unit is the gold standard against which all other diagnostic approaches and screening techniques should be measured." It is certainly imperative, they say, "in more severe cases, such as those who have failed outpatient attempts at management or for patients with seizures, suicidal tendencies, incapacitating migraine headaches, [cardiac] arrhythmias, or other problems requiring continuous vigilance." Participants in a milestone 1991 NAS workshop on MCS agreed that studies using controlled environmental units are a major research priority. In 1993, the National Defense Authorization Act allocated $300,000 for an environmental unit for testing Persian Gulf War veterans suffering from a variety of ailments that appear related to chemical exposures. It's not enough funding, but it's a start.

Environmental units, however desirable, are expensive to set up and maintain, and patients often find that their stays are not reimbursed by skeptical insurance companies—two reasons that, despite recommendations like those of Ashford and Miller, such units are scarce. Fortunately, many patients are helped without going through an environmental unit. Neither John nor I (and certainly not the restaurant manager) was ever in one. Insurance covered part of my diagnostic testing and my later stay at a detoxification clinic. (While environmental units inevitably result in the body sloughing off some toxics, their primary purpose is diagnosis, not detoxification.) Cleaning up my home environment entailed some costs, and organic food can be expensive, but now that I am much healthier, my medical expenses are minimal, my prescription drug costs almost nonexistent.

Though I may have been lucky in this respect, many of us diagnosed with EI/MCS find that we are spending less on health care than when we were trekking from doctor to doctor and spending copiously on prescription drugs. In fact, this fruitless searching may be one of the activities driving up the inordinately high costs of health care in the U.S.—what Randolph calls a "needless redundancy of medical care." According to Dr. Rogers, the average patient arriving in her office has seen a dozen doctors, has twenty complaints, has several printout sheets listing prescribed medicines, and has spent $20,000 to $40,000 in medical bills. None had found any lasting relief from their suffering, and all had wasted immense amounts of time and money.

As for the dollar cost of ineffective health care for chronic conditions, we taxpayers pay a lot of it, of course, through programs like Medicare, Medicaid, and Social Security. Whether the Clinton administration's new health care plan can reduce these unnecessary expenditures remains to be seen. Some of it is up to us: the AMA in 1993 estimated that unhealthy habits and violence cost the U.S. more than $42 billion in direct medical expenses each year, with indirect expenses such as lost productivity raising the total to $189 billion annually. But chemically induced damage to our health, other than that from smoking and alcohol abuse, probably did not figure into those totals.

Environmental Refugees

How sick can the modern environment make you? For some, the answer is "very." In the late 1970s, British pop singer Sheila Rossall, then thirty-one, was reduced to fifty-four pounds by her severe reactions to manmade fibers, plastics, processed foods, and gasoline fumes. For more than three years she was confined to a dark room in her Bristol, England, apartment, kept alive by air filters and the care of friends. Said one friend, "When we see her we have to make sure that we haven't used toothpaste or deodorant for twenty-four hours. . . . We must never wear perfume and [we must] try to make sure that our clothes are pure cotton."

In 1979, Scott Jablin, twenty-five, was spending most of his time at a friend's house in Oakland, California, sitting in a wooden chair or sleeping on a wooden table, and breathing through a cotton/charcoal mask. A sip of tap water or a whiff of the paper or ink of a newspaper could set off choking spasms, hallucinations, or seizures. "There are going to be more and more people like me," Jablin said.

"The more garbage we put into the world, the more people there will be whose bodies break down from it."

Before James J. McAdam Jr., of Woodbury, New Jersey, went to the Randolph Clinic in 1985, he would vomit as many as one hundred times a day, gasping for air and writhing in pain, in reaction to both man-made and natural substances in his environment. He is now much better, but he lives in a room lined with aluminum foil to keep out dust, plaster, and chemicals, he shaves with spring water, brushes his teeth with baking soda, and subsists on organic food cooked in spring water in a glass pot. He reads books and newspapers placed in a sealed metal-and-glass "glove box" (similar to that used to handle radioactive materials), wears only pure cotton clothes, and can watch his tiny television set for about an hour before fumes from its plastic parts sicken him. Still, "It's great. I'm almost pain-free," he told a reporter.

Obviously, these sufferers are extreme cases. They are often termed "universal reactors," because they react to almost everything in their environment. Their suffering leads to headlines like "Allergic to Life," "Allergic to the Whole World," and "Allergic to the Twentieth Century," though over the years there has been a noticeable shift in wording, from "Woman and Son Fight Obscure Environmental Illness" to "Chemical Sensitivity Spreading" and "We Are All Sick." Headline hyperbole aside, for many of those severely affected by modern toxic chemicals, the only solution has been escape—either alone to mountains or deserts, or to growing communities of chemically injured people. In 1983, Pat Canon moved from California's coast to the inland town of Mount Shasta to join a community of twenty-five EI/MCS sufferers seeking clean air and safe housing. For her, the long effort to avoid certain chemicals and foods was beginning to pay off. (Her friend Jarrold Hines, thirty-eight, also chemically sensitive, did not join her. Despairing that he would ever get better, he had shot himself to death.) In Mount Shasta, living in houses almost completely stripped of plastics and synthetics, these "escapees" sometimes react to unavoidable exposures with the usual symptoms—fatigue, depression, hyperactivity, headaches, and others—but most improve after several years in this environment.

Another EI/MCS community is in Wimberley, Texas, where

since 1978 a dozen families have located in a relatively unpolluted, no-pesticide area. Modern pioneers, each family willingly provides environmentally safe living quarters for the next family to arrive—a small guest house or space for a trailer. Janet Bennett, who like many of these residents was a patient at the Dallas environmental health clinic, now spends most of her time in a porcelain-walled trailer that she brought to Wimberley from her home in Indiana. Her son and daughter live close by to look after her, communicating mainly by intercom. In Indiana, her husband has built a ten-by-ten-foot steel room in their back yard, with porcelain walls and a ceramic tile floor, furnished only in metal and cotton, for her to live in when she is able to return. Before she was diagnosed, Janet only knew that when she walked into a store, "My legs would turn to rubber. I'd start to sweat and people told me I would get a confused, blank stare on my face. I'd have to hang onto a shopping cart or one of my kids." Later she realized that she was reacting to the pesticides sprayed on food and in the store itself. In clothing stores she reacted to formaldehyde outgassing from new clothes. "We've been married almost twenty-four years and this has to be the hardest thing we've ever gone through," said her husband.

It may have proved too hard for them, because now the Bennetts are separated. For many, having the illness has meant the loss of a spouse. Husbands, wives, other relatives, and friends often find that coping with the special needs of the person with EI/MCS is too much for them—or they may feel personally threatened by the illness, or both. Often relatives and friends react with disbelief, which is one of the hardest things for the chemically sensitive to cope with. But, to borrow from humorist Dave Barry, we are definitely not making this up.

One chemically sensitive woman, who lost not only her marriage but her Los Angeles music business after she was correctly diagnosed, moved to Potrero, California, in the high desert country near San Diego, where she founded "The Last Resort." There—with no smog, no humidity, no trees, and almost no people—she houses those who must get away from the byproducts of our civilization for periods from a few months to over a year. By living in safe housing free of pollutants, these refugees from paint fumes, pesticide spraying, perfumes, and fabric softeners hope to build up their immune systems enough for them to return to the cities they came from. Because they feel so much better there, some have decided to make Potrero their home. Potrero's original settler feels that as long as she stays in Potrero, she is completely recovered.

Housing is one of the worst problems for the chemically sensitive. In Milton, Massachusetts, Anni Waterflow suffers severe headaches, joint pain, and fatigue from chemical exposures. To avoid cigarette smoke from the downstairs neighbor in her apartment building, she began sleeping on her porch. When the weather became too cold for that, she looked into 450 different houses or apartments without finding any that would fit her medical needs or her budget. She can't work outside her home and lives on disability benefits and subsidized housing.

A Major Epidemic

Thus this illness, while seldom life-threatening, can be profoundly life-altering. No one knows how many universal reactors there are or may be, or how many have already been diagnosed with this illness. What is clear is that the symptoms and the severity of the condition differ vastly from sufferer to sufferer and that many sufferers do get much better once they know what their problem is. Maureen Lapp, a Maryland housewife affected by her suburb's lawn fertilizers and asphalt, was prone to seizures, confusion, and weakness so severe that she was often too feeble to get out of bed. Considerably improved after she and her husband built a safe, nontoxic house in the Catoctin Mountains, she says that "my priorities have completely changed: [they are now] survival and health. Two years ago I was desperate. Now there's light at the end of the tunnel. I feel much better."

Lapp's story is a familiar one to those in EI/MCS support-groups across the U.S. and in Canada and England. I first met my friend John in 1986, two years after he had taken a leading role in our area's EI/MCS support groups. Between 1984 and 1989 he counseled more than five hundred people who knew or suspected that they were reacting to chemicals in the environment; some also had candida-related complex or chronic fatigue syndrome. Many people learn what they need to know from a support group and leave it once they get better. The media, intensely competitive, like to focus on dramatic cases of EI/MCS, rarely mentioning that most people with this condition get better once they are properly diagnosed.

For many, EI/MCS is not an incurable disease, just an unusually difficult one. Yet, asked if a cure (meaning a permanently healing treatment of some sort) will ever be found, Randolph replies: "No. There cannot be a cure because new chemical hazards are multiplying faster than we can deal with them." And he is right. According to Peter Montague, of the Environmental Research Foundation (ERF), American industry doubles its annual output of organic chemicals every eleven years. In other words, every eleven-year period produces more chemicals than in all history before that period. Not all are toxic, of course, but few are tested by independent agencies for short- or long-term human health effects. The huge toxic waste dumps in New York State's now-famous Love Canal (and what they were doing to people, especially children) were discovered in 1978; by 1989 the annual chemical production by American industry was twice as large as it was when Love Canal first came to light.

According to the EarthWorks Group, today "there are more chemicals in the average American home than there were in the average chemical laboratory one hundred years ago." Slowly, subtly, chemicals have migrated from the laboratory to our homes . . . and our bodies. Even before Love Canal, the New York Academy of Sciences reported that industrial chemicals like benzene (which can cause cancer), styrene (which can cause genetic changes), and chloroform (a carcinogen and possible cause of birth defects) were present in umbilical cords of newborns. "The impact of such exposure is unknown," say the authors of the report.

Small wonder, then, that more and more of us are getting sick. In "The Paradox of Health," Harvard psychiatrist Arthur Barsky speculates about this trend: "Although the collective health of the nation has improved dramatically in the past thirty years, surveys reveal declining satisfaction with personal health during the same period. Increasingly, respondents report greater numbers of disturbing somatic symptoms, more disability, and more feelings of general illness." Though one factor, he says, is that we are living longer and are thus more subject to chronic and degenerative diseases, he attributes much of our malaise to more self-scrutiny and greater publicity about health matters, thus implying, true to his discipline, that our illness is all in our heads. Another authority, Joseph D. Beasley, MD, MPH, director of the Department of Medicine and Nutrition at the Brunswick Hospital Hospital Center, Amityville, New York, has a different answer, implied by the title of his book, *The Betrayal of Health: The Impact of Nutrition, Environment & Lifestyle on the Health of Americans.* Beasley estimates that as many as 150 million of us now have some form of chronic disease. The National Institutes of Health, the Public Health Service, and the Department of Health and Human Services (HHS) have estimated that costly and common allergic reactions and hypersensitivity diseases afflict at least 30 million Americans. Yale University's Mark Cullen, editor of *Workers with Multiple Chemical Sensitivities* (one part of the series *Occupational Medicine: State of the Art Reviews*), estimated in 1987 that "somewhere between 2 percent and 10 percent of the general population suffers from multiple chemical sensitivities and the number appears to be growing."

In fact, more and more illnesses are turning out to have an environmental cause or component. We have long recognized the many serious and even fatal conditions associated with tobacco. But consider more recent observations:

- The World Health Organization (WHO) and others believe that many modern, tightly-constructed buildings endanger occupants' health because of the concentrations of pollutants in recycled air. If you work in such a building and get sore throats, headaches, sore eyes, joint pains, nausea, chest tightness, or other "vague" symptoms, you may have sick building syndrome (SBS): you are reacting to the toxic chemicals being recirculated to you every day.

- Tobacco smoke contains thousands of chemicals, including dangerous ones like hydrogen cyanide, benzene, formaldehyde, and arsenic. A 1991 analysis by the American Heart Association estimated that 53,000 nonsmokers die every year from secondhand smoke; nonsmoking wives have a 30 percent increased risk of lung cancer if their spouses smoke. In 1993 the EPA and the Centers for Disease Control and Prevention (CDC) estimated that each year as many as 300,000 infants suffer from bronchitis, pneumonia, and other infections related to secondhand smoke, plus asthma attacks in twice that number. And, according to a study published in the February 24, 1994, issue of *JAMA*, nicotine has been found in the bloodstreams of newborn infants.

- Parkinson's disease, researchers now know, can be triggered by a specific chemical known as MPTP, while mounting evidence also links Parkinson's with multiple exposures to pesticides and other modern industrial chemicals.

- Environmental factors are also suspected in the increasing mortality rate for amyotrophic lateral sclerosis (ALS, also known as Lou Gehrig's disease), which rose substantially between 1962 and 1984.

- A major metropolitan newspaper's "family doctor," Allan Bruckheim, has written that "hay fever," meaning sneezing, sniffling, and stuffy head symptoms, can be caused by such common irritants as insecticides, cigarette smoke, plaster, newsprint, and glue.

- Asthma is on the increase, especially among children. Between 1980 and 1992 the number of children with asthma increased from 2.4 million to 3.7 million, and the American Lung Association (ALA) suspects indoor air pollution as the culprit. Since 1980 the total number of asthma patients has grown by more than 60 percent, to over 15 million; and since 1978 deaths from the disease have more than doubled. According to the National Center for Health Statistics (NCHS), in 1990 Americans spent $1.6 billion on inpatient services for asthma and $1 billion on medications; asthmatic adults lost $850 million in wages, and parents of asthmatic children lost $1 billion in order to stay home with them.

- A study of more than twenty-five hundred people, published in the *NEJM*, concluded that, contrary to widely held beliefs, almost all asthma attacks are triggered by allergies, regardless of the sufferer's age. A 1993 survey, for example, found over 70 percent of asthma sufferers attributing their symptoms to cigarette smoke, air pollution, and chemicals.

- Most participants in the 1991 NAS workshop on MCS agreed that chemical exposures can cause a variety of diseases, including autoimmune diseases like lupus, which can be triggered by the chemical hydrazine.

- Mental health experts expect panic disorder to strike more than three million Americans in their lifetimes; in 1987, a group of doctors at the University of Washington Medical School reported that "organic solvent exposure can provoke recurrent symptoms that are indistinguishable from panic attacks."

- "Mystery" illnesses have struck many Gulf War veterans. Army doctors at first blamed stress, but evidence points strongly to such exposures as diesel fuel, pesticides, kerosene heaters, and oil well fires. As with many other "mystery" illnesses, the veterans' symptoms are familiar to those with EI/MCS.

- A 1992 review of worldwide fertility studies concluded that the average sperm count in healthy men had dropped by half in the past fifty years, lending credence to speculation that environmental pollutants may damage production of sperm cells. In Costa Rica and Honduras, for example, a U.S.-made herbicide has left thousands of men sterile or impotent or both.

Headaches are also a story, though a less dramatic one. "Headache pain affects forty million Americans. Are you one of them?" trumpeted an ad for the National Headache Foundation, an organization that usually favors drug therapy for headaches. A 1992 survey published in *Internal Medicine News* arrived at an estimate of twenty-three million Americans with migraines, while interviews conducted by the CDC found that the prevalence of migraines in the U.S. increased 60 percent from 1980 to 1989. How many of us are getting headaches from toxic chemicals in our environment? No one knows, and, say the critics, no controlled double-blind tests have been done to find out.

Yet evidence is mounting. In their 1993 study "Headaches from Chemical Exposure," Richard W. Martin, MD, and Charles Becker, MD, say that though headaches are difficult to study, the National Library of Medicine Hazardous Substance Data Bank lists more than seven hundred different chemicals that cause headaches. Their review of fifty workers reporting headaches attributable to chemicals found a pattern of new, chronic headaches occurring after acute exposures in the workplace, as well as headaches that went away after low-level exposures were avoided. They plan more research in light of these provocative findings.

Tips from a Canary

If you suffer from headaches, or from any symptom of potential chemical injury, don't wait for the final tally. Start changing your environment now. You may find yourself feeling a lot better. It isn't always easy—or cheap—but the results are definitely worth it. You might even want to emulate the nineteenth-century coal miners and keep a canary in your house. According to a University of Illinois veterinarian and poison specialist, when nonstick cookware and curling irons, pressing irons, and ironing board covers coated with a common synthetic resin are overheated, the coating releases fumes that can kill a pet bird in fifteen to twenty minutes.

Yes, your pet bird *can* give you a warning, but isn't it better to protect your bird, yourself, and your family by taking a few basic steps?

- Start ridding your home of hazardous, petroleum-based products, including all scented products: let your nose be your guide. Clean air does not smell like chemicals.

- Stay informed: sample the books and other resources listed at the end of each chapter.

- Pay attention to the health clues your body gives you: find a doctor who will work in partnership with you in interpreting those clues.

- Be skeptical: don't buy heavily advertised products. There is a common myth in our society, perpetuated by advertising and public relations, that manufacturers make things for our benefit. Don't believe it.

- Don't count on the government to protect you: it is notoriously bad at that.

- Don't be discouraged: you have plenty of company and there are plenty of solutions and plenty of safe products.

- Remember the alternative: continued ill health. That's the only thing you have to lose.

                    * * * *

To get in touch with a national organization of people with EI/MCS (all are nonprofit and almost entirely staffed by volunteers):

In the United States

- Human Ecology Action League, Inc. (HEAL), P.O.Box 49126, Atlanta, Georgia 30359; 404-248-1898; the oldest national organization; gathers and provides information; publishes quarterly magazine *The Human Ecologist*, Diane Thomas, editor.

- National Center for Environmental Health Strategies (NCEHS), 1100 Rural Avenue, Voorhees, New Jersey 08043; 609-429-5358; politically oriented; provides information and advocacy; publishes newsletter *The Delicate Balance*, Mary Lamielle, editor.

- Environmental Health Network (EHN), P.O. Box 1155, Larkspur, California 94977; 415-331-9804; politically oriented; features disability rights information; publishes newsletter *The New Reactor*, Susan R. Molloy, editor.

- Share, Care, and Prayer, P.O. Box 2080, Frazier Park, California 93225; publishes newsletter; Janet Dauble, editor and executive director.

- Chemical Injury Information Network (CIIN), P.O. Box 301, White Sulphur Springs, Montana 59645; 406-547-2255; politically oriented; publishes newsletter *Our Toxic Times*, Cynthia Wilson, editor.

- Environmental Health Association of Dallas, P.O. Box 388, Forestburg, Texas 76239; provides information; publishes newsletter *20th Century Living*, Peggy Dunlap, editor.

In Canada

- Advocacy Group for the Environmentally Sensitive, 1887 Chaine Court, Orleans, Ontario, Canada K1C 2W6; 613-830-5722; publishes newsletter *AGES*, Marie Laurin, editor.

- The Allergy and Environmental Health Association, 85 Wellesley Boulevard, Toronto, Ontario, Canada M4U 1X7; publishes *The AEHA Quarterly.*

- Environmental Hypersensitivity Association of Ontario, 18 Reid Drive, Apt. 504, Streetsville, Ontario, Canada L5M 2A9; 416-826-9384; publishes newsletter *Positive Reaction,* Wanda Wilson, editor.

In England

- Environmental Medicine Foundation, c/o Mrs. Jennifer Gregson, High Orchards, Corscombe, Dorchester, Dorset BT2 ONU; provides information; features sources for patient funding; publishes newsletter.

* * * *

To locate a physician in your area of the United States who is knowledgeable about environmental influences on health, contact the American Academy of Environmental Medicine (AAEM), P.O. Box 16106, Denver, Colorado 80216; 303-622-9755.

* * * *

To Find Out More

- *An Alternative Approach to Allergies: The New Field of Clinical Ecology Unravels the Environmental Causes of Mental and Physical Ills,* by Theron G. Randolph, MD, and Ralph W. Moss, PhD, revised edition, New York, Harper & Row, 1989.

- *Chemical Sensitivity,* Volumes 1 and 2, by William J. Rea, MD, Boca Raton, Florida, Lewis Publishers, 1992, 1994 (first two volumes of a four-volume work; available from CRC Press Inc., 200 Corporate Boulevard N.W., Boca Raton, Florida 33431).

- *Chemical Exposures: Low Levels and High Stakes,* by Nicholas A. Ashford, PhD, JD, and Claudia S. Miller, MD, New York, Van Nostrand Reinhold, 1991.

- "Advancing the Understanding of Multiple Chemical Sensitivity," a special issue of *Toxicology and Industrial Health,* Vol. 8, No. 4, 1992.

- *Is This Your Child? Discovering and Treating Unrecognized Allergies,* by Doris Rapp, MD, New York, William Morrow, 1991.

- *Tired or Toxic? A Blueprint for Health,* by Sherry Rogers, MD, Syracuse, New York, Prestige Publishing, 1990.

- *The Betrayal of Health: The Impact of Nutrition, Environment, and Lifestyle on Illness in America,* by Joseph D. Beasley, MD, New York, Times Books, 1991.

- *Nontoxic & Natural: How to Avoid Dangerous Everyday Products and Buy or Make Safe Ones,* by Debra Lynn Dadd, Los Angeles, Jeremy P. Tarcher, 1984.

- *The Nontoxic Home: Protecting Yourself and Your Family from Everyday Toxics and Health Hazards,* by Debra Lynn Dadd, Los Angeles, Jeremy P. Tarcher, 1986.

- *Nontoxic, Natural, & Earthwise: How to Protect Yourself and Your Family from Harmful Products and Live in Harmony with the Earth,* by Debra Lynn Dadd, Los Angeles, Jeremy P. Tarcher, 1990.

- *Coping with Your Allergies,* by Natalie Golos and Frances Golos Golbitz, New York, Simon & Schuster, 1986.

- *The Yeast Connection,* by William G. Crook, MD, third edition, New York, Random House, 1986.

- *Chemical Sensitivity: A Guide to Coping with Hypersensitivity Syndrome, Sick Building Syndrome, and Other Environmental Illnesses,* by Bonnye L. Matthews, Jefferson, North Carolina, McFarland & Company, 1992.

- *The Type 1/Type 2 Allergy Relief Program,* by Alan Scott Levin,

MD, and Merla Zellerbach, Los Angeles, Jeremy P. Tarcher, 1983.

- *No More Allergies,* by Gary Null, New York, Villard Books, 1992.

- *The Ion Effect: How Air Electricity Rules Your Life,* by Fred Soyka and Alan Edmonds, Toronto, Bantam, 1978.

- *The Allergy Self-help Book: A Step-by-Step Guide to Nondrug Relief of Asthma, Hay Fever, Headaches, Fatigue, Digestive Problems, and Over 50 Other Allergy-Related Health Problems,* by Sharon Faelten and the Editors of *Prevention* Magazine, Emmaus, Pennsylvania, Rodale Press, 1983.

- *The Whole Way to Allergy Relief & Prevention: A Doctor's Complete Guide to Treatment and Self-Care,* by Jacqueline Krohn, MD, Frances A. Taylor, MA, and Erla Mae Larson, RN, Point Roberts, Washington, Hartley & Marks, 1991.

- *The Truth about Where You Live: An Atlas for Action on Toxics and Mortality,* by Benjamin Goldman, New York, Times Books, 1991.

- *Chemical Deception: The Toxic Threat to Health and the Environment,* by Marc Lappé, San Francisco, Sierra Club, 1991.

- *Cancer Therapy: The Independent Consumer's Guide to Non-Toxic Treatment and Prevention,* by Ralph W. Moss, New York, Equinox Press, 1992

- *Everyday Cancer Risks & How to Avoid Them,* by Mary Kerney Levenstein, Garden City Park, New York, Avery Publishing Group, 1992.

- *Silent Spring,* by Rachel Carson, New York, Houghton Mifflin, 25th anniversary edition, 1987 (still a classic).

2

Breathing Easier?

OUTDOOR AIR IS WORSE than indoor air, right? Nope. Not according to the EPA. In 1980 the EPA mounted a five-year study of twenty common toxic or cancer-causing chemicals known as the Total Exposure Assessment Methodology (TEAM) study. The investigation compared indoor and outdoor air and found that indoor air was three to seventy times more polluted than outdoor air, even in heavily contaminated areas like Los Angeles and Bayonne, New Jersey.

"It was a big surprise to us," said the head of the TEAM study, Lance Wallace, after presenting the results at the 1986 meeting of the American Chemical Society. "Personal exposure to the eleven chemicals that were present more than 75 percent of the time was much greater indoors, even though we chose what we thought were the worst outdoor levels we could find. We started this study in 1980 and we didn't really believe the results for a long time, but now they've been confirmed by Scandinavian data." Wallace added that after three hours of trying to count all the possible sources of contamination in his own bathroom, he gave up: "We're all living in a chemical soup."

Because the six hundred people participating in the TEAM study carried personal air monitors throughout a normal twenty-four-hour day, readings reflect their exposures indoors and out, in stores and other public buildings, in service stations and workplaces, as well as in their homes. The study monitored breath concentrations of such chemicals as benzene, a known human carcinogen found in cigarette smoke, and paradichlorobenzene, a related and potent animal carcinogen found in solid and aerosol air fresheners. Also monitored was tetrachloroethylene, known as perchloroethylene, or "perc," the most common dry cleaning solvent. The study found indoor levels of carbon tetrachloride (source unknown), banned from consumer products by the Consumer Product Safety Commission (CPSC), consistently higher than outdoor levels. High air levels of chloroform were thought to come from hot showers, which transform the chlorine in the water to the suspected carcinogen chloroform. Other sources of the chemicals studied were paint, sheetrock, wallpaper, carpeting, glue, cleansers, and insecticides. More than 99 percent of the exposures came from the air, with the exception of chloroform and other trihalomethanes, which were found mostly in drinking water, also tested in the homes.

The TEAM study tested for only twenty of the eight hundred known volatile organic compounds, or VOCs. Yet the EPA scientists calculated that nationwide "a typical homeowner's exposure to just six of the most common VOCs could result in as many as five thousand additional cancer cases a year—a level of risk that . . . places VOCs [third after] cigarette smoking and radon as indoor air hazards," said Wallace. VOCs are modern synthetic chemicals that evaporate quickly at room temperature. Because of this property, they are commonly used as solvents—in paints, varnishes, glues, dyes, inks, marking pens, perfumes, paint and polish removers, certain cleaning products, and anything that says "fast drying."

Yet despite a continuing accumulation of media coverage and scientific data, indoor air pollution has not found its way onto this country's regulatory agenda. Both public attention and government policy tend to focus on "big ticket" items—toxic waste dumps, the ozone layer—while ignoring the serious hazards that are, quite literally, right in front of their noses. The EPA reported in 1989 that "indoor air pollution consistently causes greater health risks than [such other sources as] hazardous waste sites, whether [in] New England, the Middle Atlantic region, or the Pacific Northwest." Yet according to the same report, "Each of the three highest health risk areas—radon, indoor air pollution, and pesticide residues—is the subject of minimal [EPA] regional program efforts. . . . By contrast, two of the low-risk problem areas—active and abandoned haz-ardous waste sites—are the subject of major regional programs."

The EPA staff's ranking of indoor air pollution as worse than outdoor air pollution and toxic waste dumps is confirmed by inde-pendent investigator Gray Robertson, an English chemist trained at the University of London and known as "the building doctor" for his work in diagnosing and treating "sick" buildings. "Most people still underestimate the problem of sick buildings," he says. "Indoor pollution is a worse environmental threat than toxic waste dumps." After examining 270 large public buildings, 90 percent of which housed offices, Robertson found that "well over half have [indoor air] problems. Sixty-four percent . . . have inadequate ventilation, and 35 percent of those operated entirely with recycled air. . . . No fresh air whatsoever. . . . That's like everyone in the same family washing in the same bath water." In Robertson's view, the greatest source of the pollution, after tobacco smoke, is synthetics and plas-tics in furnishings, carpeting, and walls, plus the detergents, pesti-cides, disinfectants, and dry cleaning chemicals used to treat the furnishings. "People get used to indoor air pollution without realiz-ing it," he warns.

Robertson's estimate is seconded by scientist James E. Woods, of the Virginia Polytechnic Institute, who agrees that as many as half the buildings in the U.S. are unhealthy. Meanwhile, according to a New York newspaper, "despite a daily barrage of inquiries and complaints from the public, no government agency has a clear man-date to do anything about indoor air pollution. . . . Trees, whales, and smokestacks of big factories aren't part of the debate over in-door pollution. Neither are environmental groups." The reason? Because rain forests, whales, and smokestacks are further from our control and thus, paradoxically, seem to need more control efforts? Because it is assumed that we can control our indoor environment and therefore must be doing so? Because of powerful commercial interests? All of the above?

At any rate, indoor air pollution does not get the funding it needs. The EPA staff has estimated that $20 million a year would be needed for indoor air pollution research. Yet for 1993 the EPA pro-jected a mere $5.9 million for its indoor air division, up from $5.5

million for 1992, a tiny percentage of the $38 billion our government budgeted for environmental protection in 1993, with a quarter of that total going for cleaning up toxic and radioactive waste dumps. Though the Clinton administration has proposed a 13 percent hike in the EPA's 1995 budget, there's little chance that indoor air's share will increase by much. Says Lance Wallace, "We concentrate on the big visible sources, chemical plants and oil refineries and outdoor air, but the true exposures are the little things under your nose."

Thus, if you have felt sick recently, consider the possibility that what made you feel that way—and what may make you feel ill for months and years to come—is the cumulative effects of the cleaning products under your sink, the padding in your sofa, the particle board in your kitchen cabinets, the cosmetics or after-shave lotion on your face, the perfume on your neck, the deodorants under your arms, the detergents and fabric softeners you use on your clothes (and the clothes themselves, if synthetic), the air "fresheners" in your bathroom, the combustion products escaping from your gas appliances. Most are petroleum-based; some, like perfumes, are designed to "outgas"; some, like synthetic clothes, outgas simply because they are made of unstable chemical compounds; others, like your gas stove, produce toxic compounds such as carbon monoxide and nitrogen dioxide as part of doing what they are supposed to do. Whatever the manufacturer's intention, toxic chemicals from such products are continuously outgassing into your personal airspace.

Products like these help make buildings "sick," and sick buildings do not come cheap, either in money or in human lives. According to Peter Berle, president of the National Audubon Society, the EPA estimates that sick building syndrome (SBS) yearly costs the U.S. economy about $60 billion, both in lost productivity and increased medical costs. The Consumer Federation of America estimates the costs as high as $100 billion a year. Indoor pollution, including secondhand tobacco smoke, may account for as many as 11,400 deaths each year, EPA researchers project. And thirty thousand more deaths a year may result from *legionella* bacteria in poorly maintained hospital systems for hot water, heating, and air conditioning, according to University of Michigan scientist Harriet Burge. "These kinds of health risks have been there [for some time].

We just haven't realized it," says John Holmes, chief of the California Air Resource Board's research division. "But slowly we're getting the results from what is a gigantic experiment," Holmes adds. "As it becomes clear what the risks are . . . society will move to reduce or severely limit those risks."

But hold on. Does it make you feel good to know that you're participating in a gigantic health experiment? Is society moving to reduce those risks? If indoor air is so much worse than outdoor air, why is so much more attention paid to outdoor air? One reason, of course, is simply visibility. You can see auto and truck exhaust, you can see plumes from smokestacks, you can see the tons of particulate matter suspended in the gray-yellow-brown smog of a sunny day in Los Angeles, just as you can see oil slicks and litter. But you can't see 4-phenylcyclohexene from carpeting, toluene from printer's ink, xylene from marking pens, formaldehyde from toothpaste, methylene chloride from paint remover.

Another reason is advertising, the billion-dollar business devoted to making us spend money we may not have for things that we may not need and that may not be good for us. Daily, in print and on television screens, we are seduced by cleverly designed commercials enticing us to buy hundreds of colorful and beautiful new products. No ad, of course, lures us to create oil slicks, to produce more auto exhaust, to build more smokestacks, or to litter. We know such things are bad. What we don't know yet, as a society, is that the "better living" we see in the ads is poisoning our indoor air and ourselves.

A third and more basic reason is denial, the way we all have of not seeing what is plainly evident or of denying it to ourselves. We want those wonderful objects we see in the TV commercials and newspaper ads. We want to have all those choices; we don't want the barren store shelves that TV shows us in Eastern European countries. We don't want to change our vaunted lifestyle—a lifestyle that sometimes seems the main asset we have left as a society, a lifestyle that makes the U.S. and other developed countries the envy of second- and third-world societies. Thus we deny any need to change the way we live, to pull ourselves back from twentieth-century "better living." If our own health isn't yet affected, or we don't fully realize what is causing our ill health, we don't want to change. It is easier to blame the people "out there"—smokestack industries, the toxic-waste dumpers, the oil companies, and the litterers—than to look into our own kitchens and bathrooms and living rooms for the toxic products we have put there . . . the products that affect our own and our children's health. In the *Wall Street Journal,* Jack Moore, director of the Institute for Evaluating Health Risks, calls the chemicals in household products a child's greatest environmental foe. It is far easier, he says, "to blame the guys who produce your food [or other products] for what they might be doing to your children than to own up to the fact that your own choices might increase their exposure to toxics."

Toxics in Our Drinking Water

Yet there is no doubt that outdoor air pollution—especially that which ends up in our drinking water—is dangerous. Take the Great Lakes, the world's largest body of fresh water. Fresh? In Lake Superior, largest and northernmost, is Isle Royale, 210 square miles of pristine wilderness, with backpacking trails, one tourist lodge, and a small, isolated inland lake—Siskiwit Lake. In the late 1970s an EPA scientist, Wayland Swain, looking for the source of toxic polychlorinated biphenyls (PCBs) in Lake Superior fish, incidentally discovered that fish in Siskiwit Lake contained not only PCBs but also toxaphene, a pesticide used exclusively in the south against cotton boll weevils. (The EPA banned toxaphene in 1982 as a suspected carcinogen.) Because Siskiwit Lake is about fifty feet higher than Lake Superior, there is no way for water from Lake Superior to get to Siskiwit Lake. Therefore the pollution must have come by air, no respecter of boundaries between land and water, or of lines between states—or nations.

DDT (dichlorodiphenyltrichloroethane) levels in the Great Lakes are another indicator of toxic fallout. In 1972 cancer-causing DDT was banned for most uses in the U.S., though it is still produced for export. At first, levels of DDT in Great Lakes fish dropped, as expected, but then they began to level off: the lakes were apparently being contaminated by DDT that blows in from Mexico and Central America, where it was—and is—still being used. In 1988 it was estimated that up to 90 percent of some toxic chemicals reach the Great Lakes by air after traveling hundreds or thousands of miles on the wind. The Great Lakes, it would seem, are gigantic sponges soaking up toxic chemicals from the entire continent. And not just the Great Lakes: according to the Minnesota Pollution Control Agency, small, remote lakes in northern Wisconsin and Minnesota have experienced a fourfold increase in levels of highly toxic mercury in the past forty years—from air and rainwater runoff. What all these lakes are telling us is that wherever we live, polluted outdoor air is reaching us in ways we may not realize: from our kitchen tap as well as in the fish we eat. Our toxic load from outdoor air is thus greater than the TEAM study indicates.

From Illinois alone, the Great Lakes are absorbing part of the toxic chemicals emitted by industries in that state. In 1987, the first year that such statistics were collected under the Toxics Release Inventory (TRI) mandated by Congress the year before, twenty-four million pounds of potentially cancer-causing chemicals were legally spewed into Illinois air, land, and water, according to Illinois Public Action, a citizens group evaluating the health effects of the chemicals covered by the inventory. About half of this toxic load went into the air. The chemicals included benzene, a solvent and component of gasoline that is known to cause leukemia; styrene, a possible carcinogen that is used to make plastics; trichloroethylene, a degreasing agent that has caused liver cancer in animals; and dichloromethane, a possible human carcinogen with many uses, including applications in making pesticides and film. In 1988, also according to Illinois Public Action, Illinois companies discharged into the environment more than seventy million pounds of pollutants that are known to cause or suspected of causing birth defects. Almost 80 percent of these emissions, including the solvents xylene, toluene, and 1,1,1-trichloroethane, went into the air, the least-regulated portion of the environment. "All the oatmeal you eat won't protect you from these emissions," said John Cameron, toxic chemical specialist for the group. And each year, such figures are only a fraction of the total emissions of toxic chemicals in Illinois or any other state— chemicals that can pose health risks other than cancer or birth defects. In 1989, for example, almost eight thousand businesses in the eight Great Lakes states discharged 751.8 million pounds of toxic chemicals into the air, water, and sewage systems—"a crime against nature," according to Tom Pollak, research director of the Citizens Fund, a national environmental group.

The Great Lakes—and your health, if you are among the forty million people living near them or eating their fish and drinking their water—are imperiled not only from the air, but from oil and chemical spills. In the 1980s more than five thousand spills were reported, nearly three times the total previously reported. Eighty percent of the spills were from land-based industries, with Detroit reporting the largest number. But bad as these facts are, they represent an improvement of sorts. Lake Erie is now cleaner—its fish have fewer tumors and birth defects—than it was in 1970, and observers agree that Lake Michigan looks better. Says Cameron Davis, of the Lake Michigan Federation, "Twenty years ago, you could see the lake pollution problems: algae and piles of fish on the beaches. Now, the [cancer-causing chemicals and toxic metals found in Lake Michigan water] have no color and no smell and the health impacts they cause don't kick in for years and sometimes decades."

According to a 1988 report by the International Joint Commission (IJC), a joint agency of the U.S. National Research Council and the Royal Society of Canada, residents of the Great Lakes area are exposed to "appreciably more toxics than residents elsewhere in North America. Yet in 1988 there was "nobody in the Great Lakes region doing [human] health effects research," said Alfred Beeton, U.S. chair of the IJC's Science Advisory Board. "It takes funding and long-term studies. We don't do that in this country." While extensive studies have been made of the apparent effects of toxic chemicals on Great Lakes wildlife, "additional studies of the health effects of lake fish on humans are desperately needed," said Theo Colborn, in 1989 with the Washington, D.C.-based Conservation Foundation. Two years later, scientists at the IJC's biennial meeting warned that toxic chemicals in the Great Lakes and other sources of drinking water may be robbing children of their ability to learn and think. Chemicals, they said, might be adversely affecting the young people's nervous systems, fertility, mental development, and immunity to disease—none of which is recorded by health agencies. In a land where the sky is falling, then, little is being done about it by those whom we would like to think are doing something about it.

In 1991 came yet another Great Lakes study, this one by a team of U.S. and Canadian environmentalists who asked for an immediate ban on up to seventy toxic chemicals and the gradual elimination of all industrial waste discharges. One member of the team, Paul Muldoon of the Canadian Institute for Environmental Law and Policy, recommended that industries find benign substitutes for these seventy chemicals; Muldoon thus became another voice for pollution prevention instead of pollution control. These investigators were optimistic about what they termed "Reilly's call to make the Great Lakes a test area for pollution prevention and other cleanup strategies." Indeed, early in 1991, then-EPA-chief William Reilly did send letters to the heads of more than six hundred U.S. companies asking them to voluntarily reduce emissions of seventeen toxic compounds and heavy metals. With forty of the firms in the Chicago area and one hundred more in the Great Lakes states together emitting more than a third of some of the most toxic pollutants being spilled in this country each year, "the region most impacted is the Chicago region, the arc that underlies the Great Lakes," said Reilly.

More voluntarism. Will it work? Only time will tell how many of these six hundred companies will stop using these seventy toxic substances, voluntarily. Even if they do, the problem remains: the first comprehensive review of air, land, and water threats to Lake Michigan, in 1992, found the most dangerous pollutants to be the toxic chemicals mercury, dioxin, dieldrin, chlordane, DDT, and PCBs. The latter four have been banned or restricted in the U.S. for years, but still persist; all except mercury also contain chlorine, putting them among the more than eleven thousand organochlorines thought to be toxic at some level. The sky, it would appear, is still falling.

Government Action and Inaction

Can we trust federal regulatory agencies to protect us against pollution—indoors or out? In the last twenty-six years, Congress has enacted the 1969 National Environmental Policy Act; the 1970 Occupational Safety and Health Act (OSHA), with its research arm, the National Institute for Occupational Safety and Health

(NIOSH); the 1970 and 1990 Clean Air Acts; the 1972 Clean Water Act; the 1973 Endangered Species Act; the 1974 Safe Drinking Water Act; the 1976 Resource Conservation and Recovery Act (RCRA), to track production and disposal of hazardous wastes; the 1976 Toxic Substances Control Act (TSCA), to regulate manufacture and use of what is now more than seventy thousand toxic chemicals; the 1978 Uranium Tailings Radiation Control Act; the 1985 Food Security Act, to protect wetlands and prevent soil erosion; the 1986 Superfund Amendments Reauthorization Act (SARA), which extended and amended the Comprehensive Environmental Response, Compensation, and Liability Act (CERCLA, or Superfund, meaning toxic waste dumps) and which included Title III—the Emergency Planning and Community Right-to-Know Act (EPCRA), whose yearly Toxics Release Inventory lets us know some of the toxic chemicals that industry is emitting; the 1988 Medical Waste Tracing Act; the 1988 Federal Insecticide, Fungicide, and Rodenticide Act (FIFRA) reform bill, mandating health and safety testing of pesticides used in the U.S.; and the 1990 Pollution Prevention Act, which attempts to expand the Toxics Release Inventory (TRI). Congress also set up three environmental regulatory agencies: the Occupational Safety and Health Administration (OSHA, 1970), the Environmental Protection Agency (EPA, 1970), and the Consumer Product Safety Commission (CPSC, 1972). SARA charged the EPA with most of the toxic waste cleanup, but it also set up the Agency for Toxic Substances and Disease Registry (ATSDR) within the U.S. Public Health Service, primarily to monitor the health effects of those toxic waste dumps on the National Priorities List (NPL).

An impressive list (got it all straight?). Since 1970 the EPA has set standards for six conventional air pollutants—carbon monoxide, sulfur dioxide, hydrocarbons, nitrogen dioxide, lead, and ozone. Every year the EPA reports the status of these pollutants outdoors, but the report omits the status in our air, indoors as well as outdoors, of TSCA's list of more than seventy thousand chemicals in commercial use, of NIOSH's list of more than four hundred toxic chemicals found in workplaces, of the TRI list of more than three hundred toxic chemicals being emitted by industry, and of the more than two hundred chemicals most frequently found in NPL toxic waste dumps (with some overlapping, to be sure). The EPA omits the status of all these toxic chemicals in our air, mainly because it does not know their status. It is not measuring their status in our air, possibly because doing so is too big a job for them or for anyone. So when the EPA tells us, as it does almost every year, that our air is getting better, we must realize that it is not telling us the whole story. In 1992, for instance, it told us that all the levels of those six air pollutants fell in the preceding ten years, with lead leading the list at 89 percent, nitrogen dioxide the lowest at 6 percent.

In reviewing environmental progress (or lack of it) from 1970 to 1989, Barry Commoner, biologist-turned-ecologist/activist, said that some outdoor pollutants are down by an average of 14 percent, with 70-to-90-percent improvement in airborne lead, DDT and related pesticides, PCBs, mercury in surface waters, radioactive fallout from nuclear bomb tests, and, in some rivers, phosphates. But the quality of our drinking water has not improved or has actually deteriorated in 90 percent of the sites tested. For the bulk of modern pollutants, Commoner says, the situation has hardly improved at all. (Of course we don't know how bad the problem would be if our government had done nothing.)

Why the improvement in these six previously major pollutants? Simply because we have stopped putting them into the environment, says Commoner. Once the pollutant is produced, it's too late. Rather, we have to take the pollutant out of the system of production entirely. This has been done, for example, in chlorine-producing plants that have substituted a semipermeable membrane for mercury in their production processes. Some paper mills now bleach with oxygen instead of chlorine, thereby reducing the production of toxic dioxin. The Model A car, manufactured before World War II, did not produce smog, according to Commoner, but the high-compression engines developed since World War II do. Therefore, he suggested in a tongue-in-cheek talk to EPA staff, the EPA should renounce regulating and turn instead to inventing.

"Environmental pollution is an incurable disease," Commoner says. "It can only be prevented." Since 1970 our government's approach to the environment has been "command and control." In an attempt to control pollution, the EPA and other agencies, when they have done anything, have tried to command (or sometimes persuade) polluters to cease and desist. But, says Commoner, once pollution gets into the environment, controls don't work. That, he says, is "the big lesson to learn in the 1990s." Recognizing this, Greenpeace U.S.A. in 1990 announced that it is shifting its activities "to a goal of pollution prevention at the local level, rather than engage in more battles with governmental bureaucracies over how much pollution is tolerable."

The big question, of course, is how much you and I will tolerate. For years U.S. industries have been dumping unknown (to us) quantities of toxic chemicals into the air, water, and land that we all share. Now we have the right to know. What has finally gotten this information to us, said Representative Gerry Sikorski, the Minnesota Democrat who sponsored the 1986 right-to-know proposal that Congress barely passed, is a kind of "heartfelt belief that people in communities have an absolute, fundamental right to know what goes into the air their kids breathe, the water they drink, and the ground they play on." (A right-to-know-more act remains stalled in Congress.)

What caught Congress's attention, of course, was the 1984 tragedy in Bhopal, India, the most terrible episode of large-scale outdoor chemical poisoning in history. It was in Bhopal that an accidental emission of methyl isocyanate in a pesticide-producing Union Carbide plant killed more than thirty-five hundred people and may have injured more than two hundred thousand people, some possibly for life. By 1991, 70 percent of 113 survivors were found to have serious lung damage and breathing impairment, as well as neurological symptoms, but no survivor had received any compensation despite an Indian court's settlement for $470 million (there were later attempts to indict Union Carbide officials for "culpable homicide"). Though it is often argued that companies are performing a public service simply by providing jobs, only a few hundred of Bhopal's residents actually worked in the plant. Most of those living in shanties near the plant came there to construct it but lost their jobs after it was finished. Now they have lost more than their jobs.

Bhopal is a long way from most Americans, but the isocyanates are no stranger to us. According to Commoner, "repeated accidents at the Union Carbide methyl isocyanate plants . . . in Institute, West

Virginia . . . have exposed workers and in some cases the neighbor-hood to this dangerous substance." In 1981, workers in another part of the country were sensitized to toluene diisocyanate by indi-rect exposure through fumes from the exhaust of a neighboring fac-tory which were sucked into their ventilation systems. In Galesburg, Illinois, long-term and acute exposures to the methylene bisphenyl isocyanate used in foam insulation disabled forty workers in a re-frigerator plant. Diagnosed with "occupational asthma," some of these workers now become ill merely by walking into fabric stores and supermarket detergent aisles. Sensitivity to toluene diisocyanate can be induced in a person with no prior history of "allergy," and that sensitivity may, in turn, contribute to an overall sensitivity to other chemicals.

Because of the EPA's yearly TRI, we now have clues as to just what is being dumped on us. In 1987 it included large amounts of toluene and xylene: what inner-city kids sniff voluntarily, we have been inhaling involuntarily. In 1988 neighbors of Kodak Co., in Rochester, New York, learned that Kodak had spewed 23.6 million pounds of sixty-five dangerous chemicals into the air the preceding year. Said one astonished neighbor who was putting his house on the market, "They are not the benevolent good neighbor we thought they were."

We also have clues as to just how much is being dumped on us. In 1988 it was 4.6 billion pounds of toxic chemicals—almost twen-ty pounds per person, many cancer-causing, more than half into the air. And emissions from small companies, government installations, auto tailpipes, and lawnmowers were not included in this total. Our government has not been setting a good example: some large federal installations have been violating clean air, clean water, and haz-ardous material laws for years, according to the *Washington Post*. The Boston-based National Toxics Campaign (now reorganized as the Jobs and Environment Campaign) has said that 1,579 Army, Navy, and Air Force bases across the country contain 14,400 sites with known or suspected contamination by hazardous material. But reform may be in sight: a 1993 executive order requires more than five hundred federal facilities to report wastes and releases under the TRI and to reduce their use of toxic chemicals.

By 1991, though total hazardous waste had increased and even though the 1990 Pollution Prevention Act had required additional reporting, such as recycling and source reduction, total releases of toxic chemicals reported in the TRI were down somewhat, to 3.38 billion pounds. (Feel any better?) Nevertheless, the EPA's 1991 report cautioned that "although the TRI includes over eighty-two thousand reports from approximately twenty-three thousand facilities each year, it captures only a portion of all toxic chemical releases nationwide." The EPA also cautioned, as it did in 1988, that TRI data alone cannot determine adverse effects on human health.

True. Take urban smog, familiar to most of us. The result mostly of factory and tailpipe emissions, urban smog is composed primarily of VOCs, nitrogen dioxide, and ozone. The latter, formed when sunlight reacts with these emissions, puts exercising and asthmatic children at risk, says Dr. Ruth Etzel, of the American Academy of Pediatrics and the Centers for Disease Control and Prevention (CDC). Though cars and factories have become somewhat cleaner over the last twenty years, industrial growth and more cars on the road have kept smog levels high. Concerned about the health effects of air pollution, the *Journal of the American Medical Association* (*JAMA*) in 1991 reported that a study of lung specimens of young accident victims in Los Angeles revealed declines in pulmonary function: "Long before clinical signs of reduced pulmonary function can be detected, there are pathological signs that may be noted." The researcher suspects ozone as a culprit. (As if outdoor ozone were not enough, calculations based on surveys of southern California homes and the fact that people spend most of their lives indoors have led to estimates of indoor ozone exposures three to four times outdoor ozone exposures.) A Harvard study of 8,111 adults followed for fourteen to sixteen years suggests that fine particles from industry, automobiles, and home heating, within governmentally set limits, are contributing to the early death of tens of thousands of people. The EPA does not even need the TRI in order to heed reports such as these.

For information on the TRI, call OMB (Office of Management and Budget) Watch, 202-659-1711, and ask for its booklet "Community Right-to-Know: A New Tool for Pollution Prevention." Unfortunately, this remarkable new tool has several grave weaknesses (in addition to the polluters not being required to report), the gravest a "recycling loophole" that enables companies to bypass some of the reporting regulations, distorting the program's totals and in the process causing serious community contamination. Toxic waste recycling is very dangerous and can by no means be considered pollution prevention. However, to find out at least some of the pollutants being emitted in your area, call the EPA at 1-800-535-0202 or 202-260-1531 for information about TRI or to learn which libraries in your area have a computerized record of TRI emissions. At least one library in every county nationwide now has access to this record. Meanwhile, beware of companies' claims of toxic chemical emissions reduction. A 1992 Citizens Fund analysis of the data revealed that only thirteen of the top fifty facilities reporting reductions between 1988 and 1989 could point to investment in pollution prevention or control as the cause. In other words, said the fund, there are few "real" reductions.

Still, we now have some idea of which toxic chemicals and how much of them are going into our outdoor environment. We also are beginning to know what toxic chemicals are going into our bodies—and staying there. By analyzing fat samples sent in by pathologists around the country, the EPA, through an ongoing study called the National Human Adipose Tissue Survey (NHATS), finds out how many of which toxic chemicals are likely to be in our body fat. In 1988, thirty of fifty-five toxic chemicals, including many carcinogens, were present in more than 50 percent of the samples tested. And this was only fifty-five out of approximately (at that time) sixty-five thousand possibly toxic chemicals. Again, VOCs head the list: xylene, from common sources like gasoline, paints, and lacquers, was found in 100 percent of the samples; toluene, also in gasoline as well as in products already mentioned, was found in 91 percent.

Yes, our bodies are now toxic waste dumps. To find out what is in your own bloodstream (these substances move back and forth between your blood and fat), your doctor can have a sample of your blood analyzed by one of several laboratories around the country. The report that you will receive may say, as one such report did, "Any level other than zero is abnormal. These compounds are foreign and serve no beneficial function to the body." That report might have added, though it didn't: "A hundred years ago, these compounds would not have been in your body. They didn't exist or weren't commonly used then." For a copy of the latest NHATS report, contact the National Technical Information Service (NTIS), 5285 Port Royal Road, Springfield, Virginia 22161; 703-487-4650.

Not only do these toxic chemicals serve no beneficial function to bodies, they may be—probably are—injuring your body. Yet concrete evidence linking small amounts of toxic chemicals to human health in the form of such illnesses as EI/MCS is only slowly being developed . . . in a medical journal article here, a book or two there. Ashford and Miller's book *Chemical Exposures* reviews the evidence for the extent of EI/MCS and concludes that "based on the increasing outbreaks of sick building syndrome, increased reporting of symptoms in contaminated communities to state health departments, increased recognition of problems in the industrial workplace, and the increasing number of physicians treating chemically related sensitivities, the existing evidence does suggest that chemical sensitivity is on the rise and could become a large problem with significant economic consequences related to the disablement of productive members of society."

In the early 1980s Congress decided that the times called for a deeper probe into the relationship between toxic chemicals and human health than had yet been done. It mandated the ATSDR to produce "toxicological profiles" for approximately 250 hazardous chemicals at Superfund toxic waste sites. These detailed but readable profiles of the chemicals, their health effects, and the ways you can be exposed to them are now available from the NTIS. Though the ATSDR's "mission is to prevent or mitigate adverse human health effects and diminished quality of life resulting from environmental exposure to hazardous substances," by 1992 it had done little to recognize or help victims of toxic waste dumps. And it took until 1993—more than forty years after the discovery of the health effect of modern petrochemicals—for Congress to give the ATSDR the princely sum of $250,000 to conduct workshops and plan a national registry for people with EI/MCS.

EI/MCS is also known informally as twentieth-century disease, for reasons that should by now be apparent. Since 1945 the nation's production of organic chemicals such as VOCs has steadily increased by more than 6 percent a year. In West Virginia's Kanawha

Valley—home to a quarter of a million people and thirteen major chemical plants—state health department records show that between 1968 and 1977, the incidence of respiratory cancer was more than 21 percent above the national average. According to EPA statistics, "a lifetime of exposure to the airborne concentrations of butadiene, chloroform, and ethylene oxide in this valley could cause cancer in one resident in a thousand." In other words, 250 residents of Kanawha Valley may acquire cancer attributable to environmental exposures. These victims are chemically injured, though they may or may not be chemically sensitive. They may or may not have become sensitized to perfumes, paints, pesticides, and supermarket detergent aisles, but their illness has been caused by alien chemicals in the environment.

Command and Control vs. Pollution Prevention

For several reasons, the present environmental policies of "command and control" and "clean up the mess" are inferior. The main reason is that they simply don't work. Using laws and regulations to "command" us to control pollutants addresses only the symptoms, not the root causes. Once the pollutants get into the environment they are uncontrollable. The EPA in 1991 estimated that eighty-four million Americans still breathe outdoor air "that exceeds limits for at least one of the six major pollutants monitored by the EPA." The National Park Service has discovered the only clean air left in the contiguous United States: an uneven, pancake-shaped area about four hundred miles in diameter, covering northeastern Nevada, northwestern Utah, and southern Idaho. On bad days, says the Park Service, "visitors can no longer see the Colorado River at the bottom of the [Grand] Canyon." Eastern parks are no better off; there the visibility is, on average, 10 percent of that in the Western parks. Power plants cause much of the smog; a 1991 agreement between the EPA and operators of a power plant near the Grand Canyon set 1999 as the target date for reducing sulfur dioxide emissions by 90 percent. That's a long time to wait to see the Colorado River.

Another reason is Congress's procrastination. In 1970 Joseph

Karaganis, an organizer of the first Earth Day, advocated banning internal-combustion engines by 1980. Now a leading environmental lawyer, Karaganis pointed out on Earth Day 1990 that autos are responsible for smog in "101 [of the] U.S. metropolitan areas that violate federal clean-air limits. . . . [Yet] the 1970 federal Clean Air Act called for smog control by 1977." Since 1970 the U.S. has repeatedly missed major environmental deadlines. The deadlines are set by Congress, but lawmakers routinely extend them because, argues Karaganis, they fail to understand the complexities of environmental issues. (Or are they failing to understand the simplicity of some?)

Even when Congress does act, the laws are often meaningless, says William Greider in his 1992 book *Who Will Tell the People: The Betrayal of American Democracy*. Congress and the executive branch enact what he calls "hollow laws"—"grand pronouncements on toxic wastes and other problems designed to sound responsive to the public, but also designed to be neutered or neglected later in the dense details of the regulatory government." Once a law is passed, agencies can foot-drag on writing the necessary but exceedingly complicated regulations; in the two years after Congress passed the 1990 Clean Air Act, the EPA missed at least sixty mandatory statutory deadlines for writing the rules to control air pollution. Or they can water them down as a result of outside pressure. (One of President Bill Clinton's first actions in office was to abolish Vice President Dan Quayle's Council on Competitiveness, notorious for its subversion of the regulatory process.) Often, says Greider, it takes good investigative reporting by major newspapers to call public attention to this corruption. "In a world of unreliable laws, the news media have become a principal agent of law enforcement," he wrote. "But . . . the media's glare is essentially a transient, accidental force." We should not have to rely on newspapers to enforce the law.

Nor on lawsuits to force agencies to do what they should be doing. After the EPA dawdled in enforcing the 1986 amendments to the Clean Drinking Water Act, an Oregon citizens' group sued the agency every time it missed a deadline, and won, despite the EPA's excuses: "We didn't know we had to do it"; "We don't agree that we have to do it"; "We don't have the money to do it"; "We don't have the time or energy to do it." In July 1993 the American Lung Association notified the EPA of its intent to sue the agency to revise its standards for particulate matter in our air. Though there is no clinical evidence yet for a cause-and-effect relationship between particulate matter—from sources such as road dust, bus exhaust fumes, tobacco smoke, fireplaces, and backyard barbecues—and increased mortality, says the ALA, studies of urban areas indicate that deaths increase in direct proportion to levels of particulate air pollution, even when levels are as low as one-third of current EPA standards.

In March 1994, the EPA again attempted command and control when it issued its final rule requiring chemical companies to upgrade their technology to prevent evaporation and leaks. Companies will get three years to cut these toxic air emissions. EPA head Carol Browner estimated that the rule would reduce such emissions by 88 percent, the equivalent of removing thirty-eight million cars from the road. But will it work? Will the EPA enforce it? The first "Annual Review of the U.S. Environmental Protection Agency," done in 1993 by the Washington D.C.-based Center for Resource Economics, concluded that while the U.S. has the world's most comprehensive set of environmental laws, it cannot ensure that American communities and industries are in full compliance with a single federal environmental law.

Unfortunately, when the EPA does take action, it sometimes makes the wrong choice. For example, it has for some time pushed incineration as a solution to the nation's toxic waste problem, despite evidence that incineration releases toxic chemicals into the air. Even if an incinerator should attain the EPA's standard of destroying 99.99 percent of the toxic chemicals being burned, there is always the possibility of human error or malfeasance, or accidents. Three such events have occurred at a toxic waste incinerator in the Chicago area. Once, the incinerator exploded because a chemical to be burned was not properly identified. On another occasion, workers deliberately disconnected air pollution monitors while overloading the incinerator with highly toxic PCBs. And once hazardous chemicals exploded during incineration, releasing an unknown amount of potentially toxic gases. In 1992 a supervisor at this notorious incinerator was indicted on charges of false material statements concerning hazardous waste, unlawful destruction of hazardous waste records, forgery, and conspiracy. The company involved, Chemical Waste Management, a subsidiary of the giant garbage-disposal firm Waste Management, Inc., has so far been fined approximately $13 million for operating violations (coincidentally only a little more than the 1990 salary of Waste Management's CEO, Dean Buntrock).

In addition to these possibilities, incineration produces a residue ash rich in toxic metals, like lead, which then pose a disposal problem. Plastics, notoriously disposed of by everybody all the time, are essentially long-lived but unstable chemical compounds that continuously outgas toxic chemicals in normal use. When burned in incinerators they produce highly toxic compounds like dioxin and furans, for which no safe limits have been established and which cannot be continuously monitored in the incinerator emissions. If you burn polyurethane, common in households, you get toxic diisocyanates. For these reasons and others, the American Public Health Association (APHA) has taken a stand against incinerating municipal solid waste, recommending instead a "federal solid waste policy rooted in resource conservation and pollution prevention."

Fine, but what about the health of Sandra Estell and her son Alex, who breathe air from the tall smokestack of the East Liverpool, Ohio, toxic waste incinerator that finally began operation in April 1993, after a long battle between opponents and supporters and after the Clinton administration insisted that it was powerless to block previous court decisions. The EPA claimed that the incinerator, one of nineteen commercial toxic waste incinerators in the U.S., did not pose a significant threat to East Liverpool or Ohio Valley residents. But the top of the smokestack is on a level with two schools and with homes like Estell's on a bluff a few hundred yards away. In Jacksonville, Arkansas, another commercial toxic waste incinerator, built to dispose of dioxin-containing waste left behind by the Vertac pesticide company in the mid-1970s, has been the subject of much controversy and several seesaw court decisions. A judge's decision to shut down the incinerator was reversed by a higher court in July 1993, despite sworn statements by Vertac employees giving vivid details of malfunctioning and possible malfeasance. Incinerators are bad news for taxpayers too, according to the

Wall Street Journal: "The current economics [of incinerators] are terrible, requiring residential and commercial customers—as well as taxpayers—to pay hundreds of millions of dollars a year over and above the going market rate for trash disposal." The 1980s incinerator-building binge now appears to be a costly mistake, as well as a health hazard.

Still another reason that command and control do not work is simply cost—not just the daunting price tag of environmental cleanup, but the draining costs of human waste and inefficiency. "We're wasting money hand over fist on the Superfund program by not clearly defining what we want," said attorney Joseph Karaganis, referring to the $10-billion program to clean up the nation's worst hazardous waste dumps. This 1980 program, the EPA's costliest, has really only just begun: of 1,218 sites requiring emergency cleanup action, only 51 had been cleaned up in the program's first *ten years!* In 1991 the *Washington Post* said that "nearly one-third of the $200 million spent by the federal government since 1988 to clean up the nation's worst toxic waste sites has been spent not to clean up anything, but to pay the administrative expenses of private contractors." By 1993, according to *Time*, $4 billion of the $20 billion spent by then had gone to lawyers and filing fees. Also in 1993, the *New York Times* reported that many scientists and public health specialists say that "billions of dollars are wasted each year in battling problems [such as toxic waste dumps or asbestos in the schools] that are no longer considered especially dangerous, leaving little money for others that cause far more harm. . . . The federal programs to clear toxic or radioactive wastes will consume more than one-quarter of the roughly $38 billion that the Federal Government spends for environmental protection this year." What did the *Times* consider more urgent problems? Mercury in lake water and lead in paint. Did it mention the toxic air we breathe indoors? No.

Given these astounding figures, is there any hope for improvement? Impressions from you, the public, are mixed. A 1989 *New York Times*/CBS poll found that 79 percent of those surveyed felt that "protecting the environment is so important that requirements and standards cannot be too high, and continuing environmental improvements must be made regardless of cost." Other polls bear this out. Yet in the 1990 elections voters rejected most environmental issues, especially California's so-called Big Green initiative that would have helped control toxic chemicals in that state. Well-financed opposition by major polluters certainly helped defeat it. Such campaigns play on voters' fears of loss of jobs, typically (and cynically) setting up a false dilemma, for example, "no spraying" means "no jobs"—failing to recognize that most environmental dilemmas have alternative solutions. Others maintain that we have to have pollution in order to stimulate the economy: a 1992 *Wall Street Journal* writer argued that "laws and regulations that force polluters to spend money on cleaning up the environment do not diminish the wealth of a nation. They transfer this wealth from polluters to polluter-cleaner-uppers and lay a foundation for greater future wealth." It may be that only when we realize that our health, not just our jobs or the environment, may be at stake, will our votes on "the environment" begin to change.

Still, there is some good news. On January 19, 1989, the EPA acknowledged in the *Federal Register* (the daily record of Washington's goings-on) that the strategy of control had failed and said that "today's notice commits EPA to a preventive program to reduce or eliminate the generation of potentially harmful pollutants." Though this is mere lip service, the notice was announcing the EPA's new, though small, pollution prevention office, now part of the Office of Pollution Prevention and Toxic Substances (OPPTS). It's a start. Remember that pollution prevention, at its best, means finding alternatives to toxic chemicals, not using smokestack scrubbers to try to remove some of them.

Meanwhile, some companies have been preventing pollution on their own. In 1975 farsighted Minnesota Mining and Manufacturing Co. (3M) adopted a formal pollution-prevention philosophy it calls Pollution Prevention Pays. The company says that it has saved $500 million "by altering processes to avoid the generation of wastes that would [otherwise] have had to be treated." In the process, the company asserts, it has avoided emitting 112,000 tons of air pollution, a billion gallons of wastewater, and 397,000 tons of sludge and solid waste. Also, according to a *New York Times* article on 3M, the company promises not to sell pollution "credits"— chits that would allow another company in its area to create more pollution—even though such credits are legal and would make money for 3M. In 1992 Union Camp Corp, in New Jersey, built a cost-effective, chlorine-free pulp-bleaching plant at its Virginia paper mill. Companies are realizing that not creating pollution in the first place is better in the long run and cheaper and healthier than cleaning it up.

At least ten states have moved toward the best form of pollution prevention, toxics use reduction, according to the 1992 General Accounting Office (GAO) report "Toxic Substances: Advantages of and Barriers to Reducing the Use of Toxic Chemicals." In 1989 Massachusetts set up a Toxics Use Reduction Institute to try to reduce toxic chemicals in production facilities in that state. Under Illinois' 1989 Toxics Use Reduction Act, large manufacturers that use any of 120 hazardous chemicals have to have a plan for reducing or eliminating those chemicals by 1994, with a "pollution prevention fee" to be levied on them until such time as the chemicals are no longer used.

Meanwhile, Indoor Air Pollution

If outdoor pollution is this bad and attention paid to it this spotty, what is to be said about indoor pollution, mainly air pollution? The short answer is that it is bad and getting worse, and little is being done. In 1987 Lance Wallace, head of the EPA's TEAM study of indoor air (remember the TEAM study?), said, "We're spending $200 million a year trying to reduce outdoor air pollution and $2 million a year on indoor air pollution. Frankly, I think it should be reversed. Air pollution is generally much higher indoors." Since the days when the TEAM study surprised a lot of people, Washington has bestirred itself somewhat. Under SARA, the Interagency Committee on Indoor Air Quality was set up to coordinate federal indoor-air activities. Indoor air quality bills have been introduced and reintroduced into both houses of Congress, so far fruitlessly. In 1991 one bill, S.455, developed by Senator George Mitchell (D-ME), passed the Senate 88–7 and later languished. In October 1993, the Senate passed another IAQ bill, but the House continues to drag its feet. Many papers have been shuffled and a few studies done.

In 1988 the EPA completed a study of indoor air in ten public buildings—homes for the elderly, office buildings, a school, and a hospital. At least five hundred VOCs, including xylene, were found in the indoor air of four of them; sources of the VOCs included building materials, consumer products, and processes such as cleaning and smoking. In two new buildings, VOCs were present in concentrations more than one hundred times greater than in outdoor air. Again the EPA cited two types of health effects that may be associated with elevated concentrations of organic gases and particles: chronic effects, including cancer; and acute effects, including "eye, nose, and throat irritation; headaches; neurotoxic symptoms such as depression, irritability, and forgetfulness; and general malaise—a group of symptoms often described as 'sick building syndrome.'" We have only scratched the surface, said the authors of the report. They called for more study.

In a 1988 report on sick buildings, the EPA cited a World Health Organization estimate that up to 30 percent of new and remodeled buildings may have such problems. (Of course, it is the unfortunate people in them who have the more important problems.) In its August 1989 report to Congress on indoor air quality, the EPA said that "sick building syndrome, building-related illnesses, and multiple chemical sensitivity are issues of potentially great significance but are poorly understood." These two remarkably understated reports bear a special irony because it was in the fall of 1987 that the EPA began renovations on its own headquarters that would later be noted for making more than 880 of its employees ill.

More and more stories of chemical injury caused by indoor air—usually the extreme cases—are reaching the media. For example, in the 1980s fifty-four-year-old Eugene Beeman, a self-employed suburban engineer, tightened his house to make it more energy efficient and added more gas-fueled appliances. The severe headaches and nausea he developed were misdiagnosed as flu. The paramedics who found him dead in his home thought he had had a heart attack, but an autopsy revealed lethal levels of carbon monoxide. He had been poisoned by the air in his own house.

Like the victims in Bhopal and the refrigerator workers in Galesburg, Illinois, a woman now living in Wisconsin found that the isocyanates can be "sensitizers"—toxic chemicals that can make a person "sensitive" to other chemicals. In the mid-1980s she, her husband, and their unborn child were exposed over a period of time to methyl diisocyanate when a solid insulating material containing it was installed in the apartment underneath theirs. Formerly an editor with a promising career, she says: "I am totally and completely disabled from doing anything except dishes, laundry, and housecleaning (with safe products). I cannot leave my home, not even to walk outside or sit in my yard. I cannot read a book, watch TV, listen to the radio, play a cassette tape. I have no forms of entertainment or mental diversion. . . . I cannot have anything with ink or printed matter in the house, including cereal boxes and monthly bills. If my husband or daughter want to watch TV or read, they must go outside or in the garage to do so. I cannot tolerate a mattress or pillow and am sleeping alone in a room stripped of everything but a metal box spring and one forty-year-old wool blanket. My daughter can have neither new nor used toys in the living quarters. I cannot have guests in my home unless they use my shampoo and soap for one week before they visit, shower when they arrive, and wear my or my husband's clothes. I am often ill the next day from lingering scents of commercial shampoo in their hair. It literally takes me twenty-four hours to recover from a one-second exposure to something as innocuous as a photograph. The way I feel the next day is as though I had singlehandedly consumed a pint of vodka. My disability is about as profound as it can get. My system has been so ravaged by isocyanates and workplace chemicals that I have no defense against even the most minute exposure to chemicals. I have blood tests showing an immune system in disarray."

Her EI/MCS symptoms, mainly neurological, include altered vision, a "hung-over" feeling, numbness and tingling, weakness, and chronic fatigue. Her husband also became chemically sensitive, though not so severely; he is able to continue working. Her daughter, who has been chemically sensitive since birth, must have been exposed to chemicals through the umbilical cord. The lives of all three have been profoundly altered by indoor air exposures.

In sick buildings, ventilation systems are often a large part of the problem. A five-year study of several million U.S. Army trainees found that the incidence of flu and colds was at least 45 percent greater among those housed in new barracks than among those housed in old barracks. Researchers attributed the discrepancy to modern, energy-saving heating and cooling systems that recirculated as much as 95 percent of the air in the new, tightly constructed buildings. The study did not pinpoint any chemical cause, though it seems likely that what was being recirculated was a soup of alien chemicals, and that the trainees in the tight buildings experienced a form of environmental illness.

Ventilation problems in sick buildings can be solved, but the solution is almost always expensive. More than half the workers in a new building at the University of Florida in Gainesville were getting headaches, rashes, and other symptoms. The problem was finally diagnosed: fungi from a nearby horse barn had entered the ventilating system. Repairs were expected to cost $6 million, half the original cost of the building. An out-of-court settlement of a lawsuit cost the owners of a new office building in Goleta, California, $600,000 when an employee successfully traced loss of consciousness and permanent brain injury to formaldehyde fumes in the building. Cheaper remedies would include installing exhaust hoods over copy machines or adjusting partitions to permit a freer flow of air.

At Appalachian State University, in Boone, North Carolina, in 1992, faculty members blamed their headaches, dizziness, sinus problems, and cancers on a "sick" two-year-old classroom building. "The administration here does not give a damn about the faculty and staff who are in buildings which have problems," charged economics professor Fred Wallace. In Illinois, employee health problems forced affluent Du Page County to close its new $53-million courthouse for much of 1992. The county spent $3.5 million on improving ventilation after 450 employees complained of headaches, nausea, respiratory problems, rashes, fatigue, and sore throats. Several workers became chemically sensitive. A report by a team of medical experts recommended, in addition to better ventilation, reducing chemicals used in cleaning and maintenance, banning smoking, reducing carpeting, and checking perfume bottles and other aerosols at the front door. Lawsuits were filed against the architects, engineers, and general contractor by both employees and the county. Similarly, workers in the Tax and Finance building in Albany, New York, suffered a variety of ailments, including EI/MCS, caused by inadequate maintenance and poor ventilation.

Millions of dollars were spent on cleanup costs. "NIOSH Deluged by Sick Building Complaints" headlined a 1993 *Indoor Air Review* article identifying most of the complaints as coming from Florida, where an $11-million courthouse plagued with moisture problems may cost more than $3.5 million to rehabilitate.

Some poorly ventilated or "tight" buildings create temperature inversions indoors (atmospheric conditions like those that trap pollutants over industrialized cities), says Dr. William Rea, whose Environmental Health Center has investigated and modified thousands of sick buildings in the U.S. and abroad. In one such building, the only outside air intake was "in the loading dock, and all of the diesel truck exhaust was being taken in," said Rea. By routes like this, emissions from outside sources become trapped inside, where they mingle with recirculated fumes from cigarettes, copy machines, laser jet printers, typewriters, cleaning products, the various components of new furniture, and people's petroleum-based clothing and grooming products—with serious health effects to many.

Who is looking after ventilation in the nation's public buildings—offices, factories, stores, hospitals, nursing homes? One set of standards available to government and industry has been established by the American Society of Heating, Refrigerating, and Air-conditioning Engineers (ASHRAE). In 1989, on the basis of its research since 1981, ASHRAE tripled its recommended minimum fresh-air-supply rate, from five cubic feet per minute per person (cfm/person) to fifteen cfm/person; the recommended maximum is twenty cfm/person.

These rates are based on providing ventilation to satisfy 80 percent of a building's occupants or visitors, mainly by keeping them from smelling tobacco smoke. But what about the 20 percent who are offended? What about those of us in buildings that do not follow ASHRAE's recommendations? They are, after all, only voluntary. Local building codes, according to the EPA, provide for "less ventilation than is now believed required to maintain indoor air quality." And should all this attention to ventilation be the only approach? A 1993 study of almost two thousand Canadian workers reported in *NEJM* got the surprising result that bringing in more outside air made no difference in the number of health complaints. When *can* we breathe any easier?

Risk Assessment

Setting ventilation standards is an example of a technique increasingly used by government agencies to answer the question: how safe? This technique is *risk assessment*. Right now government and industry experts are busy deciding how much risk you will take. Have you been asked whether you want to take a one-in-a-million risk of cancer from eating certain raw or processed foods? The EPA calls this a "negligible" risk, but what if you or a loved one is the one in a million? Have they asked you whether you want to take a three-in-a-million risk of getting cancer from eating almonds, grapes, peanuts, corn, wheat, and other foods that have been sprayed with EBDC (ethylene bisdithiocarbamate) fungicides? The EPA calls this "not an unreasonable risk." Have they asked whether a 2.4-in-a-million risk of getting cancer from the dioxin in paper products that leaches into food is OK with you? The EPA said in 1987 that this poses "no significant health concerns." In 1989 an EPA spokesman said that "air emissions [of dioxins and furans from U.S. municipal-waste incinerators] contribute from two to forty cancer cases per year." Do you want this contribution? The figures begin to add up.

Who really knows what the risks are? What kind of system produces results that vary by a factor of twenty, as in the dioxin and furan emissions statistics just given? One EPA spokesman, while admitting that toxic air is perhaps a thousand times riskier than living near a toxic dump (that is, he said, as long as you have a safe source of drinking water), attempted to put things into perspective. Breathing toxic air, he said, is "far less dangerous than driving a car; there are two chances in a hundred that you will die in a car accident in your lifetime." Wonderful. Even the newly invigorated (1990) Clean Air Act declared that an "'ample' margin of safety for toxic emissions is one that causes cancer in one of every ten thousand 'most exposed' individuals." Is this margin ample enough for you? Did they ask? Do you know if you are one of the most exposed individuals?

By now, you can see the primary flaws in current risk assessment techniques:

- You are not being asked. If you want to drive or ride in a car, that is your decision. If you want to go white-water rafting (which in 1989 caused one death in 269 million people visiting the U.S. park system), that is your decision. If you want to be a smoker, that is your decision. But with governmental risk assessments, others are making the decision for you. And they are the same people who gave us DDT, dieldrin, chlordane, heptachlor, asbestos, PCBs, urea formaldehyde foam, and flame retardants in children's pajamas, telling us that the risks were insignificant. Most of these toxics have now been banned, at least for use in the U.S. If risk assessment were a wholly neutral activity, you would expect the risks to be overestimated as often as they are underestimated. Many chemicals have been found to be less safe than originally claimed; but according to public health expert Earon Davis, "virtually no chemical has been found to be safer than originally claimed by industry and government."

- No one works to add up the risks or try to find out what happens when a person is exposed to more than one (or one hundred) toxic chemicals at once. What are the effects of combinations of chemicals and what happens when chemicals in land and water degrade over time, i.e., change to other chemicals?

- Methods of determining risk are still crude and often based on animal studies, which may or may not apply to humans. Yet our government has for years funded animal studies to determine risks to humans, even though "so much evidence has accumulated that chemicals frequently have wholly different effects in animals and humans that officials throughout government and industry often do not act on the studies' findings," said the *New York Times* in 1993. At a more basic level, "scientists do not have a solid scientific basis about low-level toxicity," said a toxicologist at a 1989 American Chemical Society (ACS) panel discussion, "The Risks/Benefits of Chemicals in Our Lives." The ACS has since elaborated, pointing out that "detection of a chemical in human tissue does not provide insight into the time or magnitude of exposure; present analytical methodology is inadequate for surveillance of some chemicals; and the bioavailability of a substance depends on many different factors, such as its characteristic properties and the route of exposure." Under these circumstances, how can anyone evaluate risk?

- The standard format for risk assessment considers only cancer and obvious chronic effects, ignoring more subtle effects on the human reproductive, nervous, and immune systems, as well as on fetal development. For example, though most pesticides are neurotoxins (nerve poisons), the EPA does not test pesticides for effects on the nervous and immune systems. Why is this huge health effect being ignored? EI/MCS, only grudgingly acknowledged by governmental authorities, is entirely left out of the figures used to establish health risk. Headaches? Just endure them: don't be chemophobic—the chemical industry's word for the chemically sensitive.

- Risk assessments are usually averages that ignore the different impact of toxic chemicals on different groups, though health risks are known to be higher for fetuses, children, the elderly, the chronically ill, and workers in certain occupations.

- Perhaps most important, assessments of risk to health exist for only a tiny portion of the chemicals now in use by industry. Professor Ross Hume Hall, formerly of Canada's McMaster University, pointed out that of the more than sixty thousand chemicals in industrial use in 1990, we have "absolutely no information whatever" on forty thousand of them. Studies aren't being done, he says, and without studies, how can we conclude that there is no problem?

At best, then, risk figures are only educated guesses that are easily manipulated by industry and government to suit their own interests. In 1983 the EPA decided to allow some industries to do their own risk assessments of their toxic wastes; when environmentalists and local people protested, EPA retreated, saying that it would prepare all risk assessments in the future. Thus most of the twenty-five hundred premanufacture notifications that the EPA receives each year have few risk assessments done by the submitting company, and little or no toxicity data.

Industry says that it is up to government to find "safe" levels of chemicals, but the EPA has taken more than twenty years (since the Clean Air Act of 1970) to set standards for only six outdoor air pollutants. How long would it take to set standards for the hundreds of toxic chemicals in our outdoor air—let alone the air in our homes? "It's difficult to take on these chemicals case by case," said EPA spokesman David Kee. "We should shift the burden to industry."

There you are. Each wants the other to take responsibility. Evasions by industry and government leave environmentalists like Peter Montague, of the Environmental Research Foundation, John O'Connor, of the Jobs and Environment Campaign, and Lois Gibbs, of the Citizens Clearinghouse for Hazardous Wastes (CCHW) "urgently arguing that the strategy of attempting to regulate and control each separate chemical, with the premise that each toxin is innocent until proven guilty, is both chemically and politically bankrupt." The EPA, already overwhelmed, knows that the cost of more extensive assessments would be astronomical. According to the National Toxicology Program (NTP), a "preliminary assessment of the combined effects of just twenty-five contaminants in drinking water would require thirty-three million experiments at a cost of about $3 trillion." Looking at costs another way, the OMB tried in 1991 to estimate the cost of enforcing current rules for each premature death apparently averted. Two examples: the benzene exposure limit for workers, $8.9 million; 1.2-dichloropropane limits in drinking water, $653 million.

How much better—and cheaper for society—to find safer alternatives for these chemicals. Again, pollution *prevention*—the reduction of toxic pollution at its source—is the solution of choice. Prevention would require major and possibly wrenching adjustments by industry, but there is little doubt that it could be done. In the words of Greenpeace writer Joe Thornton, "benign alternatives exist for virtually every polluting technology." Business writer William Neikirk has suggested that the government set anti-pollution taxes and tax penalties so high that a company would have to pay "more to pollute than it would to invest in environmental measures and equipment." (And if a company developed less-toxic alternatives for some of its basic materials, pollution-control measures would not even be needed.) This philosophy has worked in some states. As the result of a federal lawsuit filed in 1990 under RCRA, United Technologies Corporation, Connecticut's largest private employer, began serious efforts to reduce hazardous wastes and agreed in 1993 to pay $5.3 million in penalties for previous hazardous-waste mishandling. Louisiana, highly polluted by emissions of all sorts from its petrochemical plants, became in 1991 the first state to enact a law linking tax penalties to a company's pollution record. The Worldwatch Institute, a leading environmental research group, agrees that governments should impose heavy taxes on "products and activities that pollute, deplete, or otherwise degrade natural systems."

Consider how emissions, waste, and illness would plummet if we adopted Peter Montague's "gold standard." Of approximately "3 billion Troy ounces of gold mined during the past six thousand years," he says, only a tiny fraction is now lost—sunk at sea, buried in tombs, or otherwise irretrievable. A "waste gold" problem we do not have. Montague wittily envisions that as society applies his "gold standard" to polluters, "zero discharge of their poisonous wastes will . . . allow them to retain what they already have and cherish: their good names, the absence of leg irons, and the uninterrupted flow of life fluids between their shoulders and their heads."

Unfortunately, risk assessments in their present form have gained acceptance because their victims are unknown and anonymous, as are most of the perpetrators of the pollution that victimizes them. An ancient Venezuelan legend concerned itself with just such a situation. Making a bargain with the devil in order to recover his family's lost fortune, a young Argentinian named Alejandro stuck a pin at random in a map of South America, on an island named Margarita, with the result that a young Venezuelan fisherman named Luis did not return to the island from the storm-tossed sea. Though the devil had promised Alejandro that since he did not know his victim his hands would not be stained with blood, the young rich man suffered so much remorse that he finally gave half his fortune to the poor people of Margarita and went to live the simple life of a fisherman on the island. Gradually Alejandro changed into a humble and generous person, and one day Luis returned to the island. Recovering from severe illnesses on the European-bound ship that had rescued him, Luis had had a nightmare in which the devil had tried to take his soul, a crucial part of the devil's bargain with Alejandro. But because of Alejandro's transformation, the devil lost. In the modern world, if it were known that Person A suffered cancer or nerve deterioration or asthma from what Person B had done, everything would be different. Damages would be assessed, lawyers would have more business, and people would be jailed.

To make the present situation a little more specific, North Carolina's Agricultural Resources Center (ARC), tongue in its collective cheek, is setting up the National Cancer Volunteer Registry (NCVR), also known as the "adopt-a-chemical" plan. Under this plan, you may choose any of the more than seventy cancer-causing chemicals from the EPA's list of suspect and cancer-causing pesticides to be your very own toxic chemical. Volunteer! Be a point of light! It's the American Way. As our population approaches 250 million, it will take only 250 volunteers, says the Center, for each cancer-causing chemical to reach the cancer goal of the "negligible risk" standard of one cancer in a million. You can be the one to sacrifice your life for other Americans.

Actually, however, far more than 250 volunteers are needed. With more than seventy carcinogens registered as pesticides for use on food, the NCVR needs 17,500 volunteers just to get started toward that negligible risk standard. The Center warns that it will accept only "Americans who are healthy (both physically and mentally) and eighteen years of age or older. Youngsters may qualify but they must have parental consent. In fact, children are needed to fill important quotas in such categories as childhood leukemia, one of the many cancer risks deemed 'acceptable' by the government and the chemical industry." But don't be discouraged. Remember, the NCVR is talking only about pesticides. There are plenty of other toxic chemicals, so that no one need feel left out. (To volunteer, call the NCVR at 919-967-1886.)

Despite ironic comments like these, however, risk assessment appears here to stay. In 1989 then-EPA-chief William Reilly said that "despite the inherent uncertainties . . . comparative risk assessment is still one of the best indicators of where we should be directing resources." In 1993 the Clinton administration officially made risk assessment the "philosophy of regulation" for all government regulatory agencies. If only the scientists on the EPA's Science Advisory Board could persuade the American public—and our government—that indoor air pollution should be first (as they think) instead of seventeenth (as the public believes) on the list of risks, risk assessment might help us breathe a little easier.

Taking a Deep Breath

Finally, here are a few simple things to keep in mind: The nation's production of organic (carbon-containing, mostly petroleum-based) chemicals is doubling every eleven years. With more than seventy thousand chemicals now registered under the Toxic Substances Control Act (add a thousand more each year) and with more than two hundred on the Superfund list, the EPA has set outdoor air pollution standards for only six contaminants. Many of these thousands of chemicals are incorporated in consumer products, including modern drugs, most of which are derived from petroleum and all of which have side effects. Some, like the mercury in the "silver" fillings in your mouth, are known poisons. Most are untested for human health effects. Without question, their adverse effects can build up slowly, the result of many small exposures. Many of these modern, petroleum-based consumer products end up in homes and workplaces, outgassing. We spend about 90 percent of our time indoors. Indoor air is much worse than outdoor air. We live and work in a chemical soup. To be chemically injured is to be damaged by chemical exposures. To be chemically sensitive is to react to seemingly infinitesimal exposures to toxic chemicals.

Can you possibly breathe any easier? There *are* ways. Here are a few general suggestions (for more specific advice see the end of other chapters):

- Unless the outdoor air smells really polluted, air out your house or apartment at least once a day; it's worth the few extra pennies.

- Rid your home of as many petroleum-based products as possible: start with fabric softeners, detergents, air "fresheners," mothballs, deodorant soaps, paints, paint thinners, perfumed cosmetics and personal grooming products (actually, anything chemically scented), synthetic cleaning products, synthetic and treated fabrics, pressed-wood furniture, and "solvent"-based marking pens. Plant-based, water-based products and processes are safer. You're going to get some toxic chemical exposures no matter what, so minimize your own risks by controlling those you *can* control.

- Realize how much you have been seduced by advertisements, which tell you that the only way to keep your house and body clean is to douse them with chemicals—chemicals that are dangerous not only to you but to those around you. Germ phobia inside and pest mania outside have ruled us for too long.

- Demand that the chemical content of every product on the market be fully given on labels. Manufacturers can tell us what chemicals are in products and still maintain "trade secrets"—by not disclosing the amounts they used. If we are going to assess our own risks, that is the least we can expect. For too long we have been massively uninformed; we should accept nothing less than a policy of informed consent.

- Government and private researchers will always call for more studies. Research is their livelihood. Of course "good" science is important (it has been quipped that "bad" science is all science not funded by industry). Meanwhile, however, people are falling ill and dying. More studies, yes, but while you're waiting, protect yourself.

- Until government gives up its ineffective and dangerous command/control and risk-assessment policies in favor of pollution prevention, realize that to a large extent your health lies in your own hands. And your health doesn't mean as much to anyone else as it does to you.

- Be aware that anyone can become chemically sensitive at any time. One additional chemical exposure, added to all the rest, may give you this difficult-to-handle illness. If you are now bothered by perfumes or by walking into fabric stores or down supermarket detergent aisles, you are beginning to become chemically sensitive. People frequently show up at EI/MCS support group meetings, angry, frustrated, and baffled, asking, "What happened to me? Why didn't anyone warn me?" "Why isn't the government doing anything about this?" "Why didn't I know?"

* * * *

To Find Out More

- *The Toxic Cloud,* by Michael H. Brown, New York, Harper & Row, 1987.

- *Making Peace with the Planet,* by Barry Commoner, New York, Pantheon, 1990.

- *Chemical Exposure and Human Health: A Reference to 314 Chemicals, with a Guide to Symptoms and a Directory of Organizations,* by Cynthia Wilson, Jefferson, North Carolina, McFarland & Company, 1993.

- *Who Will Tell the People: The Betrayal of American Democracy,* by William Greider, New York, Simon & Schuster, 1992.

- *1991–1992 Green Index: A State-by-State Guide to the Nation's Environmental Health,* by Bob Hall and Mary Lee Kerr, Washington, D.C., Island Press, 1991.

U.S. Environmental Protection Agency (401 M Street SW, Washington, D.C. 20460)

(You can call the EPA Public Information Center at 202-260-7751, the EPA User Support Service at 202-260-1531, the EPA Indoor Air Quality Information Clearinghouse at 1-800-438-4318, or the EPA Safe Drinking Water Hotline at 1-800-426-4791, but be warned that getting to the right office in Washington can be exasperating.)

- "The Total Exposure Assessment Methodology (TEAM) Study," EPA/600/S6-87/002, September 1987 (Project Summary available from the EPA's Office of Acid Deposition, Environmental Monitoring, and Quality Assurance at the above address).

- "The Inside Story: A Guide to Indoor Air Quality," EPA/400/1-88/004, September 1988 (co-published by the EPA and the CPSC).

- "Comparing Risks and Setting Environmental Priorities," PM-220, 1989.

- "Reducing Risk: Setting Priorities and Strategies for Environmental Protection," 1990.

- *Building Air Quality: the EPA's Guide for Building Owners and Facility Managers,* published by NIOSH, December 1991.

- EPA Pollution Prevention Hotline: 202-260-1023.

Indoor Air Publications
(Primarily for Professionals)

- *Indoor Air and Human Health,* revised edition, by R. B. Gammage and S. V. Kay, Boca Raton, Florida, Lewis Publishers, 1990.

- *Indoor Air Pollution Control,* by Thad Godish, Boca Raton, Florida, Lewis Publishers, 1989.

- *Indoor Air Quality Directory 1992–1993,* Bethesda, Maryland, IAQ Publications, 1993.

- *Indoor Air Review: The Newspaper of the Indoor Air Quality Industry,* IAQ Publications, Inc., 4520 East-West Highway, Suite 610, Bethesda, Maryland 20814; monthly, $72/year.

- *INvironment: The Newsletter of Building Management and Indoor Air Quality,* Landis and Gyr Powers, Inc., 1000 Deerfield Parkway, Buffalo Grove, Illinois 60089-4513; quarterly, $95/year.

- *Indoor Air Quality Update,* Cutter Information Corporation, 37 Broadway, Arlington, Massachusetts 02174-5539; monthly, $207/year or try your local library.

- *Indoor Pollution News*, Buraff Publications, 1350 Connecticut Avenue NW, Washington, D.C. 20036; biweekly, $417/year or try your local library.

- *Indoor Pollution* and *Indoor Pollution Law Report*, Leader Publications, 111 Eighth Avenue, Suite 900, New York, New York 10014-0158.

Laboratories That Test for Toxic Chemicals in the Human Body (Primarily for Physicians)

- ACCU-CHEM (part of Enviro-Health), 990 North Bowser Road, Suite 800, Richardson, Texas 75081; 214-234-5577 (tests blood, urine, and fat).

- Pacific Toxicology Laboratories, 1545 Pontius Avenue, Los Angeles, California 90025; 213-479-4911; in California 1-800-23-TOXIC; outside California 1-800-32-TOXIC (tests blood, urine, and fat)

- Doctor's Data, P.O. Box 111, 30 West 101 Roosevelt Road, West Chicago, Illinois 60185; 1-800-231-3649; in Illinois 708-231-3649 (tests blood, urine, and hair).

- Serammune Physicians Lab, 11100 Sunrise Valley Drive, AMSA Building, 2nd floor, Reston, Virginia 22070; 703-785-0610 or 1-800-553-5472 (tests blood for mercury and pesticides; also uses ELISA-ACT, which tests for immune-system reactions to 235 foods, pesticides, and other environmental chemicals).

- Antibody Assay Laboratories, 1715 East Wilshire #715, Santa Ana, California 92705; 1-800-522-2611 (tests for chemical exposures and antibodies).

- Immunosciences Lab. Inc., 1801 La Cienega Boulevard, Suite 302, Los Angeles, California 90035; 310-287-1884 (tests for immune-system impairment).

- Citizens Environmental Laboratory, 1168 Commonwealth Avenue, Boston, Massachusetts 02134; 617-232-5833 (technical support for grassroots groups).

Organizations Working Toward Pollution Prevention

- Jobs and Environment Campaign, 1168 Commonwealth Avenue, Boston, Massachusetts 02134.

- Citizen's Clearinghouse for Hazardous Wastes, P.O. Box 6806, Falls Church, Virginia 22040; publishes *Everyone's Backyard.*

- Environmental Research Foundation, P.O. Box 5036, Annapolis, Maryland 21403-7036; publishes *RACHEL'S Hazardous Waste News.*

- Silicon Valley Toxics Coalition, 760 N. First Street, San Jose, California 95112; publishes *Silicon Valley Toxics News.*

- Washington Toxics Coalition, 4516 University Way NE, Seattle, Washington 98105; publishes *Alternatives.*

- Institute for Sick Buildings, P.O. Box 546, Auburndale, Florida 33823; 813-967-6791.

- Greenpeace USA, 1436 U Street NW, Washington, D.C. 20009.

- Citizens for a Better Environment (Midwest), 407 S. Dearborn Street, Suite 1775, Chicago, Illinois 60605; publishes *Environmental Review.*

- United States Public Interest Research Group Education Fund, 215 Pennsylvania Avenue SE, Washington, D.C., 20003-1107; 202-546-9707; publishes *Working Notes on Community Right-to-Know.*

3

Warning: Your Job May Be Hazardous to Your Health

WHEN CONNIE ARTHUR STARTED her new job at Du Pont's Belle plant in West Virginia's Kanawha County in 1979, she was thinking mainly of how her salary would augment her family's income. Like millions of women in the U.S., she knew that she needed to work to help support her family. What she didn't know was that her new job was going to ruin her health. Though she worked in an office—and offices were then generally thought to be safe workplaces—chemical fumes from the plant were being drawn through the ventilation system and concentrated in her office. After a year she had continuous urinary tract infections and heart palpitations (premature ventricular contractions that feel like missed heartbeats); later she became so weak that she couldn't even grasp a pencil. "We weren't designed to be toxic waste dumps," Arthur says. "My body almost completely shut down before I realized what my problem was."

In May 1988 Dr. Allan Lieberman, medical director of the Center for Environmental Medicine in Charleston, South Carolina, tested Arthur and diagnosed her with EI/MCS. That summer, still trying to work, she was exposed to pesticide spraying in her office—it proved to be the final drop in her chemical rain barrel. When she returned to her office after the spraying, she became so sick that she called her husband and said, "You're going to have to come and get me." Totally unable to function, she spent several weeks in bed. Having by then lost her job, she could not afford the next step—

detoxification at Dr. Rea's Dallas clinic. But members of her church, seeing her suffering, offered to help. Du Pont co-workers also pitched in with expenses. (Her company-issued insurance policy, which considered the detoxification treatment "experimental," refused to cover it, and her application for permanent disability from Du Pont had been denied.) In Dallas she underwent a sauna detoxification program that has enabled her to live safely in her home, which she and her husband have stripped of all potentially toxic materials. "As long as I stay in a controlled environment," she says, "I can function. It's sort of like a checker game. You have to calculate every move. It's turned our life upside down. We [she and her husband and son] can't just take off and go on a vacation. We can't just go to McDonald's, or go shopping. At times, it's sort of like being a prisoner in your own home."

Arthur's home now bears a large black-and-yellow sign: CAUTION: STRONG CHEMICALS CAN BE LIFE-THREATENING TO RESIDENT. Newspapers are banned unless they have been baked or aired out. Everything that enters the house, including food, is carefully screened for chemical content. Visitors must avoid perfumed products such as after-shave or scented deodorant. On her rare trips outside her home, she wears a white surgical mask. "Who's out there protecting human life?," she asks. "This happened to me, and I thought I was protected."

Not so. Most people do not recognize chemical dangers within the workplace, and doctors often misdiagnose chemical injury. Compounds like the ones Arthur was exposed to in her office "have the ability to disregulate all of the body's regulatory systems," says Dr. Lieberman. "Many of these common chemicals are neurotoxic and may produce irreversible damage to the brain and nervous system. For this reason, many of the signs and symptoms of the chemically injured patient are referred to the nervous system, causing erroneous diagnosis of emotional or psychological disease or disorder." Hence the statement commonly made to chemical victims: "It's all in your head."

Is this example of work-related illness an isolated case? Unfortunately, not so. In 1986 a young woman, trained in biology, found that her work in a university immunology laboratory made her so ill with headaches, nausea, spaciness, and lack of motor control that she had to quit her job. At work she was exposed to toxic solvents like toluene and benzene, to formaldehyde powder, to a gas-fired Bunsen burner, and to a malfunctioning hood. (Laboratories usually have vented metal hoods over potentially dangerous work areas.) Seeking safer employment in an outdoor setting, she took a job driving an open-air sightseeing tram at a botanic garden. When that made her sick also, she switched to an office job at the garden—it was just as bad. The garden itself, with its repeated pesticide sprayings and its use of other toxic chemicals, indoors and outdoors, was making her ill. Diagnosed with EI/MCS, she quit that job and for several years was unable to find any other workplace that she could tolerate. Social Security disability payments became her primary means of support.

In Maine, Kathryn Buck's health problems began in her early twenties, also with chemical exposures in a laboratory job. By age thirty, her anxiety attacks and other physical problems had progressed to total physical disability and a seizure disorder. After leaving her job, she spent most of her time researching the illness, which by then she knew was EI/MCS, and cleaning up her home environment. Free of anxiety attacks, she still takes anticonvulsant medicine every day, and has to take more when she goes out. Going out, for her and for her son Michael, who is also chemically sensitive, is infrequent and must be carefully planned. "I don't waste my trips out," she says. "I go to the grocery store once a month, and it nearly kills me. But every Friday I go to the health food store and to a tea shop for lunch. . . . If someone sits next to me with perfume on, I have to leave. I would never ask anyone to move for me." To the people who still don't believe that EI/MCS really exists, she replies, "Do you really think I would live this way if I didn't have to?"

Three young women in three different parts of the country—all sick from chemical exposures in the workplace. Is the chemical industry aware of these people and their illness? In a 1990 letter in *Chemical & Engineering News*, former chemist W. Alfred Mukatis, now a law professor, said, "I became a victim of chemical susceptibility over twenty years ago from exposure to chemicals in the workplace. I have had to give up exposure to chemicals in any job setting, but still have continuing health problems because total avoidance is not possible, and my sensitivities spread during the years I continued to practice chemistry." Concerning the tragic toll this illness exacts on health, families, and careers, Mukatis appealed to the American Chemical Society to educate chemists and industry in the dangers of EI/MCS and to assist ACS members with the illness to "collect on disability insurance policies so that they can retrain before they become chronically ill and permanently disabled. . . . For too many years," he said, "this illness that affects chemists and the general public alike has not received adequate attention—primarily because of the lack of appropriate diagnostic methods and the medical community's general reluctance to accept any medical condition as real if its tools are inadequate to recognize [the condition]. We chemists, as scientists, are all familiar with the long resistance of the orthodox medical community to accepting the germ theory of illness."

At least one scientist is alert to the problem. Stephen Hall, professor of toxicology and chair of the Department of Occupational Health at the Medical College of Ohio, has another view of the worker who has what he calls "chemical hypersensitivity syndrome." In the professional journal *Pollution Engineering*, Hall wrote, "Occupational health and safety professionals frequently encounter one or more individuals in a plant with a remarkable ability to detect chemical leaks, the escape of any solvent vapor or any toxic fumes, or breakdowns in the exhaust system. These individuals can detect the presence of chemicals in the air long before anyone else notices them. . . . They have increased susceptibility to being overcome by solvents or chemical odors. They feel lightheaded and queasy, and experience headache, nasal congestion, and throat irritation following the least exposure to a variety of chemical odors. They are barely tolerated by their co-workers and are sometimes regarded as being crazy. These individuals, in fact, suffer from the chemical hypersensitivity syndrome." Poor souls, if Hall is correct about co-workers' reactions—these twentieth-century chemical victims not only must suffer physically, they can also suffer rejection for serving as an early warning system for their scoffing co-workers.

In Hall's own state, however, one employee feels appreciated. Working in a General Motors paint shop in Lordstown, Ohio, Alberta Faber experienced blackouts, dizzy, spells, bleeding at the mouth, and other symptoms. "I worked right by the oven," she said, "so . . . at night when the fumes came back, they watched to see when my eyes rolled back and I painted the wrong colors. Then we were relieved. . . . I felt like a canary in a coal mine, really."

Underrecognized, Underreported, Undercompensated, Understudied, and Underprevented

Scoffing workers take note: an estimated 350,000 *new* cases of illness occur among workers each year from toxic exposures on the job, according to leading public health researcher Philip Landrigan, of the Mount Sinai School of Medicine in New York City; and some 71,000 thousand Americans a year are estimated to die from job-related disease, according to an independent study by the Chicago-based National Safe Workplace Institute. After a two-year study published in 1990, the Institute concluded that occupational disease is "the most neglected public health problem in the United States . . . [and] one of the great 'unders' of American health care—under-recognized, underreported, undercompensated, understudied, and underprevented. Almost everyone involved in occupational disease, from victims to physicians, from companies to government officials, has failed to respond adequately to the challenge." Death from occupational disease, the Institute's figures revealed, is "1.5 times more common than deaths from motor vehicle crashes, 3.4 times greater than from murder, and 5.3 times greater than from AIDS." While not greater than deaths from smoking, in 1990 more than 350,000 a year in the U.S., job-related deaths are the leading "nonvolitional" cause of preventable death in this country, according to Joseph Kinney, the Institute's director. For while we presumably have a choice with smoking, too often we have little or no choice as to where—or whether—we work. And where we work may be adversely affecting the health of as many as 20 million U.S. workers, estimates Joel Butler, professor of psychology at the University of North Texas. Add that to those who are exposed at home, he says, and the numbers could be staggering.

The National Safe Workplace Institute was started in 1987 by Kinney, a former Congressional staff member who became con-

cerned after his brother died in a preventable construction scaffold-
ing accident. His independent and highly respected research has led
him to propose his "two lung" theory. EPA and OSHA, he says,
have two different standards: "the acceptable level for lead at work
is thirty-three times higher than the level legally allowed in the general environment; for carbon monoxide it's four times higher, for
particulates (dust) one hundred times higher, and for sulfur dioxide
it's 62.5 times higher." One set of lungs for factory workers, one for
everyone else. The same is true for enforcement: the government
spends sixty times as much protecting the environment as it does
protecting workers. "More than 125 individuals have been sentenced under federal environmental laws to more than a thousand
collective years in jail; over the same two decades only two employers were successfully prosecuted under federal job safety laws for a
total of forty-five days in jail." And while Finland and Sweden
spend more than twelve dollars per worker per year on job health,
the U.S. spent sixty-three cents per worker in 1990. "We have a corporate culture, a business culture," says Kinney, "that removes decision makers from any kind of responsibility." Paying fines is
usually cheaper than making workplaces safe. "We've got expendable and vulnerable populations who are intuitively exploitable,"
he said, especially young blacks, Hispanics, and new immigrants.

By 1990 the American Chemical Society had registered more
than ten million chemicals, with nearly six hundred thousand new
chemicals reported every year. Industrial and academic laboratories
are busy synthesizing new chemicals, primarily from petroleum or
coal tar, though most of them are not studied or used outside the
laboratory. Of the Toxic Substance Control Act's (TSCA's) contin-
ually expanding list of toxic chemicals in commercial use, the Office
of Technology Assessment's (OTA's) *Neurotoxicity* says that "since
few of these chemicals have been tested to determine if they adversely affect the nervous system, no precise figures are available on
the total number of chemicals in existence that are potentially neurotoxic to humans." Thus, unknown to most of us, our workplaces
are exposing us to thousands of new chemicals that did not exist before this century—or even before World War II. "People are working with chemicals whose hazards simply are not known," says Dr.
Landrigan. "The government has relied on industries to decide

whether new chemicals should be tested and what tests should be applied to new chemicals. Industry reviews the literature and claims there is no need to test."

Some occupational health researchers have been sounding the alarm about unsafe workplaces for years. In a 1974 talk on health hazards in the arts and crafts, Dr. Bertram Carnow said that there is "a continuous struggle between humans and their environment, which is essentially hostile. . . . A new chemical is discovered every twenty minutes and no good way has been devised to determine whether or not it may have long-term effects on people." In 1980 the National Toxicology Program woke up and contracted with the National Research Council, or NRC, research arm of the National Academy of Sciences (NAS), for a study of toxicity testing. By 1984 the researchers came to the shocking conclusion that some 80 percent of the sixty-five thousand industrial chemicals then in use had "*no toxicity information available*" [emphasis added]. (Alarmed at what his committee had turned up, Dr. Richard Thomas, director of toxicology, epidemiology, and risk assessment for the NAS, said, "There is no doubt that a lot of things in our environment cause illness. . . . I think in a lot of cases there are illnesses that are just coming to light.") By 1990 the number of chemicals used or manufactured in U.S. workplaces had increased to about sixty-eight thousand, and the General Accounting Office (GAO) issued a report with the revealing title, "Toxic Substances: EPA's Chemical Testing Program Has Made Little Progress," which said that "the health and environmental effects of thousands of chemicals remain unknown." By 1992 the number was about seventy thousand, with less than 10 percent tested at all for neurotoxicity, according to the NRC. Since World War II this rate of increase has been consistent. Like compound interest, our exposure to untested chemicals can increase amazingly fast.

What are some occupational diseases? According to the Institute's study, exposure to toxins, indoor air pollution, stress, and other causes of occupational disease caused deaths in up to 10 percent of cancers [at least twenty-four thousand people], up to 5 percent of nervous-system disease, up to 3 percent of heart disease [at least nine thousand people], 100 percent of all lung diseases attributed to inhaling dust, up to 4 percent of other lung diseases, up to 3 percent of kidney disease, and up to 5 percent of birth defects. While many of these illnesses represent chemical injury, chemical sensitivity is not mentioned—another set of statistics that has over-looked its existence. Yet Ashford and Miller say that "the range of indoor air pollutants affecting industrial workers is enormous. Seemingly, almost any process involving chemicals appears to have the potential for initiating chemical hyperreactivity via long- or short-term exposure."

In Ohio's Mahoning Valley, site of huge steel and auto plants, workers did their own research into suspicious numbers of illnesses and deaths. Forming a group called WATCH (Workers Against Toxic Chemical Hazards), they went through obituaries printed in local newspapers and found that in just eighteen months, seventy-five of their co-workers, average age fifty-six years, had died of can-cer, leukemia, and kidney and heart diseases. Local news coverage embarrassed both the United Auto Workers and General Motors and led them to sponsor an official study that confirmed the work-ers' unofficial one. It found that "the death rate from cancer among the auto workers at Lordstown's two assembly plants was nearly 40 percent higher than normal." Plant workers, fearful of complaining, had for years endured "red dirt" and fumes from lacquers and open tanks of acid.

Given the nation's prolific use of toxic and untested chemicals, the wonder is that we have not experienced a few Bhopals here. We have come close, however. Over the last twenty-five years, seven-teen potentially catastrophic industrial accidents in the U.S. released deadly chemicals in volumes and levels of toxicity exceeding those that killed thousands of people in Bhopal, India, in 1984, according to a 1989 EPA report, "Acute Hazardous Data Base." "Only through luck have we managed to avoid a catastrophe," says Debo-rah Sheiman, of the Natural Resources Defense Council (NRDC). In response, Kyle Olson, associate director for health and safety of the Chemical Manufacturers Association (CMA), asserted, "When you look at the millions of people involved in the manufacture, han-dling, storage, and use of chemicals, I think the chemical industry's safety record continues to look pretty good." To the industry, ap-parently, slow death doesn't count.

Nor does neurotoxicity. Neurotoxic pesticides and solvents are common sources of exposure for workers in industry and agriculture, according to the OTA's neurotoxicity report: "NIOSH has identified neurotoxic disorders as one of the nation's ten leading causes of work-related disease and injury. . . . Approximately 9.8 million workers are exposed to solvents every day through inhalation or skin contact. Acute exposure to organic solvents can affect an individual's manual dexterity, speed of response, coordination, and balance; it can also produce feelings of inebriation. Chronic exposure to some organic solvents can result in fatigue, irritability, loss of memory, sustained changes in personality or mood, and decreased learning and concentration abilities; in some cases, structural changes in the nervous system are apparent." Organic solvents, the OTA continues, "are components of a variety of products, including paints, paint removers and varnishes; adhesives, glues, coatings; degreasing and cleaning agents; dyes and print ink; floor and shoe creams, polishes, and waxes, agricultural products; pharmaceuticals; and fuels. . . . Organic solvents are of particular concern because most are toxic in different ways and to varying degrees. . . . The increase in the number of available organic solvents and the development of new processes utilizing them present major occupational health challenges."

Indeed. Biochemist Bambi Batts Young, former director of the environment and behavior program of the Center for Science in the Public Interest (CSPI), says that NIOSH has studied 588 major industrial chemicals known to be hazardous. Of these, "167 have documented neurotoxic effects, 115 are known to affect the lungs, and 9 are linked to cancer. For the two hundred most prevalent industrial chemicals, NIOSH estimates one million workers are exposed to each one. Of these two hundred industrial chemicals, sixty-five have shown evidence of neurotoxicity." By this estimate, as many as sixty-five million workers are today at risk of damage to brain and nerve cells. In one of the few controlled studies of workplace exposures to neurotoxins, researchers in 1988 found neurobehavioral dysfunctioning, nausea, headaches, and "subjective distress" in workers with a history of solvent exposure.

"The worldwide spread of chemicals continues to threaten us all," wrote toxicologist/internist Janette Sherman, MD, in her book *Chemical Exposure and Disease.* Having carefully evaluated the health records of eight thousand workers over a period of seventeen years, she dedicated her book to the "vast number of workers who labored under the false impression that they were being protected against chemicals in their environment that would ultimately ruin their lungs, hearts, kidneys, and livers, resulting in untold misery and early death." One of her discoveries: though "much rides on the information given on death certificates," often the cause of death is given as stroke or heart attack without any indication of the poisonous chemicals that the victims had been exposed to in their workplaces. Because doctors rarely ask questions about patients' occupations, health statistics are skewed in favor of the final death-triggering event. Regarding a fifty-year-old agricultural worker whose death she investigated, "If the precipitating cause of [his] death was clearly parathion poisoning [as the hospital record indicated] and not recorded on this death certificate [where the cause of death was given as a "cerebrovascular accident," or stroke], then one may question how many other cases of pesticide and other toxicologically related deaths go unreported." In another case, a man developed severe headaches after his company introduced a paper-treating process using formaldehyde. After five years of headaches, of testing "normal" on numerous cardiac-function and other sophisticated tests, and of taking a great variety of prescription drugs, including one that constricts blood vessels, he suffered—at age forty-five—the first of several heart attacks. "Failure to determine the cause of his headaches led to his being treated with a number of drugs that, like all medications, carry side effects," says Dr. Sherman. "Because he was not removed from the cause of his headaches, and the medications were continued, he suffered a significant side effect: a heart attack." Her conclusion: "Chemical agents have joined parasites, bacteria, and viruses as documented and common causes of illness and death."

Meanwhile, we should not be "using the American worker as a testing laboratory for toxic chemicals," warned Robert Balster, a psychologist and toxicologist testifying before a Senate subcommittee in 1989. Also testifying was Dr. Gordon Baker, a Seattle physician who has treated over a hundred aerospace workers for toxic chemical exposures. The exposures caused a variety of serious health problems, but "the worst by far are those related to the central nervous system," he said.

Human Testing Laboratories

What are some of these human testing laboratories for toxic chemicals? Could you be working in one of them? In the nebulous and shifting area of risk assessment, no one knows for sure which workers are most at risk. There are a few statistics, a few opinions, and many personal stories. The OTA says that "there is so little agreement about the number of workplace-related illnesses that OTA does not take a position on the controversy about the 'correct' number. Most deaths and injuries occur one at a time or in small numbers in the nation's more than 4.5 million workplaces. . . . Arguments about the number of occupationally related diseases may obscure the important fact that occupational illness is preventable." Instead, workers often must change or leave jobs because of health or occupational hazards. A study of ninety patients seeking workers' compensation included nineteen office workers, thirteen transportation workers, twelve in electronic manufacturing, eleven in medicine and social work, eight teachers, eight in other manufacturing, four in the food industry, and three hairdressers; the most common causes given for claims were exposure to paint (and thinner), smoke, organic solvents, and pesticides. Certain occupations—in the rubber, oil, chemical, plastics, and machine-tool industries—and professions—pathology, hematology, cosmetology, veterinary medicine, and embalming—have been found to pose higher-than-average risks for brain cancer. Researchers led by Aaron Blair of the National Cancer Institute (NCI) have found that farmers are at heightened risk to several malignancies, including leukemia, Hodgkin's disease, non-Hodgkin's lymphoma, and cancers of the brain, stomach, prostate, skin, and lip. A 1993 Canadian study, reported in the *American Journal of Epidemiology*, found that the number of acres sprayed with herbicides significantly increased farmers' risk of prostate cancer mortality. (So much for the healthy outdoor life.) And Dorothy Nelkin and Michael S. Brown, in *Workers at Risk: Voices from the Workplace*, include among endangered workers "the 4.6 million employees in chemical and chemical prod-

ucts industries, along with others who use chemical products in occupations as varied as fire fighting, glass making, fine art, gardening, scientific research, food production, nursing, and maintenance
work."

Also at special risk for chemically induced illness, because they
deal with complex mixtures of chemicals, are hazardous waste
clean-up workers, including those injecting toxic chemicals into
abandoned oil wells. Being poor and black is another risk: Luke
Cole, one of three full-time environmental poverty lawyers in the
U.S., sums up a huge problem when he says that "poor people and
people of color bear the brunt of environmental problems because
they have the dirtiest, most toxic jobs and live in the dirtiest neigh-
borhoods, next to industries." It's no wonder that, according to
professor of occupational medicine Samuel Epstein, blacks have
lower cancer survival rates than whites.

Curiously, some of the most dangerous places to work appear to
be locations in the health care industry: hospitals, nursing homes,
and dentists' and physicians' offices and laboratories. Such locations abound with toxic chemicals used for treatment, research, and
cleaning. In Syracuse, New York, five hospital X-ray technicians
sued a hazardous waste removal firm in 1990 for permanent respiratory injuries caused, they say, by noxious fumes from the hospital's chemical waste storage tank. The firm was cleaning the tank
one floor below the hospital's radiology department. Used as a de-
pository for chemical wastes from the hospital's laboratory and radiology department, the tank contained highly toxic cyanide,
toluene, benzene, xylene, and other volatile organic chemicals.
Since then, said one technician, "My health has been terrible. . . .
I've had days when I just couldn't breathe."

Dentists and dental assistants routinely work with the highly
toxic element mercury—and put it in our mouths. "Silver" fillings
contain silver—about 30 percent—but are at least 50 percent mercury. According to the Foundation for Toxic-Free Dentistry, approximately 14 percent of dental offices in the U.S. have mercury
vapor levels above 50 micrograms per cubic meter, some as high as
180 micrograms per cubic meter, three times the limit recommended
by NIOSH. Several studies have suggested a relationship between
the use of mercury and health problems of dental workers. One

study reported three dentists with high blood levels of mercury and typical mercury-poisoning symptoms such as hand tremors, a metallic taste, muscular weakness, slurred speech, and loss of motor control. Another study found ninety-eight dentists scoring much worse than fifty-six control subjects on tests of memory, concentration, and motor skills. A forty-two-year-old dental assistant with a twenty-year history of exposure to mercury developed a "rapidly fatal" kidney illness and died; a high level of mercury was found in her kidneys. In pregnant women working in dental offices, mercury has been found to cross the placenta into the fetus. A 1993 University of Georgia study found that when monkeys' teeth were filled with mercury amalgams, bacteria in the monkeys' intestines became resistant not only to mercury but to commonly used antibiotics as well.

Mercury is not the only hazard in dental offices and in laboratories. Shortly after a Chicago woman began working as a dental technician, she noticed frequent heart palpitations that became increasingly frightening to her. Getting little relief or understanding from her regular doctors, she finally sought help from Dr. Randolph. In his office she tested strongly positive to ethanol and to natural gas—and with this knowledge started back on the road to health. At her workplace she had worked for years with Bunsen burners in a small, poorly ventilated room and had used countless ethanol-based products—sterilizing and disinfecting solutions, hand soaps, and hand lotions (ethanol is also the base for most perfumes and colognes). Once she was able to avoid these items or find substitutes, her almost constant palpitations dwindled within a few days to one or two a week. Now she notices only an occasional skipped beat—cause unknown.

Palpitations also afflicted resident physicians working in the pathology department of Boston City Hospital in 1974. One young resident pathologist died suddenly of a heart attack before investigators were able to link the unusual number of palpitations affecting department workers with a fluorocarbon being used as an aerosol to speed up the preparation of frozen tissue sections.

Strong cleaning solutions, so prevalent in infection-conscious hospitals and nursing homes, increasingly pose serious problems for personnel. Barbara O'Connor, formerly a nurse at Marin General

Hospital, in California's Marin County, has become so injured by chemicals in her work assignments—especially ammonia in floor cleaners and formaldehyde in mattresses—that she can no longer work. Marin Hospital's changes in its new wing—baking out (heating to one hundred-or-so degrees for several days and then airing out for a day) the wing to dissipate chemical fumes, instituting a smoking ban and perfume bans for nurses and hospital volunteers, using less-toxic cleaning supplies—have apparently come too late to help her.

More hospitals need to read the Centers for Disease Control's startling guidelines for hospital housekeeping: "the actual physical removal of microorganisms by scrubbing is probably as important as any antimicrobial effect of a cleaning agent, *if not more so* [emphasis added]." Hospitals, says the CDC, should choose cleaning agents solely on the basis of price and safety. And use more elbow grease. Or safer, simpler products. "In America we clean for appearance. We don't clean for our health," said Joseph Latiburek, a Massachusetts building consultant, explaining that industrial strength formulas are often overkill. "Except for major projects, like washrooms, a little lemon and vinegar in water can take care of many cleaning jobs." Indeed, industrial-strength cleaners used in washrooms *have* killed: in 1989 two Chicago workers died from inhaling fumes from an industrial-strength cleaner called "Seal-Off," which is 90 percent methylene chloride. They were using the product to strip wax from a men's room floor. Later an OSHA spokesperson said that the type of mask given to the workers was inadequate for use with methylene chloride. Too late.

Even soaps can pose dangers—to personnel and patients alike. According to Debra Lynn Dadd, in *Nontoxic and Natural: How to Avoid Dangerous Everyday Products and Buy or Make Safe Ones*, "The most popular and most heavily advertised soaps are the antimicrobial 'deodorant' soaps. An FDA advisory review panel has questioned the safety of using these potent germ-killers on a regular day-to-day, year-after-year basis."

Intensive care nurses may be among those most at risk. Sandy McCabe, an intensive-care nurse for twenty years at San Francisco General Hospital Medical Center, experienced dizziness and headaches that forced her to work only part time. Now chemically sensitive, she places at least some of the blame on exposure to chemicals in the hospital. "[EI/MCS] can be so severe, but it's really an invisible illness," she says. "You'd never know it to look at us. Unless you've known somebody with it or had it yourself, you don't know about it."

"Epidemics are not usually discussed in terms of contact allergy, but we are in the midst of one to natural rubber latex," says Dr. Ronald Brancaccio of New York University's Medical Center, referring to the 7 percent of surgeons and 5 percent of operating room nurses who find themselves allergic to the latex in their surgical gloves. Even more alarming in its implications is a 1991 report that eight children operated on for deformed spines developed severe, anaphylactic reactions later determined to be caused by the latex products used during the surgery. Said Dr. Mary A. Setlock, "We now question all patients about possible allergy to rubber products." Even brief exposures to rubber products can be seriously affecting: a chemically sensitive but otherwise healthy Oregon woman vomited immediately after unwrapping crutch grips that she had previously wrapped in plastic because of their disagreeable smell.

Construction is another hazardous industry. In the words of Kitty, an industrial painter, from *Workers at Risk*, "I've found out some pretty horrendous things about epoxy [paint]; it makes you bleed through your pores, it burns your lungs, burns your eyes, gives you ear infections, and . . . can kill you. . . . It's funny how few of the journeymen know what the dangers are that you can run up against, what the chemical will do to you or what's really in it. If you refuse to use it, you might get laid off, fired, or suspended . . . so most guys don't want to rock the boat. I guess they figure ignorance is bliss."

Though most new paint no longer contains lead (since 1977) or mercury (since 1990), it can contain toxic volatile solvents like toluene, xylene, and benzene, as well as poisonous fungicides and mildewcides. Such compounds can have many serious health effects, especially central nervous system diseases, according to Dr. Baker, who has treated many afflicted workers, including painters, with symptoms like nausea, dizziness, headache, disorientation, and increased violent behavior. In fact, a Swedish study of prisoners has found a higher incidence of violent crime by painters than by all other workers. Baker's observation is that painters and carpet gluers tend to be alcoholics. They develop "severe headaches as a result of solvent exposure, so that they have alcohol in increasing amounts to relax and anesthetize themselves, and thus end up poisoned with alcohol in addition to solvents." Painters' immune systems can be affected: a 1982 Polish study of 108 seemingly healthy workers in contact with organic solvents in paints and varnishes found immune-system suppression (depressed levels of T cells, part of the body's protective mechanism), which, it was thought, could predispose the workers to allergies and cancer.

Painters are also exposed to the highly toxic isocyanates, which can induce asthma. Actually, asthma is a risk in twenty-eight different occupations, many of them involving materials used in construction. After a homeowner got symptoms from newly installed particle board, Connecticut architect Paul Bierman-Lytle reported that carpenters on that job suffered from itchiness, fatigue, headaches, and skin and eye irritations. "Carpenters . . . say that's fairly common, that being sick and uncomfortable goes hand in hand with the job," he said. Worse than being sick and uncomfortable, the "average construction worker has a life expectancy ten to twelve years less than the average," according to John Moran, a safety expert formerly with NIOSH. "In Indiana, the average construction worker dies at sixty—before he even collects Social Security."

Workers in the printing industry are similarly exposed to toxic chemicals. In New York State, where occupational disease is the fourth leading cause of death, Rick Hayden can no longer work, read, ride a bicycle, or do math problems. His central nervous system is damaged, his doctors say, from exposure to solvents at his job at the Morrill Press, near Syracuse. Though the company's insurance carrier repeatedly warned of excessive worker exposures, employees' clothes were often soaked with solvents. The company, while maintaining that workplace solvents did not cause Hayden's problems, claims to have finally put in place all of its insurer's recommendations for worker safety.

Fifty-one-year-old printer Don Snyder, a resident of Madison County in upstate New York, began finding himself so dizzy by the end of the work week that he could hardly drive. He was afraid that he was going to have a heart attack. At home, tired, aching, he would rest and gradually revive himself for the start of the next work week. Finally consulting Dr. James Miller, a specialist in environmental medicine, he learned that he has EI/MCS and that the "inks, solvents, and other tools of his trade were making him sick." The illness has cost him his job. "I never knew," Snyder said. "I always handled that stuff with my hands when I worked the machines. I didn't know it was bad for you. I had no idea." The printing and publishing industries use many toxic chemicals whose emissions they are now required to report under the 1986 Emergency Planning and Community Right-to-Know Act—chemicals such as toluene, xylene, glycol ether, methyl ethyl ketone, tetrachloroethylene, and 1,1,1-trichloroethane. Provisions of the Act refer to companies' outdoor emissions of toxic chemicals into air, water, and land, but Don Snyder's experience tells us that the chemicals are a hazard to workers indoors as well.

A Canadian psychiatry professor, Ernest McCrank, has speculated as to the cause of a rare neurological disorder, progressive supranuclear palsy, in three of his patients. Because all three had worked as lithographers at the same printing plant, he suspected the organic solvents used at the plant. Speaking to the Canadian Psychiatric Association in 1987, McCrank remarked that this devastating disease is often misdiagnosed as depression, dementia, or Parkinson's disease and suggested that "medical people should be watching and noting whether there is any connection between symptoms and solvents in their patients."

Chemicals used in the garment industry also put many workers at risk. New York City fashion designer Doris Brundza discovered this the hard way. Having first developed chemical sensitivity from large doses of antibiotics, she began reacting to the formaldehyde finishes on fabrics, and now must work out of her home on untreated fabrics only. Her problem was compounded by working in a garment district building with sealed windows, where co-workers' smoking often made her weak, sleepy, and dizzy.

One of the worst examples of worker poisoning and societal indifference occurred at a small fabric-coating factory, called Uretek, located in the basement of what looked like an abandoned building in New Haven, Connecticut. According to *Hartford Courant* writer

Gary Dorsey, who investigated the story in 1987 and titled his article "The Poison Factory," the place was "a natural draw for untrained, transient Hispanic workers. At Uretek, you didn't need special skills to mix and pour chemicals or to run fabric-coating machines. You didn't have to speak English. You didn't need an education or, necessarily, proof of American citizenship." The pay was good if you worked overtime, even though the chemical stink made some of the men vomit. They used to bet on how long a new man would last around a coating machine.

In 1986 workers from the factory began showing up in the emergency room of the local hospital with nausea, headaches, and abdominal pain. Tests revealed liver damage. The emergency room doctor contacted Dr. Mark Cullen, a young Yale University professor and physician who directs the Yale-New Haven Occupational Medicine Program, known as one of the best private occupational medicine clinics in the country. Cullen, who was at the time editing a book, *Workers with Multiple Chemical Sensitivities*, was immediately suspicious of possible workplace exposures. He contacted Uretek's owners, who, to his surprise, proved cooperative. Thus began an investigation that eventually found noninfectious hepatitis in eleven workers and led to the the conviction of Uretek and its vice president and chief chemist, John Andrews, for mishandling hazardous wastes—leaking, rusted, unlabeled drums on Uretek property, filled with toxic chemicals like methyl ethyl ketone (which can cause skin, eye, and respiratory problems), toluene (which can cause nausea, headaches, and eye irritation), and dimethylformamide (which can cause liver damage). In his defense Andrews wrote, "The exact chemical composition of the coatings is unknown to us, as the suppliers consider the coatings as proprietary. I have been assured, however, that the compositions do not contain any unduly hazardous or toxic chemicals."

Curiously, the criminal charges said nothing about workers or their health. And OSHA, one of the two agencies charged by Congress with protecting workers, failed these victims as it has failed many others, one reason being that OSHA had only one full-time doctor on staff for the entire country. (A physician at the Yale Clinic had tried to get help from OSHA for workers at a dry-cleaning establishment—another human testing laboratory—only to be met by stifling bureaucratic indifference.) Shortly after the court case ended, a Puerto Rican organizer for the International Ladies Garment Workers Union organized the factory in seventy-two hours, took the workers out on strike, and "blew [the situation] wide open" by contacting the media. By then, 78 percent of Uretek's production workers had fallen ill. Many got worse during the strike; some simply vanished. The ones who remained in the area during the strike were left only with the hope that a union contract would bring safer working conditions.

"We were horrified by this particular outbreak," Cullen said, "but we were not particularly surprised by it. It is not, in essence, an isolated experience." Commenting on his reasons for starting the Yale Clinic, he observed that workers' illnesses are often misunderstood or overlooked: "The disease could look like any other disease, but the source wouldn't be identified because doctors aren't trained to think about the workplace. The ball is dropped." In eight years at the Clinic, Cullen treated about two thousand patients with work-related disease—all, he says, "100 percent preventable."

Meanwhile, in Illinois two landmark toxic chemical cases also involving blue-collar workers are making their way through the courts. In one, three former executives of a suburban film processing company, Film Recovery Systems, were charged with murder in the death of a Polish emigrant employee poisoned by the cyanide he used in the recovery of silver from X-ray film. In the other, executives of Chicago Magnet Wire were accused of knowingly exposing forty-three workers to toxic chemicals used to coat wire with enamel and plastics.

Many modern chemicals are used in what used to be thought "clean" industries—aerospace and computers. At least 160 workers at Lockheed's Burbank, California, Stealth bomber plant suffered health problems ranging from nausea and minor rashes to disorientation, memory lapses, and cancer, believed by the workers to be caused by chemicals used in the plant's secret projects. In 1988 a number of afflicted employees sued the company, and in 1989 OSHA fined Lockheed $1.49 million for failing to adequately inform its workers of health hazards from chemicals. Writing in *The Human Ecologist*, Dr. Baker described "aerospace workers' syndrome" as a "disease of our advanced technology," one resulting in part from the use of phenol-formaldehyde resins in the manufacture of aircraft parts. Baker has treated a number of patients with this syndrome, including one young man, previously healthy, who lost his job, his savings, and his health. Bitterly, he said that his company (a major aerospace firm), "has been [my family's] whole life, and now it isn't helping me with my disability. It doesn't care at all." Baker's comment: "The unfortunate victims of these chemical poisons should be properly cared for and should not be subject to harassment, demotion, or termination, or forced to continue working in unhealthy environments until they can work no more."

In the mid-1980s in Silicon Valley, California, home of major computer firms, hundreds of electronics workers developed a "mystery disease," characterized by headaches, memory problems, and physical reactions to cigarette smoke, car exhaust, perfumes, household bleach, and supermarket detergent aisles. They had acquired EI/MCS, apparently traceable to toxic chemicals in their workplace. "No other industry on Earth uses nastier chemicals than the semiconductor industry," said Don Rose, publisher of *Electronics Materials*. Some of the afflicted have been able to obtain workers' compensation benefits. IBM, one of the Silicon Valley firms, has since switched from a toxic—and ozone-depleting—cleaning solvent to a water-based one. This is the kind of pollution prevention that companies and workers need more of, but the change came too late for some women working with glycol ethers in the electronics industries; several studies have shown higher rates of miscarriages for these workers. Another study found abnormal liver enzyme levels in 44 percent of heavily chemically exposed electronics workers and in only 4 percent of lightly exposed workers employed at the same plant.

Another "mystery illness" has affected thousands of workers in the military "industry"—the Persian Gulf veterans. Symptoms included headaches, nausea, rashes, muscle weakness, chronic fatigue, hair loss, disorientation, and chemical sensitivity. While some army doctors at first blamed stress-related adjustment problems, there is a growing consensus that these persistent symptoms were the result of such exposures as pesticides used to control sand flies, diesel heaters in tents, and diesel-contaminated water. One Gulf veteran, Steve Buyer, a freshman congressman from Indiana, who had been "completely physically fit" before the war, developed multiple physical complaints, allergies, and asthma after the war. "It's crazy," he said. "The Gulf War changed my life and my body; that's a fact."

An earlier twentieth-century war has affected the health of members of our armed forces. In 1993 the Department of Veterans Affairs finally extended disability benefits to Vietnam veterans with cancers of the lung, larynx, and trachea, and with multiple myeloma. This belated ruling came several months after a thousand-page NAS report linking these and other health problems to herbicides used in Vietnam, including the deadly Agent Orange.

One of Agent Orange's deadliest components was dioxin, a term used for seventy-five chlorine-containing chemical compounds—and for a hazard that remains with us still. Today, dioxin is commonly found as a byproduct of chlorine-based industries or processes such as paper and pesticide manufacture, garbage disposal and incineration, and wood preserving, oil refining, and metal smelting. As a byproduct, dioxin, which the EPA in 1985 called "the most potent carcinogen ever tested in laboratory animals," makes its way into our water, soil, and air.

One study, reported in the *NEJM*, of workers exposed to dioxin found significantly increased mortality from soft-tissue cancers and respiratory cancers in a subgroup of workers that was most exposed to the substance. Since this study was done, however, industry spokespersons and government officials fostering a dioxin "backlash" have claimed that dioxin is not the villain previously thought. *New York Times* environmental reporter Keith Schneider effectively detoxified dioxin by saying it was no more risky than "spending a week in the sun." Schneider later admitted to the *American Journalism Review* that no scientist ever told him that: he and his editors simply made it up. While industry research purports to show few adverse health effects in humans, an EPA scientist, Cate Jenkins, has charged fraudulent research by at least one chemical company. In 1993 the EPA took another look at dioxin; its draft (preliminary) review of all data linking dioxin to human health effects concluded that four separate studies of workers exposed to dioxin revealed an overall increased mortality from all malignancies combined.

Office work does not exactly constitute an industry, but new, sleek-walled, tightly constructed, energy-conserving, inadequately ventilated buildings that are making some of the workers in them sick may be the biggest workplace hazard of all. It has been estimated that "at any one time ten to twenty-five million workers in 800,000 to 1.2 million commercial buildings in the U.S. will have symptoms of the sick building syndrome." These workers, mostly women, now spend forty or more hours a week in buildings with recirculated air, often using computers whose long-term health effects from outgassing and electromagnetic radiation are unknown. Copiers are frequently in unventilated closets; new carpeting and other furnishings exude unpleasant and dangerous fumes, cleaning fluids contain hazardous chemicals; paint is often new and toxic; poorly-maintained air conditioners spread mold and bacteria; smoking is still permitted; and disagreeable perfumes and personal grooming products abound. You want to open a window, but you can't.

Little wonder that surveys reflect worker dissatisfaction with the air they breathe. One study by Honeywell Technalysis found that a fourth of six hundred workers in various buildings said that there were air quality problems in their offices; another study found 60 percent of Chicago office workers complaining about their indoor air. These are not just idle complaints. In 1988 *JAMA* published a report of two women who suffered hoarseness, coughing, itching, and rashes after contact with carbonless carbon paper. The paper contained a chemical—alkylphenol novolac resin—that the researchers thought could have caused a potentially fatal swelling of the larynx. Exposure to a laser printer was found to be the cause of a fifty-one-year-old insurance company employee's developing severe nasal congestion, a burning sensation on his skin, headaches, and stomach pain, according to a letter in the May 3, 1990 *NEJM*. As little as ten minutes' work with the printer would produce his symptoms.

A Washington, D.C., legal secretary, Madeline Abbene, gradually fell ill as workers were putting three coats of finish on her boss's floor in their tightly closed building, and finally fainted. Further renovations increased her respiratory, muscle control, and memory loss problems; she became so debilitated that she could no longer work. Seven years later she was still ill with these symptoms—and with EI/MCS. "Just as some people are more susceptible than others to certain diseases," notes Robert K. McLellan, director of the Center for Occupational and Environmental Medicine at Hamden, Connecticut, "some of us are more vulnerable to chemicals. . . . The person gets sick and then, for reasons no one yet understands, becomes more and more ill in response to progressively lower and lower levels of exposure to the same or other chemicals. Symptoms come and go, depending on the exposure." But the problem of sick buildings will get worse, says Dr. John Spengler, of the Harvard School of Public Health, because another generation of "pathologic" buildings is already on the drawing board.

Some of these buildings' architects should listen to George Bourassa, partner in the Chicago engineering firm of Flack and Kurtz, which has been working to cure sick buildings: "The best way to deal with this is by prevention, not after it occurs." Architects who remodeled the Natural Resources Defense Council building in New York did listen to Flack and Kurtz. The result: a 50 percent saving in energy costs—and happier workers. Said interior designer Kirsten Childs, "You can tell the difference at the NRDC. Workers benefit; the air feels good all the time."

A variety of occupations are functioning as human testing laboratories. As you might expect, landfill and toxic waste workers are also at special risk. Mike Galvin, at thirty-two a casualty of his employment at an Oswego County, New York, landfill, was exposed to toxic chemicals like toluene and benzene and an unknown "white gas" that came out of boxes he accidentally ran over with his truck. The gas burned his throat and chest. But his worst symptoms are nausea, headaches, dizziness, and amnesia. "One thing that kind of scares me right now," Galvin said, "is my lack of being able to concentrate . . . [or] to follow simple directions. I have to read [them] several times." According to his wife, "He forgets things all the time now and he's very moody. He tries to keep busy but he can't do the things he used to do." His doctor, also Dr. Miller, has diagnosed him as having EI/MCS: "He's not thinking straight. This is common to guys with solvent injuries—they can't think straight. They can't remember. They can't figure things out. They drive past their exits. They get to the store and can't remember what they went there for." Yes, we all do things like this occasionally, but for some people these chemically caused "failings" are so severe as to be disabling, perhaps permanently.

Workers at a toxic waste incinerator run by Caldwell Systems, Inc., in Lenoir, North Carolina, experienced similar problems after working for years with dozens of toxic chemicals that they were never warned about or trained to handle. Unsuspecting, they "waded in chemicals up to their ankles and entertained themselves with toxic sludge-ball fights," according to a June 1990 report by the North Carolina Department of Environment, Health, and Natural Resources. Finally, suffering burns, dizziness, disabling headaches, vomiting, hallucinations, and violent mood swings— symptoms that persisted—some of them ended up in the office of local doctor Marc Guerra. One of them, said Dr. Guerra, "walked into the office and looked like a leper covered with rashes, shaking like a leaf. He couldn't remember from one moment to the next." A San Francisco occupational health specialist, Dr. James Cone, who examined some of the former Caldwell workers, said, "These are some of the most affected people I've ever seen in workplace exposures." Yet Caldwell president Charles Foushee Jr. said that these things are "blown way out of proportion. We don't believe these are serious illnesses." Guerra says that at least sixteen Caldwell workers have "significant brain damage." Guerra is also treating residents of the area who have been exposed to the incinerator's toxic emissions. The plant is now closed, and the EPA, which sent toxic wastes to the incinerator but did not supervise the work, may make it a toxic waste site qualifying for emergency assistance. Considering its reputation for dealing—or not dealing—with toxic waste, the EPA may deserve the joking appellation given to it by some environmentalists: Evade, Procrastinate, and Avoid responsibility.

Burning modern chemicals often creates deadly fumes. An Earth Day 1980 explosion and fire at a hazardous waste facility in New Jersey left some fire fighters with respiratory ailments and an unusual number of other health problems. Ten years later a newsletter from the New Jersey Environmental and Occupational Health Sciences Institute commented laconically, "The actual chronic health effects experienced by the firefighters will become more apparent with time." In 1992, near Syracuse, New York, a volunteer fire fighter, William L. June Jr., walked into a toxic pesticide cloud thought to be a fire and now suffers from chronic fatigue, an over-sensitivity to chemicals, and a tingling sensation in his arms and legs. Unable to work at his two jobs, he filed a $9 million lawsuit against the farmer and the pesticide manufacturer involved. Nationally, fire fighters have much higher rates than average of certain cancers, with the evidence pointing to burning plastics as the biggest culprit. Though thousands of chemical combinations are involved in fires and are thus hard to study, one researcher found benzopy-rene, a known human carcinogen, in every one of the twenty-four fires that he monitored.

A controlled study of workers exposed to hazardous perchloro-ethylene in dry-cleaning shops found kidney abnormalities suggesting that they are at risk for chronic kidney failure. Because of this and other studies, the EPA has begun evaluating the alternative cleaning methods already tested by millions of people for hundreds of years: biodegradable soaps, heat, steam, and pressing.

Even working with plants can be hazardous. Jeff Arbogust, owner of Forever Green Tropicals, in Austin, Texas, accidentally sprayed himself with the highly toxic pesticide chlordane, before it was banned in 1998. His symptoms of tremors, stomach pains, and severe headaches and his fat levels of chlordane and DDE (a metabolic product of DDT) were reduced by treatment at HealthMed, the detoxification center in Los Angeles. (Most ornamental plants and cut flowers have been sprayed with pesticides; to confirm, call your local florist or nursery.)

Finally, one company has taken stringent environmental measures—to protect not its workers, but its product. The Chrysler plant, in Toledo, which manufactures Jeeps, forbids its workers to use certain anti-perspirants. It seems that flakes of aluminum, chlorine, and silicon from these deodorants were falling on the cars and leaving tiny craters in the paint, causing thousands of dollars in damage. When will companies forbid such products in order to protect the health of vulnerable workers?

OSHA and NIOSH: A Goddam Joke?

What exactly have OSHA and NIOSH—Occupational Safety and Health Administration and National Institute for Occupational

Safety and Health, our government's two occupational safety agencies—been doing to protect the health of American workers? Not enough, obviously. Part of the problem is understaffing and underfunding. Another part is that these two agencies set up different standards. NIOSH's standards consider only the health of the worker; OSHA's standards have to consider costs and technologies and must go through a public rule-making process. This conflict between the ideal and the possible—or what appears possible after interested parties have a go at it—leads to confusion. NIOSH busies itself publishing "current intelligence bulletins" like "Organic Solvent Neurotoxicity" (1987), "Toluene Diisocyanate (TDI) and Toluenediamine (TDA): Evidence of Carcinogenicity" (1989), and "Environmental Tobacco Smoke in the Workplace: Lung Cancer and Other Health Effects" (1991), but whether these publications actually affect the workplace is dubious. As for OSHA's effectiveness, the odds of its eight hundred inspectors catching up with companies' violations of its standards are very small, according to William Greider. When violators *are* cited, fines are so small that leading safety expert John Moran called them "a goddam joke. In construction, nobody worries about OSHA any more. They don't take it seriously."

Another problem, according to federal scientists and inspectors testifying at 1988 Senate hearings about OSHA, was the Reagan administration's emasculation of these safety and health standards. "I stay awake thinking of the people who are dying," said Dr. Susan Harwood, director of OSHA's health standards programs. OSHA's political appointees stalled regulations and pressured inspectors to inflate performance records. Reagan's Office of Management and Budget often cited excessive costs as the reason for vetoing proposed OSHA rules, such as one governing workers' exposure to formaldehyde, which can cause cancer. In 1984 President Reagan ignored a request by Ralph Nader and Dr. Sidney Wolfe, of Public Citizen's Health Research Group (PCHRG), that more than two hundred thousand endangered workers be notified of NIOSH's study showing them to be at increased risk of cancer, lung disease, heart disease, and other health problems. A budget request for funds to do the notification was turned down, even though a NIOSH pilot study of 586 workers working with betanaphthylamine (BNA), known to cause bladder cancer, had found thirteen workers with bladder cancer and twenty-six workers with possible premalignant changes. Before they were notified, 74 percent of these workers were unaware that BNA is harmful. A decade later, with less than 30 percent of the original two hundred thousand workers notified, PCHRG wrote to President Clinton urging a speeding of the process—the results as yet unknown. In other ways, both the Bush and Clinton administrations have failed the worker. In 1992 OMB ruled that imposing stricter health standards in the workplace could make workers poorer and, therefore, sicker, using the convoluted reasoning that such standards could lead to layoffs and reduce hazard pay. In 1993 the Clinton administration, without explanation, declined to appeal a court decision throwing out or weakening OSHA's air quality standards (permissible exposure limits, or PELs) for nearly four hundred hazardous substances. The court had rejected the standards as lacking sufficient supporting evidence. To some scientists, however, the very concept of "safe" exposures to any chemical is inherently unscientific, because of limited measurement tools. "Discarding the term 'threshold limit' [on which PELs are based] is," they say, "a necessary first step in correcting this false ideology of the past."

To circumvent government inaction, safe workplace advocates around the country have since 1972 been organizing local Committees on Occupational Safety and Health. In response to their pressures, OSHA in 1985 issued a workers-right-to-know standard requiring better labeling of hazardous chemicals, the provision of material safety data sheets (MSDSs) to workers, adequate training of workers in the handling of chemicals and other risks, and worker access to employers' programs for hazard communication. On paper, then, workers have rights, but, said Rick Engler of the New Jersey Industrial Union Council, "even if OSHA tripled the number of inspectors, which would be good, there's a limit to what they can do." Ultimately, workplace safety and health are a power struggle, and OSHA often proves a weak fighter. According to environmental writer David Moberg, "OSHA currently [in 1989] refuses to act on more than 90 percent of the cases in which workers complain they have been fired for exercising their rights to a safe workplace." And since 1980 only "thirty cases of job fatalities were turned over by OSHA to federal authorities, only four of those were prosecuted, and no corporate official was imprisoned (although there have been a handful of successful state prosecutions)," according to a report by the Bureau of National Affairs. Its data were based on a 1988 Congressional committee report entitled "Getting Away with Murder in the Workplace: OSHA's Nonuse of Criminal Penalties for Safety Violations."

Once again, it looks as if your health, if you work outside your home, is going to have to be, as much as possible, in your own hands. First of all, you need accurate information. Can you rely on the national media for this? No, says Moberg, in his series of articles "Danger: People at Work." When a Rutgers University team studied media coverage of environmental risks, it concluded that "if coverage were proportionate to risk, during the study period the major networks would have aired about 360 times more coverage of just three well-known environmental risks than of airplane accidents. Instead, the airplane accidents received eight times the coverage of the environmental risks."

The team also found that "an occupational death is roughly one-tenth as newsworthy as an environmental death." Moberg finds numerous reasons for this: few reporters are assigned to occupational health or even to labor issues; blue-collar and ethnic workers tend to get slighted or ignored by advertisers and reporters with middle-class views; the subject can be too technical; the big tragedies are emphasized, rather than the slow deaths with multiple causes; reporters may be prejudiced against unions; chemical hazards "become newsworthy only when they affect the wider public"; hazards can be considered "just part of the job"; reporters don't see workplace accidents and illnesses as preventable; press coverage tends to rely too much on government pronouncements rather than labor-union criticism; and during the 1980s our national economic obsession was how to keep up with foreign competition, not how to make our workers happier or safer. Yet, says Moberg, "workers die in other industrialized countries at one-fifth to three-fourths the rate they do in the U.S., while those countries' products outsell American goods. Even more telling, if the U.S. had Sweden's workplace-fatality rate, the country would save $12 billion a year." Thus Moberg sees our media as failing to cover a major story: "the dangers of the environment in which more than one hundred million Americans spend one-third of their lives."

Off to Work You Go

If you are one of those spending one-third of your life in a workplace provided by your employer, especially if you suspect that your health problems may be related to the workplace environment, consider doing the following:

- Ask your employer for the chemical names of the chemicals you are exposed to and for the MSDSs for those chemicals. Though MSDSs can be hard to fathom and sometimes withhold chemical names as trade secrets, you may find out something useful.

- Call NIOSH at 1-800-35-NIOSH for information about ordering the *NIOSH Pocket Guide to Chemical Hazards*, published in 1985 and updated in 1990. You may find the chemicals in your workplace listed there, with their health hazards and recommended precautions. But chemical names are tricky: you may have to look several places. For example, betanaphthylamine is listed under "N," not under "B." "Target organs" for BNA are bladder and skin; "carc" (for "carcinogen") is given under symptoms. Now you have a clue.

- For information on sick building syndrome (SBS), call NIOSH at 1-800-35-NIOSH to order its *Guide to Indoor Air Quality*. Be aware that when your building has a central ventilating system, your symptoms may be caused by businesses in your building—dry cleaners, beauty salons, print shops, copy shops, and medical offices and laboratories.

- NIOSH can also provide a Health Hazard Evaluation of your workplace. Call 1-800-35-NIOSH; you can ask to remain anonymous.

- Your local OSHA office will also inspect your workplace. Again, you can ask to remain anonymous.

- Ask your employer if your workplace has ever been monitored for chemical exposures. If so, request the results. Under OSHA's Access Standard, they must be provided to employees.

- Contact Public Citizen for a copy of "Communities and Workers' Right to Know," Publication #1006, March 15, 1985 (Public Citizen Health Research Group, 2000 P Street NW, Washington, D.C. 20036; 202-833-3000). It has other suggestions for action. Also ask for Public Citizen's 1994 report *Workplace Health Hazards* (send $10) and its 1985 *Health Letter Special Supplement*, which lists the names and locations of workplaces with increased risks of cancer, lung disease, heart disease, and other health problems.

- Find out if your state has an occupational health hotline. Between 1981 and 1986, California's hotline received more than eight thousand inquiries on over three thousand hazardous chemicals.

- Realize that safer substitutes exist for many toxic chemicals: soy ink instead of petroleum-based inks; oxygen instead of dioxin-creating chlorine in paper-bleaching processes; borax instead of dangerous pesticidal cleaning products.

- Above all, think in terms of pollution prevention instead of pollution control. In Chicago, leaders of the highly polluting electroplating industry are beginning to use less-toxic materials in order to avoid expensive but required pollution-control measures. Around the Great Lakes, local groups calling themselves the Zero Discharge Alliance are working together to ban toxic discharges into the Lakes, beginning with a ban on chlorine. If paper and pulp industries can no longer dump dioxin-producing chlorine into the Lakes, they may be forced to switch from chlorine to less-toxic oxygen for bleaching. Thus chlorine and its byproducts will be kept out of workers' bodies, out of the atmosphere, out of water, out of fish, and out of our diets—the best kind of pollution prevention.

In the late 1970s many American companies began to exclude fertile women from high-paying jobs, ostensibly to protect them and their unborn children from birth defects caused by exposure to toxic industrial chemicals. Such policies, which coincided with the "right to know" movement, permitted companies to go on using toxic chemicals without cleaning up workplaces; instead, workers were "allowed" to know the names and some of the properties of the toxic chemicals they worked with. In 1991 the U.S. Supreme Court invalidated these well-meaning but misguided fetal protection policies as sex discrimination. As it becomes better known that many toxic exposures harm male as well as female reproductive systems, society may be moved to reduce the use of toxic chemicals so that the unborn will not suffer from either parent's chemical exposures. All of us—workers and others—will benefit from this kind of pollution prevention.

* * * *

To Find Out More

- *The Expendable Americans*, by Paul Brodeur, New York, Viking Press, 1974.

- *Office Hazards: How Your Job Can Make You Sick*, by Joel Makower, Washington, D.C., Tilden Press, 1981.

- *How to Survive in Your Toxic Environment: The American Survival Guide*, by Edward J. Bergin, with Ronald E. Grandon, New York, Avon, 1984.

- *The Nontoxic Home and Office: Protecting Yourself and Your Family from Everyday Toxics and Health Hazards*, by Debra Lynn Dadd, Los Angeles, Jeremy P. Tarcher, 1992.

- *Toxic Work: Women Workers at GTE Lenkurt*, by Stephen Fox, Philadelphia, Temple University Press, 1991.

- *Chemical Exposure and Disease: Diagnostic and Investigative Techniques*, by Janette D. Sherman, MD, New York, Van Nostrand Reinhold, 1988.

- *Workers at Risk: Voices from the Workplace*, by Dorothy Nelkin and Michael S. Brown, Chicago, the University of Chicago Press, 1984.

- *Retreat from Safety: Reagan's Attack on America's Health*, by Joan Claybrook and the Staff of Public Citizen, New York, Pantheon, 1984.

- *The Health Detective's Handbook: A Guide to the Investigation of Environmental Health Hazards by Nonprofessionals*, M.S. Legator, B.L. Harper, and M.J. Scott, editors, Baltimore, Johns Hopkins University Press, 1985.

- *Clinical Toxicology of Commercial Products*, fifth edition, by Robert E. Gosselin, Roger P. Smith, and Harold C. Hodge, Baltimore, Maryland, Williams & Wilkins, 1984 (in library reference rooms).

- *Chemical Hazards of the Workplace*, second edition, by Nick Proctor, James P. Hughes, and Michael L. Fischman, Philadelphia, J.B. Lippincott Company, 1988.

- *Sax's Dangerous Properties of Industrial Materials*, eighth edition, by Richard J. Lewis Sr., New York, Van Nostrand Reinhold, 1992.

- "Toxic Chemicals Bibliography," Public Citizen Publication #1058, April 1986 (write Public Citizen Health Research Group, 2000 P Street NW, Washington, D.C. 20036).

- *Indoor Air Quality and Work Environment Study: EPA Headquarters Buildings, Vol. I: Employee Survey*, by EPA, NIOSH, Westat, Inc., and the John E. Pierce Foundation Laboratory at Yale University, November 1989; also *Indoor Air Quality and Work Environment Study, EPA Headquarters Buildings, Supplement to Vol. I: Additional Employee Adverse Health Effects Information*, by the National Federation of Federal Employees Local 2050 (P.O. Box 76082, Washington, D.C. 20013; 202-382-2383) and the Federation of Government Employees Local 3331, November 20, 1989.

- *Workers with Multiple Chemical Sensitivities*, Mark R. Cullen, MD, editor, Vol. 2, No. 4, *Occupational Medicine: State of the Art Reviews*, Philadelphia, Hanley & Belfus, 1987.

- *Problem Buildings: Building-Associated Illness and the Sick Building Syndrome*, James E. Cone, MD, MPH, and Michael J. Hodgson, MD, MPH, editors, Vol. 4, No. 4, *Occupational Medicine: State of the Art Reviews*, Philadelphia, Hanley & Belfus, 1989.

- *Is Work Making You Sick?: Information for Workers Handling Hazardous Materials*, by the Labor Occupational Health Program, University of California at Berkeley, 1989. This forty-page booklet is in both English and Spanish; for copies, contact the Labor Occupational Health Program, University of California at Berkeley, 2521 Channing Way, Berkeley, California 94720; 415-642-5507.

- *Turning Things Around: A Women's Occupational and Environmental Health Resource Guide*, by Lin Nelson, Regina Kenen, and Susan Klitzman, 1990, available from the National Women's Health Network, 1325 G Street NW, Washington, D.C., 20005; 202-347-1140.

- *The Work-at-Home Sourcebook*, by Lynie Arden, 1990, available from the New Careers Center, P.O. Box 339-UB, Boulder, Colorado 80306; 1-800-634-9024.

- *Silicon Valley Toxics News*, newsletter published by the Silicon Valley Toxics Coalition, 760 North First Street, San Jose, California 95112; 408-287-6707.

- *Voice*, newsletter published by Washington State's Chemically Disabled Workers, P.O. Box 1328, Renton, Washington 98057.

- *Workplace Safety and Health*, newsletter published by the National Safe Workplace Institute, 54 West Hubbard Street, Suite 403, Chicago, IL 60610; 312-661-0690.

- "Air Pollution in the Office Building," a one-page flyer available from the American Lung Association, 1740 Broadway, New York, New York 10019-4374; 212-315-8700.

- Desert Storm Veterans 24-Hour Hotline: 812-948-9366.

4

Warning: Your Home May Be Hazardous to Your Health

H OME. THAT WONDERFUL PLACE you go to relax, be
yourself, be comfortable, be safe. No place is like it. And no
place is more likely to be dangerous to your health.

Yes, according to the EPA, your home, like your body, is a repository for dozens of dangerous chemicals, most of them substances that didn't exist a hundred years ago. As taxpayers, we pay the EPA to find out these things and tell us about them—though maybe the EPA hasn't been telling us enough, often enough. Or maybe it doesn't have the resources to keep up with modern technology's "miracle" products and what those products outgas into the air of your home. The EPA can barely keep up with estimates of deaths from indoor air pollution by natural and manmade substances in our homes: yearly (as reported in 1990), five thousand to twenty thousand deaths from radon; six thousand from secondhand tobacco smoke; four hundred sixty from benzene, known to be a human carcinogen; and nearly eight hundred from five other suspected carcinogens—chloroform (from chlorine in water), carbon tetrachloride (source unknown), paradichlorobenzene (from moth balls and air "fresheners"), and tetrachloroethylene (perchloroethylene, or "perc") and trichloroethylene, two common dry-cleaning solvents.

Most of us spend at least one-third of our lives in our homes; for many of us it's more like two-thirds, for some three-thirds. A hundred years ago, when the U.S. and the rest of the world were mostly agricultural, people spent far more time outdoors. Now we live in artificial environments—behind glass in our homes, cars, and offices, in artificial light, eating artificial (partially manufactured) food, and breathing air filled with artificial (synthetic) gases. The six possible carcinogens just mentioned are a tiny fraction of the toxic chemicals we breathe, drink, and eat every day; and cancer is only one of a number of adverse health effects these chemicals can cause.

Healthy Buildings

Your home can be hazardous to your health in many ways. Take the buildings themselves. The construction industry has changed enormously in the last hundred years, with glue replacing nails, particleboard replacing solid wood, plastic pipes replacing metal pipes, chemically treated wood replacing untreated wood, synthetic, wall-to-wall carpeting replacing wool and cotton area rugs, and toxic insulation materials being added for energy efficiency. What health effects have these and other changes caused?

In the 1980s homebuilder Kurt Reetz and his family felt sick as soon as they moved into a new house in a Chicago suburb. Both he and his wife, Susan, became chronically tired; she would wake up with swollen eyes, feeling as if she had a hangover. Their son became hyperactive and developed rashes and respiratory infections. After six months she seemed worse, so the couple consulted Dr. Randolph, who told them to move out of the house as soon as they could. When they did, she was immediately better. The main culprit was determined to be formaldehyde, for the last thirty or so years a ubiquitous component of building materials like particleboard and glues and of furnishings like carpeting, draperies, upholstery fabrics, wallpaper, and wood furniture. (Particleboard, commonly found in cabinets, wood furniture, and other wood products, consists of compressed and glued wood shavings.) Health problems, Reetz discovered, can also stem from the stain-repellent and flame-retardant chemicals used to treat fabrics and mattresses, from insulation materials, from latex paint, and from mothproofing chemicals. Since that experience, Reetz has not only built his own nontoxic home, but also begun to specialize in building safe homes for others. To his clients he recommends electric instead of gas kitchen stoves and warns against tightly constructed houses. "You don't want to build an airtight house," he says. "If you do, you're killing yourself."

Near Ottawa, Canada, Rafael and Virginia Salares knew that they needed special housing for two of their children. Three-year-old Aileen, healthy at birth, had developed asthma and eczema, possibly from molds. Seven-year-old Rachel had been born with severe skin rashes, violent allergies to most common foods, and an incredible sensitivity to odors and airborne chemicals. Though on a limited budget, the Salares were lucky to find a trio of architects—Greg Allen, Oliver Drerup, and Elizabeth White—who had already built one nontoxic home and who were willing to cooperate with the family in its special needs. As the frame went up, a sign was posted on the building site, a site chosen to be far from city pollution: "Notice: Chemical Sensitivity. Absolutely no materials are to be used or stored in this building without prior approval of Allen-Drerup-White, supervisor. No smoking." Smoking inside the frame was prohibited because smoke can be absorbed and retained by wood, to be released later into house air. To avoid basement molds, the house was built on a concrete slab, which had to be free of all chemical additives and smooth enough for the family to live with until they could afford to install ceramic tile. Virginia Salares, trained as a research chemist, evaluated proposed building materials by the "sniff test": she put a small sample of each material in a large, covered glass beaker for several days and then sniffed it herself before letting the children try it. Substitutes had to be found for almost all commonly used building materials. The finished house, though kept small because of extra costs, has proved comfortable and safe for the two girls, whose symptoms have diminished. The house even includes a separately ventilated greenhouse for growing organic vegetables. Was all the trouble worth it? Definitely, say the Salareses.

In Indiana, Lynn Bower became chemically sensitive after her husband, John, restored their nineteenth-century home in Lafayette, using paint-stripping chemicals. Now living in the woods in a safe house that her husband built, she is homebound, unable to tolerate car fumes or the chemical odors on other people. When her husband, who is not chemically sensitive, returns home from the outside world, he must immediately toss everything he is wearing into the washing machine to remove the perfume and cigarette smoke residues that might make her sick. Before they moved, she recalls, "I thought I had Legionnaire's disease. I couldn't move. I couldn't breathe. I couldn't swallow. I had a temperature and a bladder infection. It affected my joints. It was just devastating. My whole body fell apart." Actually, her husband goes through a "hangover-like withdrawal" when he returns from extended trips and his pollutant-ridden body has to readjust to the pure atmosphere of their home.

The passive-solar-heated house that John Bower built for his wife has a metal frame, metal siding, and metal roof, to avoid any need for termite spraying. The floors are ceramic tile, the cabinets solid wood, the kitchen counters stainless steel with no plywood underneath to outgas. The furniture is mainly metal without upholstery; cushions are filled with washed cotton blankets. On the floors are washable cotton rag rugs. "The principles of building a safe house are eliminate, separate, and ventilate," says Bower. Carpeting is the most important thing to eliminate. Not only does it emit toxic gases—as many as a hundred, he says—the synthetic dust it gives off can create hydrogen cyanide when it gets into a furnace and burns. In their house, Bower has separated insulation from living space and, by means of a glass door, cooking odors from the rest of the house. (For insulation, he particularly warns against the use of cellulose, which is originally a plant product, wood, in the form of ground-up newspapers. By the time it is blown into house walls and ceilings, however, it is saturated with chemicals from printer's ink, dyes, resins, varnishes, pigments, insecticides, fire retardants, and other toxic additives and treatments. The fine dust it creates has caused health disasters for several families.) The Bowers' ventilation system can exchange outside air for the entire house air in an hour, with a heat-recovery system transferring warmth from the stale air to the fresh air. Both heating costs and cleaning time have been reduced to a minimum. Extra construction costs for a healthy house, Bower says, "can range from zero to 25 percent, depending on how carried away you want to get." Based on their experiences, Bower has produced several helpful books and a video, "Your House, Your Health," available through health or video stores. His advice:

"You have to be selective with what you want from the twentieth century."

Careful selection was exactly what Patricia Prijatel did in building a healthier house for herself and her chemically sensitive children in Des Moines, Iowa. Doing that turned out to be simpler and less expensive than she had thought: only $2,400 out of a total cost of $142,000 for 1,980 finished square feet, an increase of less than 2 percent. In their new home the family are breathing easier, relieved of asthma, headaches, and unusual fatigue.

Money was no object for a New York couple who were clients of Connecticut architect Paul Bierman-Lytle. A safe, healthy environment was. For them Bierman-Lytle, whose environmental awareness began when he realized that building materials were causing his headaches, coughing, and sneezing, designed and built a house with a romantic tower on an island off the Atlantic coast. This handsome modern house, featured in the *New York Times* Living Arts section, contained "insulation derived from a mineral mined from sea water, 'natural' grout, and wood finishes made from linseed oil, citrus peel oil, juniper berries, and rosemary." More conventionally, Bierman-Lytle practiced his usual avoidance of synthetic and treated wallpaper, solvent-based glues, formaldehyde-based plywoods, and wall-to-wall carpeting. To most clients he recommends "natural floor coverings, usually cotton, wool, or goat-hair rugs over untreated jute [or] vitreous tiles, linoleum, cork, stone, brick, and solid wood." He favors "full-spectrum light bulbs (closer to natural light), tropical wood from controlled-timbering areas, and a heat-recovery ventilator that draws out stale air and brings in fresh." Because many of the materials that Bierman-Lytle uses are specially prepared or imported from Europe, where the "bau-biologie" (literally "building biology," more loosely translated as "healthful housing") movement has taken hold, construction costs for his buildings can run 25 to 35 percent higher than normal.

Costs may decrease, however, after Bierman-Lytle opens his planned "twenty-first century lumberyard" in Los Angeles. There he hopes to sell more than five thousand environmentally sound American-made building products. Also, *U.S. News & World Report* predicts that comparative costs may flip-flop as "class-action suits in the hundreds of billions of dollars are filed against paint

manufacturers, architects, and developers for the public health hazard posed by toxic building practices." The American Institute of
Architects, sensing a new trend, has begun work on an environmental resources guide that will provide chemical analyses of commonly
used materials and list less toxic alternatives. In 1993 Susan Max-
man became not only the first woman president of the American Institute of Architects but the first AIA president to give top priority to
environmental concerns. It's about time.

Environmental organizations have also begun to catch on. In
New York, architect William McDonough designed for the Environmental Defense Fund a less-toxic building, one with solid wood
rather than plywood and particleboard, with carpets tacked rather
than glued, with beeswax- rather than polyurethane-finished floors,
and with windows that open. Also in New York, the National
Audubon Society has renovated a building that may even be safe for
human canaries. Audubon's chief scientist, Jan Beyea, was astonished by the results: "A month before we moved in, I'm walking
around, and they are painting the walls and laying down the carpet
and I can't smell anything. That shows we did our job."

Safe homes need not look much different from unsafe ones. By
doing a few relatively simple things, Linda Mason Hunter, author
of *The Healthy Home*, and her husband, Bob, made their new (to
them) eighty-year-old house in Des Moines, Iowa, much safer than
it had been. Yet it looks completely "normal," the only possible
giveaways being an activated-charcoal water filter, mostly bare
floors, and a locked backyard shed containing toxic paints and automotive supplies. Older houses, built with untreated, solid wood
and plaster instead of drywall (which can contain toxic adhesives),
are easier to make safe. For those in newer houses, Hunter recommends that formaldehyde-emitting pressed wood in cabinets or
under countertops be sealed with a safe sealer. "The same high-
powered chemistry that makes modern building products perform
so well also makes them potentially hazardous to our health,"
Hunter wrote.

Another wood to beware of is wood that has been pressure-
treated with chemicals—chromated copper arsenate, creosote, or
pentachlorophenol, all highly toxic or carcinogenic—to reduce susceptibility to decay, rot, or termite attack. The EPA and the Na-

tional Coalition Against the Misuse of Pesticides warn that such wood should be used only with great care: wear protective clothing and use a dust mask when sawing it; do not use where it would come in contact with drinking water or food, as in picnic tables and vegetable gardens; do not burn scraps in bonfires, wood stoves, or fireplaces; do not walk barefoot on a pressure-treated deck; and do not use unsealed pressure-treated wood where children will come in contact with it. A good alternative is wood treated with borates, derivatives of boric acid, a less-toxic pesticide.

Unlike our ancestors, we spend most of our days (and nights) in artificial light, behind car, house, and office windows. Yet we need full-spectrum natural light for the regulation of our body chemistry. Ultraviolet light, essential for the production of vitamin D by our bodies and important for calcium metabolism, is filtered out by glass. While too much ultraviolet light may cause eye damage and skin cancer, not enough can lead to a condition that John Ott, who performed pioneering studies of the relationship between full-spectrum light and human health, calls "mal-illumination," the environmental counterpart of malnutrition. "The long-term solution is obvious," says John Banta, owner of Healthful Hardware, a Prescott, Arizona, store. "Halt the release of pollutants that decrease light levels and destroy ozone, spend more time outdoors, and build homes and work places using materials that will admit natural full-spectrum light." Health-conscious architects are beginning to do just that—and to use properly shielded, properly constructed full-spectrum lighting fixtures. However, while fluorescent light sources like Vita-Lite and the Ott-Light can approximate sunlight, the world is still awaiting bona fide "full-spectrum" incandescent bulbs.

Rachel Salares, Lynn Bower, and the Prijatel family have EI/MCS. The Reetz family, the Jones family, and Paul Bierman/Lytle were on their way to acquiring EI/MCS. Dr. Rea has the following advice for homebuilders and homeowners, from the Summer 1990 issue of *The Human Ecologist*: Build away from electric power lines and waste dumps, preferably on a hill, not in a valley, where pollution gets trapped. Use copper water pipes and foil-backed fiberglass insulation. Locate gas or oil furnaces outside the house, with metal ducts and no air supply in contact with motors, pumps, or fuel sources. (This issue of *The Human Ecologist* also has an article on selecting and installing safe home-heating systems, by Mary Oetzel, a Texas-based consultant on environmentally safe building practices.) Use solid hardwood and as little plywood as possible, with walls of sheetrock, glass, tile, plaster, or porcelain and floors of wood, tile, terrazzo, marble, or "hard-brittle" linoleum. Avoid petrochemical-based glues, caulks, grouts, or varnish. Minimize radon exposure by adequate design and ventilation. Install water and air purification equipment, copper wiring, full-spectrum lighting with a radiation shield, and, where possible, electric appliances. (If a gas kitchen stove must be used, vent it to the outside.) Use furnishings of solid wood, glass, metal, and natural, unsprayed, untreated fabrics. Safe homes, says Rea, "are the result of knowledgeable people exercising wise choices. To create and maintain a healthy home is to create and maintain a healthy body. There is no other safe alternative for this decade or for the next century."

For apartment dwellers (or apartment hunters), the same issue of *The Human Ecologist* has a checklist by Louise Kosta designed to help readers make wise housing choices. The checklist rates by +, -, or 0 such factors as the neighborhood, indoor public areas, ventilation, the presence of odors, and air quality room by room. To get a copy of this issue, contact the Human Ecology Action League at P.O. Box 49126, Atlanta, Georgia 30359; 404-248-1898.

Healthy Furnishings

Once you have selected or built your house or found your apartment, what do you put in it? Which products should you use, and what should you beware of? Fortunately, many alternative products have appeared in the market, especially since Earth Day 1990. "Green" is now a popular color; recyclable catalogs of "environmentally safe" products are becoming as common as compost piles. While some caution is still in order even with "green" products (see Chapter 13), there is much you can do today to outfit a healthy, nontoxic home. Let's look at yours from the bottom up. Your heating system and laundry are probably located in your basement or, if you are an apartment dweller, in a separate utility area. Each of these systems can be safe if installed and used properly. Unfortunately, careless installation and improper use can make each a threat to health. Gas furnaces should, ideally, be located outside the house in order to avoid the buildup of harmful combustion products. If this is not possible, they should have sealed combustion, should be carefully vented, and should heat outdoor air rather than recycling "old" indoor air. Many common laundry products—from strong, synthetic detergents to stain removers to fabric softeners— are highly toxic, particularly when released into the home through poorly vented dryers. Fabric softeners in particular, developed since World War II to prevent "static cling" with synthetic fabrics, are highly nauseating (i.e., toxic) to the chemically sensitive and should be avoided as both ineffective and dangerous. If you live in a high-rise apartment building with in-apartment dryers, you can get unwanted fumes from other people's dryers that vent into common ventilating shafts. To avoid this pollution, consider installing in your own dryer a metal, flexible exhaust vent with an automatic closing damper.

If your heating system is a kerosene space heater, consider scrapping it. Dr. Alfred Zamm, author of *Why Your House May Endanger Your Health*, has said, "A kerosene space heater? Can you believe that someone would invent such a crazy idea? That they would have combustion inside the home without a chimney?" A better alternative would be a ceramic radiant heater especially for the chemically sensitive, designed not to outgas anything (see the resources at the end of this chapter).

If ground water is leaking into your basement and you are thinking of using an outdoor water sealer indoors, realize that there have been nineteen incidents of consumers suffering symptoms such as headaches, nausea, dizziness, and breathing difficulties after being exposed to water sealers, according to the Consumer Product Safety Commission. Two people died.

Your auto may be in an attached garage leading into a utility area (actually, chemically injured people are wary of attached garages, whether in houses or apartment buildings). If the ethylene glycol in your anti-freeze gets inside your car or gets tracked into the house, through a spill or leak, it can cause headaches, asthmatic symptoms, fatigue, muscle soreness, depression, and one-sided pupil dilation. Also, your dashboard may be lighted with radium at possibly toxic levels; turning down the brightness can reduce the radiation effect.

Your garage or your basement may contain old or new cans of paint, thinner, or paint stripper. Oil-based paint does not usually contain the toxic chemical mercury, used as a pesticide, but latex paint manufactured before August 20, 1990, does. A study published in the *NEJM* found that people who had recently painted their homes with mercury-bearing paint had more than four times as much mercury in their bodies as did people who did not use the paint. Mercury was banned in interior latex paint when a four-year-old Detroit boy developed severe nerve and motor problems after inhaling mercury from paint in his home. Because most of us are increasing our mercury levels by eating mercury-tainted fish and by inhaling vapors from silver/mercury tooth fillings, it would be wise to decrease your mercury levels by avoiding latex paint containing mercury, which may still be on store shelves or your shelves. For information on specific paints, call the EPA's pesticide hotline: 1-800-858-7378. Volatile organic compounds, found in most paints, are now recognized as a problem under the Clean Air Act, and paint manufacturers are beginning to clean up *their* act. Glidden, for instance, plans to eliminate all solvents by the year 2000.

Though highly toxic methylene chloride is now banned in hair sprays, it is still a common ingredient in paint strippers. The CPSC advises extreme caution in using this substance, which can cause cancer and heart attacks. In 1985 the CPSC calculated that "three of every thousand people who used a methylene chloride-based paint stripper once per year . . . (for three hours each time in a closed work room) could develop cancer as a result"—the highest cancer risk the CPSC had ever calculated for a household chemical. Immediate signs of overexposure include nausea, headache, dizziness, and lightheadedness.

Every home has a kitchen with at least two appliances, a stove and refrigerator, and possibly many more. If you have a gas stove, know that carbon monoxide and nitrogen dioxide levels from a natural-gas stove in a vented kitchen can become as high as those in Los Angeles during a smog attack; if the kitchen is not vented, the levels can rise to three times the Los Angeles smog level at the same period, according to research done at California's Lawrence Berkeley Laboratory. Yes, an electric stove would be healthier—except that we now know that most appliances generate electromagnetic fields (emfs).

Electromagnetic radiation is an area crying out for more research. The twentieth century has brought us countless electrical appliances, and existing research on their health effects is tentative, controversial, and inconsistent. While the magazine *Consumer Reports* advised in 1989 that children and pregnant women should avoid electric blankets and pads because of possible danger from emfs, in 1990 AMA vice president Dr. William Hendee said that there are no major risks associated with using video display terminals, which also produce emfs. Hedging, he added, "I don't know of anything that's without risk." A preliminary, utilities-sponsored study reported in 1991 that "youngsters who live near power lines, often use hair dryers, or frequently watch black-and-white televisions may be twice as likely to develop leukemia as other children." Pending more conclusive evidence, you may want to heed the advice given by physicians Robert O. Becker, author of *Cross Currents*, and George E. Shambaugh: don't sit close or let your children sit close to a television screen; don't put your television set against a wall that has a bed or crib on the other side (electromagnetic radiation goes through walls); use incandescent rather than fluorescent bulbs (fluorescent bulbs create twenty times as much electromagnetic radiation as incandescent ones); use battery-operated rather than plug-in clocks by your bedside (they create less electromagnetic radiation); don't put a crib near an electric heater, whether baseboard or portable; do not use electric blankets or heat rooms with electric cables in the ceiling; do not live within a hundred feet of a television or radio tower, especially if you have children. According to these doctors, exposures to electric stoves, electric razors, and hand-held hair dryers are dangerous only if prolonged.

Wanting to explore the subject for themselves, the staff of the magazine *Green Alternatives* conducted their own electronic safari. Buying two gaussmeters (the unit for measuring emfs is the "gauss," named after German mathematician Karl Gauss) and testing for electromagnetic fields their own homes, their office, their cars, a restaurant, a computer lab, and under high-tension wires, they got some surprises. The latter two had only moderate readings; the highest were the cars, the restaurant, and appliances such as dishwashers, television sets, electric shavers, hair dryers, and anything with a transformer. All fields dropped off quickly with distance.

This doesn't mean that you need to scrap your electric stove or all those toasters, blenders, mixers, toaster ovens, corn poppers, or whatever; just remember to stand close to them only as much as necessary to do your cooking.

Lead, now known to be more ubiquitous and dangerous than previously thought, is present in expensive as well as inexpensive china and glassware, where acidic foods can leach it out. After the British medical journal *Lancet* reported that wine and spirits can leach lead from crystal, the FDA recommended that food and beverages not be stored in lead crystal, that children and women of child-bearing age do not drink from it, and that it be used infrequently. For a list of several hundred patterns of safe china, send a self-addressed envelope with fifty-two cents postage to the Office of the Attorney General, Press Office, 1515 K Street, Sacramento, California 95814. Before lead was banned in paint in 1978, the paint industry heavily promoted the use of high-lead paint, at the same time that medical journals were publishing articles warning that children were being poisoned by the lead paint in their homes. Now millions of older homes have lead not only in the paint itself but leached into the wood under it. Fortunately, you can now find inexpensive lead-testing kits for both dishes and wood in your local hardware store.

Also, if you buy bread in plastic, printed bread wrappers, don't turn them inside out and use them for storage. Lead may be contained in paint on the outside of the wrapper, according to Dr. Bernard Goldstein, director of the Environmental and Occupational Health Sciences Institute in Piscataway, New Jersey.

Kitchen soap pads can be dangerous to your health. A chemically sensitive Louisiana woman neglected to read the label on the soap pads she used to clean her oven. Two hours later she experienced three migraine auras (visual disturbances) in a row, followed by a severe, prolonged headache. The labels listed "dyes and perfumes." After reporting her experience to the CPSC, she called the manufacturer to try to obtain more specific information as to the ingredients.

The company spokeswoman, calling it "proprietary information," would only play a guessing game: she would say "yes" or "no" to specific chemicals. The complainant never did find out what was in the product. To register a complaint about unsafe products other than food, drugs, cosmetics, health care products, cars, or baby car seats, call the CPSC hotline—1-800-638-CPSC.

The taps in our kitchens and bathrooms provide us with drinking water. Unless we filter it, the water many of us drink contains traces of at least eleven common—and toxic—VOCs, like benzene, toluene, xylene, and styrene, according to Enviro-Health Laboratories. Water quality in the U.S. varies widely, but no matter where you live or where you get your water, you are probably drinking some chemical contaminants. Iowa farmers are drinking well water contaminated with nitrates and pesticides at levels exceeding federal health standards, which are probably too high anyway. During the late 1970s and early 1980s, Des Moines, Iowa, residents drank water with levels of TCE—trichloroethylene, a suspected carcinogen—that were anywhere from two to ten times the amount permitted by federal standards in 1988. A local company had used TCE as a degreaser and then sprayed the residue on their parking lot and dumped the rest into a drainage ditch. Wells in Los Angeles and its suburbs are also contaminated with TCE, causing some residents to have high levels in their blood and to have neurotoxic symptoms such as headache, dizziness, nausea, irregular heart beat, fatigue, and decreased mental acuity. Of nearly one thousand contaminants in drinking water, the EPA by 1988 had set enforceable limits for only thirty. In 1993 the NRDC documented some 250,000 violations of the Safe Drinking Water Act in 1991 and 1992, violations committed by 43 percent of the water systems serving about half of the American people.

Since the early 1970s, $100 billion has been spent on sewage treatment plants across the country. Have they contributed to decontaminating the environment? Not much, according to Steven Skavroneck, water quality engineer for the Milwaukee, Wisconsin, Metropolitan Sewerage District. The new plants were designed to treat sewage, not remove chemical toxins, though industries routinely dump toxic wastes into sewer systems. "Conventional treatment just moves the toxic [waste] around—in the water, in the sludge, or into the air," he says. "The only sane way to deal with [toxic waste] is to keep it out of the waste stream in the first place." Skavroneck believes businesses are learning that "it is better to prevent pollution, rather than try to clean it up, and maybe save money doing it"—by recovering and reusing chemicals.

While many toxic chemicals arrive in our drinking water through industrial waste disposal, others are simply formed from the chlorine added to "purify" our water supply. And, according to the *New York Times*, officials are particularly worried about a group of studies that link cancer to chlorine—the very chemical used to disinfect drinking water for more than 200 million Americans. "It's a very painful dilemma," says Dr. David Ozonoff, a Boston University epidemiologist. "It's more complicated than the average hazardous waste issue. We're also getting a great deal of benefit from the use of chlorine. It's a real risk-risk situation." Some cities and towns are adopting new water-purifying technologies, such as ozone and activated charcoal, but until your local water-supply systems do, you would be well advised to purchase water filters; make sure they remove chlorine.

Lots of chemicals reside in your bathroom; recall from Chapter 2 that after Lance Wallace headed the EPA's TEAM study of indoor pollution, he spent three hours in his bathroom and finally gave up trying to count all of the possible sources of contamination. Take air "fresheners": after a cleaning firm finished off its vacuuming of a house's air ducts with a heavy spray of "freshener," family members became so ill that they had to move to another house, according to the Rachel Carson Council, which says that several of the components of air fresheners are known carcinogens, and that other components "have a wide range of immediate and long-term toxic effects on vital organs. What the total effect is of whatever mix occurs in a particular product is unknown, even to the producers." In 1962, in her now-classic *Silent Spring*, Rachel Carson alerted the nation to the dangers from pesticides and other toxic chemicals. Since her death in 1964, the organization bearing her name continues her efforts to warn people. Also since her death, air "fresheners" have begun to appear bolted to the walls in public washrooms, often timed to squirt toxins at regular intervals.

In the 1980s a British psychiatrist saw a patient with palpitations, insomnia, and feeling of unreality; the psychiatrist could find no cause for these symptoms in the patient's life or personality. When the patient reported feeling worse in her bathroom, the doctor suggested removing the air freshener in the bathroom; the symptoms disappeared. Calling this an "air freshener syndrome," the psychiatrist went on to discover that thirty-two patients with feelings of unreality (16), headache (12), tremor (11), nausea (9), lassitude (9), mucosal irritation (7), giddiness (6), and anxiety (5) improved when "fresheners," including all forms of deodorant sprays and fabric conditioners, were removed from their houses.

Take disinfectants: an EPA study has found that the active pesticide in a leading disinfectant is among the five pesticides most commonly pervading the households studied. The manufacturer of this disinfectant recently admitted to covering up the fact that the disinfectant was contaminated by highly toxic dioxin. On the subject of disinfectants, the GAO in 1990 told the EPA that as much as 60 percent of the EPA's disinfectant data may be "inaccurate or incomplete." Disinfectants, designed to kill bacteria, whether on bathroom walls or on our bodies, are considered pesticides by the EPA—and, like all pesticides, are dangerous to living organisms. Don't we want our government to know all about disinfectants and what they may be doing to us?

Take diapers, often changed in bathrooms: cloth diapers, touted as environmentally preferable to disposable diapers, may not be preferable for babies' bottoms. If you use a diaper service, here's what the president of one says: "We don't just launder diapers, we clinically process them" with anti-bacterial additives (read "pesticides") and fabric softeners. (Pesticides and other toxic chemicals are more dangerous for children than for adults.)

Take after-shave lotion: during the Persian Gulf war, the U.S. armed forces, fearing chemical warfare, purchased not only atropine-containing syringes for counteracting chemical exposures but also a number of Chemical Agent Monitors (CAMs), hand-held devices for detecting "deadly agents." These sensitive CAMs can be "pre-set to detect not only mustard [gas] or nerve agents, but even after-shave lotion," reported columnist David Evans. Better keep your atropine handy when you shave!

Many people have carpets in their living room. Yet studies reported at the Fifth International Conference on Indoor Air Quality and Climate, in 1990, showed that "home carpeting can become a dramatic reservoir of toxic pollution—much of it apparently tracked in from outdoors," according to *Science News*. (This pollution is, of course, in addition to the toxic chemicals that are already in the carpet from manufacturing materials and processes.) Typical lead levels exceeded those at toxic waste dumps. At the Sixth International Conference, in 1993, John W. Roberts, a Seattle consulting engineer, reported his team's finding that dust vacuumed from carpets in eight homes in Columbus, Ohio, contained detectable levels of seven potentially carcinogenic polycyclic aromatic hydrocarbons (PAHs, a subgroup of VOCs). Unbelievably, total PAH levels in the homes "far exceeded the one part per million limit requiring cleanup of residential soil at hazardous waste sites in Washington State." Another study of house dust revealed that rugs can hold up to one hundred times as much of the fine debris as a bare floor. Some of this debris included residues of toxic wood preservatives (from outside decks) and pesticides, like DDT, banned many years before the study.

If you are chemically sensitive or simply environmentally aware, you may find it best to buy used or antique furniture, avoiding any that has been recently stripped and refinished or sprayed with pesticides (storage companies often spray routinely). One disadvantage of used furniture, however, is that it may have absorbed perfume or other chemical odors from its previous home. Before buying, give it the sniff test.

If you buy new furniture, realize that the entire store has a chemical smell. Look for furniture made of solid wood; if the clerk doesn't know whether a given piece is solid or not, run your fingers along the bottom edges. If they feel rough, that means particleboard (also known as pressed wood). A chemically sensitive writer forgot to do this when she was buying two attractive wood desks for her new computer and printer. Soon after the pieces were delivered, she realized her mistake. The new-furniture smell had been masked in the store; and as she worked at the computer, she began feeling dizzy. Suspecting formaldehyde, she put aluminum tape over the rough bottom edges, and the dizziness stopped. However, when she developed a severe, all-day headache and nausea after a few hours at the computer, she knew the problem had not been completely solved. Next step: hiring someone to apply four coats of a sealer that she first sniff-tested for possible reactions. Now the furniture is safe for her.

In your living room or family room you may have a TV and VCR, and you may not know that such appliances can give off chemical fumes. An Ohio woman noticed that her new VCR gave off a bad odor when she was using it. She also began feeling "unwell," with headaches increasing until, after using the VCR for twenty-six days, she felt so sick that she thought she was having a heart attack. After four doctors ridiculed her suspicions, she took the VCR to a laboratory in Pittsburgh. Using NIOSH methods for analyzing emissions, the laboratory found that the VCR was giving off fumes of acetone, benzene, and toluene—all highly toxic chemicals. No wonder she was sick! The laboratory speculated that the fumes came from an overheated electronic part, probably a resistor.

In your living room or family room you may want to look at a photo album. Listen to this company's insert for its plastic photo-album pages, which touts the fact that its pages (unlike most) contain no polyvinyl chloride: "PVC or vinyl pages contain plasticizers, solvents, and residual catalysts that volatilize. The volatile elements cause the most serious damage when they are in direct contact with photos, such as photo album pages, and can even cause damage to photographic materials by contaminating the air in their immediate vicinity." No mention of what might happen to humans in their immediate vicinity. A small exposure, no doubt, but exposures do add up.

Computers—in your family room, bedroom, or study—can be a problem too. Alerted by Paul Brodeur's meticulously researched book *Currents of Death: Power Lines, Computer Terminals, and the Attempt to Cover Up Their Threat to Your Health*, the magazine *Macworld* has prodded the Apple company, maker of the popular Macintosh computers, into a belated acknowledgment of the possible hazards from electromagnetic radiation emanating from computer screens. Apple announced in 1990 that it supports "the development of industrywide safety standards," according to the *Nation*. Until steps are taken to make computers safer, however, if you use a computer regularly at home or at work you would be wise to sit no closer than twenty-eight inches from the front of your monitor or four feet from the sides and back of someone else's. There are also safe shieldings available for computer screens; for a fact sheet giving sources, send a stamped, self-addressed envelope and $1 to *VDT News*, P.O. Box 1799, Grand Central Station, New York, New York 10163.

Take insect repellents: in 1990 two popular insect repellents, Deep Woods OFF! and Cutter's, were voluntarily withdrawn from the market by their manufacturers after the EPA advised consumers not to use products containing a possibly dangerous chemical known as R-11, listed on products as 2,3,4,5-Bis(2-butylene) tetradyro-2-furaldehyde. But R-11, which has been used in these insect repellents for about thirty years, is not the only possibly dangerous chemical in such products. In 1991 the EPA warned of possible birth defects from another chemical, 2-ethyl-1,3-hexanediol, found in several insect repellents. The chemical N,N-diethyl-meta-toluamide (deet), the main active ingredient in some bug sprays, has been associated with "central nervous system problems, allergies, and other ills, especially in small children," according to Martin Wolfe, the physician who runs the Washington, D.C.-based Travelers Medical Service. *Consumer Reports*' July 1993 issue warns of health problems from the overuse of deet repellents and suggests alternatives. Though this widely-read magazine has long been oblivious to many of the hazardous ingredients in the household products it rates, it made a start in its November 1993 issue with a two-page article, "Toxic Chemicals at Home."

Take Christmas decorations: according to Jane Elder, Midwest representative for the Sierra Club, most live Christmas trees are sprayed with chemicals, some even with green paint. "Pesticides and other chemicals are as much a part of the Christmas tree industry as other agricultural products," said one purveyor of Christmas trees. Some brands of spray-on snow contain perchloroethylene, which, according to the nonprofit National Environmental Law Center, may cause cancer, birth defects, and sterility. The Center also warned about the use of mothballs, spray paint, and fingernail polish. "With most environmental laws focused on controlling pollution at the end of the pipe, the millions of pounds of toxic chemicals that are put into consumer products are often overlooked," said a Center research scientist.

Paper and cloth products can be found in every room of your home. When it comes to fabrics, whether used as draperies, upholstery, clothes, or towels, chemically sensitive people act as canaries for the rest of us. Dona Shrier, of Richardson, Texas, found that her heart palpitations and joint pains cleared up in an environmentally controlled unit of a Dallas hospital. Though she got rid of her foam mattress when she went home, her symptoms returned when she slept on a specially made 100-percent-cotton mattress. Correctly concluding that pesticide residues in the cotton were the culprit, Shrier found someone who would grow organic cotton for her and started a thriving mail-order business offering organic, 100-percent-cotton futons, pillows, quilts, and comforters.

Not only are cotton fabrics heavily treated with chemicals, cotton itself is heavily pesticided, even as seeds. In 1980 cotton farmers were the third largest users of herbicides in the U.S., after corn and soybean growers. (The term "pesticides" is generally used to include herbicides, fungicides, miticides, rodenticides, and bacteriocides—all designed to kill living organisms.) Things are not much better overseas: while Egyptian cotton is still hand-picked and thus less pesticided, Brazil subsidizes pesticides for cotton, and in India 60 percent of all the pesticides used in that country (including DDT, banned for most purposes in the U.S.) are applied to cotton crops. Here, then, is one more source of pesticides, to be absorbed through our skin and added to the pesticides we eat and breathe.

As for other fabrics, be aware that silk is often treated with formaldehyde to prevent water-spotting and that undyed linen and wool generally contain fewer chemicals than cotton, though wool is likely to have been mothproofed with toxic chemicals like paradichlorobenzene. Clothing can be a major problem for the chemically injured, who often must settle for less-than-ideal fabrics and repeated laundering of new or used clothing items with baking soda before wearing them.

A few tips for those who want to avoid as many toxic chemicals as possible:

- Because synthetic dyes can be quite toxic, avoid dark colors (especially burgundy), for they require more dye; "garment-dyed" and "yarn-dyed" clothes tend to be safer than "printed" ones.

- Be aware that most imported clothes are fumigated with pesticides on board the ship that brings them to the U.S. (this may apply to carpeting as well).

- Instead of commercial bleaches, try using food-grade hydrogen peroxide in your wash instead (available in health-food stores).

- Wash clothes and other fabrics in cold water instead of hot water; heat accelerates chemical reactions and "locks in" chemicals, especially with hairy, absorbent fibers like cotton.

For your safe bedroom, one source for untreated wool and wool products like futons, mattresses, comforters, and pillows is a small company called Heart of Vermont (see the resource section at the end of this chapter). "We take in so much pollution, so many toxins during the day," said a California carpenter, "it's important to be as healthy as you can while you sleep." If you want a mattress that has not been treated with toxic chemicals for flammability, you can try one with wool stuffing, which is fire-resistant, or cotton batting treated with relatively nontoxic boric acid, but you will need a doctor's prescription. For pillows, quilts, and comforters, a prescription is not needed. Other safe, natural substances are now being used in bedding: kapok, millet hulls, buckwheat hulls, and milkweed—yes, milkweed fluffs, those lovely, light, white things you used to try to catch in your hands in late summer. Says Herb Knudsen, head of the Ogallala Down Comforter Company, manufacturer of cotton-covered quilts stuffed with 70 percent down and 30 percent milkweed, "It's a tricky crop to harvest. . . . If you let it go too long, it can really get away from you—gone with the wind."

Most paper in the U.S. is bleached with chlorine, though substitutes such as oxygen and hydrogen peroxide are available and are being used in Sweden and other countries. Chlorine bleaching produces up to a thousand chlorinated compounds—dioxins, furans, and polychlorinated biphenyls. The most toxic of these is 2,3,7,8-TCDD, commonly called dioxin and considered by some to be one of the most toxic chemicals known. According to the environmental organization Greenpeace, dioxin is present not only in pulp and paper industry wastes, but also "in everyday consumer paper products such as diapers, sanitary napkins, paper plates, toilet paper, coffee filters, food packaging, and writing paper." Also, says Greenpeace, concentrations of dioxin in breast milk are "already so high that a nursing infant is exposed to levels that exceed standards set by the World Health Organization."

A Few Helpful Tools

You may need help in tracking down sources of your symptoms. Several books are useful for both homes and workplaces. The *NIOSH Pocket Guide to Chemical Hazards* lists up to ten adverse effects each for 398 chemicals commonly found in workplaces—and you can bet that many of these chemicals end up in the products that end up in your home. Take, for example, a glycol ether that NIOSH lists by its chemical name, 2-ethoxyethanol (trade name Cellosolve solvent). Found in "cruelty-free" household cleaners and commonly used in leather-finishing and paint, dye, and ink manufacturing, this chemical, according to NIOSH, can cause eye irritation, as well as liver, kidney, and lung damage. Further, finding that this glycol ether caused testicular atrophy and sterility in male animals (so much for "cruelty-free"), NIOSH suggested in 1983 that manufacturers inform workers *and customers* about the adverse reproductive effects on both men and women.

Shouldn't manufacturers also warn customers about other health effects? In 1990 a chemically sensitive Kentucky woman bought a handsome—but smelly—pair of leather boots, aired them out for months in her basement, finally wore them, and, figuring they must be "gassed out" by then, kept them in her front hall. Increasing bouts of nausea puzzled her until she connected them with the boots, which still smelled. Now the boots are back in her basement and she is feeling better. Did the boots come with a warning? Have you ever seen a health warning on boots? In 1992 a non-chemically-sensitive woman bought an expensive Italian leather purse and developed an itchy, bright-red rash on the hand that held the purse. When the itching progressed to her legs, she put the beautiful purse back in her closet. Did the manufacturer of these products possibly use a leather-finishing spray containing "petroleum distillates" that in 1992 sickened more than four hundred unsuspecting customers nationwide who bought the spray, Wilson's Leather Protector? Complaints included coughing, shortness of breath, tightness or burning in the chest, headache, nausea, and fever. The manufacturer has recalled the product.

For information about ordering NIOSH's handy little book, call 1-800-35-NIOSH. Or try Cynthia Wilson's 1993 book, *Chemical Exposure and Human Health: A Reference to 314 Chemicals*, with a Guide to Symptoms and a Directory of Organizations (McFarland & Company, Box 611, Jefferson, North Carolina 28640; 919-246-44650) or *Toxics A to Z: A Guide to Everyday Pollution Hazards*, by John Harte, Cheryl Holdren, Richard Schneider, and Christine Shirberg (University of California Press, 1991). Your local public library's reference room probably has the 1984 *Clinical Toxicology of Commercial Products*, a useful but large volume that indexes toxicity information in several ways. There you can, for example, look up triclocarban, which some popular deodorant soaps list on their labels as an ingredient. You will find that triclocarban has a toxicity rating of 2, meaning slightly toxic, on the basis of animal studies. It is highly unlikely that it has been formally studied on humans. Informally, of course, we are all participating in toxicity studies. Another chemical, triclosan, is a "topical disinfectant and fungicide" in other popular soaps; it has a toxicity rating of 3— moderately toxic.

You may or may not find a list of ingredients, toxic or otherwise, on labels of common products like soaps. Ingredients in cleaning products, unlike ingredients in processed foods, do not have to be listed on the product label. If a substance has been found to be toxic to humans, the CPSC requires one or more of the following warnings on the label of a product containing that substance: "toxic" or "highly toxic" (poisonous if eaten, inhaled, or absorbed through the skin); "extremely flammable" (will catch on fire if near gas heat or flame); "corrosive" (will eat away your skin); "irritant" (will cause redness and rashes of skin and inflamed mucous membranes); or "strong sensitizer" (will provoke allergic reaction). If you must purchase a toxic product, remember also that one that says "caution" or "warning" is somewhat less toxic than one that says "danger" or "poison." None of these labels, of course, takes into account long-term health risks. And realize that "use only as directed" protects the manufacturer, not you. Such disclaimers don't allow for tolerance levels that may have been set too high, as they have been for lead, or that are based on insufficient or fraudulent data on human health effects.

So if you suspect that the soap (or any other product) you are using is the cause of any chronic symptom you are experiencing—not just a skin condition: it could be nausea or dizziness or muscle weakness or extreme fatigue or headaches—write down any ingredients given on the product's label, go to your local public library, and look up either the ingredient or the product itself in *Clinical Toxicology*. If the ingredients are toxic, you have a good clue. Changing to a product that doesn't have toxic ingredients is a good deal cheaper and pleasanter than spending money on drugs (i.e., more chemicals) and spending time in a doctor's office—or continuing to suffer.

A Few Helpful Suggestions

By now you are probably depressed or anxious or baffled or angry or frustrated—or all of the above. The message is clear: unknown to most Americans, pollutants abound in our water, indoor air is worse than outdoor air, and even our homes are not safe havens. The good news is that because it's your own home that is contaminated, you can do something about it. And you had better take it on yourself, because industry's sorcerers will go on doing *their* thing—making new and "better" products from new, untested chemicals and spending billions to try to get you to buy them—and government, though parts of it are struggling to help, is overwhelmed by the magnitude of the problems that modern technology has created. The sorcerer's apprentice simply can't keep up with the growing flood of chemicals that are affecting your health and mine.

What can I do? you ask. Plenty, and it's not as hard as you may think. First, don't be discouraged. Clean up your home one step at a time. In fact, a good place to start is with cleaning products. If you are already sick, discard (safely, if possible) those petroleum-based products you have, and switch to simple, inexpensive, old-fashioned ones like Arm & Hammer baking soda (sodium bicarbonate, a good deodorizer and all-purpose cleaner); Arm & Hammer Super Washing Soda (sodium carbonate, cuts grease, removes stains, disinfects, softens water; but avoid perfume-containing Arm & Hammer Ultra-Fresh); distilled white vinegar (full strength dissolves mineral buildup on chrome, porcelain, and metal—mixed half and half with water, it cleans glass beautifully); Bon Ami (nonchlorinated cleanser—an old standby); Twenty Mule Team Borax (mixed with hot water, a good disinfectant and mold-remover—another old standby); and sodium hexametaphosphate (for use in dishwashers or as a bleach, available only from chemical supply houses—look in your telephone directory). All except hexametaphosphate are available in your local supermarket. All are currently free of dyes, pesticides, and perfumes, but always check labels carefully. Other fairly safe cleaning products, such as Granny's unscented liquid soaps, are available commercially. Liquid soaps do not contain phosphates. In general, soaps are safer than detergents, which are manmade, and mainly petroleum-derived, and which pollute the environment in addition to causing health problems for the chemically sensitive and adding to everyone's buildup of toxic chemicals. For more specific information about cleaning products, write Buyers Up, P.O. Box 53005, Washington, D.C. 20009 for a copy of its "Chemically Free Cleaning" or the Human Ecology Action League, P.O. Box 49126, Atlanta, Georgia 30359, for its list of safe cleaning products. Or locate one of the excellent books listed at the end of this chapter.

A word about using plants to detoxify your home. Based on the work of B.C. Wolverton, scientist at the National Aeronautics and Space Administration (NASA), the media have been recommending the use of houseplants such as spider plants and philodendron to remove toxic chemicals from indoor air (NASA had discovered that the synthetic materials inside Skylab emitted more than a hundred chemicals). While such plants do remove some pollutants like formaldehyde, Thad Godish, director of Ball State University's Indoor Air Quality Research Laboratory, has cautioned that when Wolverton infused formaldehyde into a spider-plant-occupied test chamber, he was testing a one-time exposure only, not the continuous exposure that formaldehyde-laden products infuse into a house. Godish's experiments with continous exposure found the small amount of formaldehyde control (up to 20 percent) by spider plants counterbalanced by greater formaldehyde emission caused by the plants' humidity. Plants may not be the lifesavers that they had appeared to be.

The sources listed at the end of this chapter will give you specific information to help you maintain your health in a chemicalized world. Here are a few simple, general suggestions to help you learn to live, breathe, and eat in a more natural, less toxic, less damaging way.

- Be very careful what you put in your body, on your body, and near your body. You don't want to be sorry later. Any person with EI/MCS would tell you, "If I had known then what I know now, I would not have gotten so sick."

- Don't read ads or watch commercials, read labels instead—both front and back. Though our present laws permit ingredient information to be incomplete or missing, you may learn something useful.

- Invest in air filters and water filters, activated-carbon ones that remove chemicals such as formaldehyde and chlorine, not particulates (though you may need filters that do that too).

- Don't be fooled by words like "all natural" or "naturally." The list of ingredients—if there is one—is what counts.

- When ingredients are given, buy products that contain only things that sound as if they came from plants, such as eucalyptus, pennyroyal, aloe vera gel, or vitamin E oil, not things that sound as if they came from a chemistry lab, such as FD&C red no. 40, c-10-30 carboxylic acid sterol ester, or methylchloroisothiazolinone. Numbers in an ingredient are almost always a giveaway that the substance has been synthesized from petroleum. Word length also helps. You don't have to know chemistry; with a little practice you can tell.

- Resist using product coupons: most of the stuff they promote will ultimately cost you more in medical bills than the pennies you'll save.

- Dry-clean as few things as possible (labels are often overprotective). Take newly dry-cleaned items out of the plastic bag as soon as possible and air them out as long as possible and as far away from people as possible.

- Realize that whenever you buy any product, you are signaling the producer or manufacturer to make another one. Each of us can affect the market, and we do.

- Don't be misled by experts saying that because no one knows if something is harmful, you might as well go on using it. Wouldn't it be more prudent to say that because no one knows if something is harmful, you won't go on using it, but will look for a better alternative? Think about it.

* * * *

Books on Healthful Housing

- *The Healthy House: How to Buy One, How to Cure a "Sick" One, How to Build One*, by John Bower, New York, Lyle Stuart, 1989.

- *Healthy House Building: A Design & Construction Guide*, by John Bower, Unionville, Indiana, The Healthy House Institute, 1993.

- *Why Your House May Endanger Your Health*, by Alfred V. Zamm, MD, and Robert Gannon, New York, Simon & Schuster, 1980.

- *Sunnyhill: The Health Story of the 80s*, by Bruce and Barbara Small, Goodwood, Ontario, Canada, Small and Associates, Publishers, 1980.

- *Your Home, Your Health, and Well-Being*, by David Rousseau, William J. Rea, MD, and Jean Enwright, Berkeley, California, Ten Speed Press, 1989.

- *The Healthy Home: An Attic to Basement Guide to Toxin-Free Living*, by Linda Mason Hunter, Emmaus, Pennsylvania, Rodale, 1989.

- *The Natural House Book: Creating a healthy, harmonious, and ecologically sound home environment*, by David Pearson, New York, Simon & Schuster, 1989.

- *Healthful Houses: How to Design and Build Your Own*, by Clint Good with Debra Lynn Dadd, Bethesda, Maryland, Guaranty Press, 1988.

- *The Smart Kitchen: How to Design a Comfortable, Safe, Energy-Efficient, and Environment-Friendly Workspace*, by David Goldbeck, Woodstock, New York, Ceres Press, 1989.

Books About Cleaning Up Your Home Environment

- *Nontoxic & Natural: How to Avoid Dangerous Everyday Products and Buy or Make Safe Ones*, by Debra Lynn Dadd, Los Angeles, Jeremy P. Tarcher, 1984.

- *Buyer's Guide to Water Purification Devices*, a booklet by Debra Lynn Dadd, 1989 (P.O. Box 279, Forest Knolls, California 94942).

- *Nontoxic, Natural, & Earthwise: How to Protect Yourself and Your Family from Harmful Products and Live in Harmony with the Earth*, by Debra Lynn Dadd, Los Angeles, Jeremy P. Tarcher, 1990.

- *The Nontoxic Home and Office: Protecting Yourself and Your Family from Everyday Toxics and Health Hazards*, by Debra Lynn Dadd, Los Angeles, Jeremy P. Tarcher, 1992.

- *Clean & Green: The Complete Guide to Nontoxic and Environmentally Safe Housekeeping*, by Annie Berthold-Bond, Woodstock, New York, Ceres Press, 1990.

- *A Consumer's Dictionary of Household, Yard, and Office Hazards*, by Ruth Winter, New York, Crown, 1992.

- *Computer Health Hazards*, Volumes 1 and 2, by Marija Hughes, Washington, D.C., Hughes Press, 1990/1993.

- *Success in the Clean Bedroom: A Path to Optimal Health*, by Natalie Golos and William J. Rea, MD, Rochester, New York, Pinnacle Publishers, 1992.

- *Healing Environments: Your Guide to Indoor Well-Being*, by Carol Venolia, Berkeley, California, Celestial Arts, 1988.

- *House Dangerous: Indoor Pollution in Your Home and Office—and What You Can Do About It!*, by Ellen Greenfield, Vintage, 1987.

- *Residential Air-Cleaning Devices: A Summary of Available Information*, U.S. Environmental Protection Agency, February 1990 (ANR-445; EPA 400/1-90-002); also *Indoor Air Facts No. 7: Residential Air Cleaners*, (ANR-445; EPA 20A-4001). For these booklets and information on drinking water, pesticides, radon, and indoor air, contact the EPA Public Information Center, 401 M Street SW, Washington, D.C. 20460; 202-260-7751.

Helpful Periodicals

- *Informed Consent: The Magazine of Health, Prevention, and Environmental News*, Jack Thrasher, editor, P.O. Box 1984, Williston, North Dakota 58802-9900.

- *Green Alternatives for Health and the Environment*, Annie Berthold-Bond, editor (with contributions by Debra Lynn Dadd and John Bower), Greenkeeping, Inc., 38 Montgomery Street, Rhinebeck, New York 12572; 914-876-6525.

- *Healthy Home & Workplace*, newsletter published by Healthy Home & Workplace, 248 Lafayette Street, New York, New York 10012.

Information About Safe (or Unsafe) Buildings

- *Indoor Air Pollution and Housing Technology*, by Bruce Small and Associates, prepared for the Planning Division, Policy Development and Research Sector, Canada Mortgage and Housing Corporation, August 1983 (spiral bound, 295 pages, available from Technology and Health Foundation, R.R.#1, Goodwood, Ontario, Canada, L0C 1A0).

- *Healthy House Catalog: First-ever national directory of indoor pollution resources*, produced by the Environmental Health

Watch and Housing Resource Center, 1990 (this book and audio tapes are available from Environmental Health Watch, 4115 Bridge Avenue, Cleveland, Ohio 44113; 216-961-7179).

- *Safe Home Resource Guide*, published by Lloyd Publishing, Inc., 24 East Avenue, Suite 1300, New Canaan, Connecticut, 1992.

Consultants for Healthy Buildings

- John Bower, The Healthy House Institute, 7471 North Shiloh Road, Unionville, Indiana 47468; 812-332-5073.

- Clinton Good, AIA, Box 143, Lincoln, Virginia 22078; 303-530-7077.

- Hal Levin, research architect, 2548 Empire Grade, Santa Cruz, California 95060; 408-425-3946.

- The Masters Corporation, P.O. Box 514, 12 Burtis Avenue, New Canaan, Connecticut 06840; 203-966-3541.

- Mary Oetzel, Environmental Education and Health Services, 3202 West Anderson Lane #208-249, Austin, Texas 78757; 512-288-2369.

- Bruce Small, P.Eng., R.R.#1, Goodwood, Ontario, Canada L0C 1A0; business phone 416-294-3531.

A Few Sources for Safe (or Safer) Building Materials
(for information only, not as a recommendation)

- Air Krete, Weedsport, New York; 315-834-6609 (for an insulation made of magnesite, cement, air, and water).

- Pace Chem Industries, Inc., 779 S. La Grange Avenue, Newbury Park, California 91320; 1-800-350-2912 (for sealers and finishes).

- AFM Enterprises, Inc., 1140 Stacy Court, Riverside, California 92507; 714-781-6860 (for paints, sealers, clear finishes, strippers).

- Eco Design Co., 1365 Rufina Circle, Santa Fe, New Mexico 87501; 505-438-3448 or 1-800-621-2591 (source of Livos waxes and other plant-based paints and finishes; catalog "The Natural Choice").

- Miller Paint Co., Inc., 317 S.E. Grand Avenue, Portland, Oregon 97214; 503-233-4491 (for low biocide/no fungicide paints).

- Auro Natural Paints, Sinan Company, P.O. Box 181, Suisun City, California 94585; 707-427-2325 (for alternative wood preservatives and natural building products).

- Old Fashioned Milk Paint Company, 436 Main Street, Groton, Massachusetts 01450; 508-488-6336 (casein-based, no VOCs).

- Glidden Spred 2000, 925 Euclid Avenue, Cleveland, Ohio 44115; 1-800-221-4100 (water-based, no VOCs).

- Preserva-Products, Inc., P.O. Box 744, 2955 Lake Forest Road, Tahoe City, California 95730-0744 (for wood and concrete preservatives and sealers).

- Environs Control and Containment Products, Inc., 1400 Brook Road, Richmond, Virginia 23220; 804-649-0007 (for citrus mastic removers).

A Few Sources for Safe (or Safer) Household Products and Clothing
(new products and catalogs appear almost every day; addresses and phone numbers can change; remember that "natural" does not always mean "nontoxic")

- Heart of Vermont, The Old Schoolhouse, Route 132, P.O. Box 183, Sharon, Vermont 05065; 1-800-639-4123 (for chemical-free wool bedding, organic cotton, unfinished hardwood furniture).

- Dona Designs, 825 Northlake Drive, Richardson, Texas 75080 (for furnishings of pure, organic cotton).

- Ogallala Down Comforter Company, Box 830, Searle Field, Ogallala, Nebraska 69153; 308-284-8403.

- Jantz Design, P.O. Box 3071, Santa Rosa, California 95402; 1-800-365-6563 (for organic cotton clothes and natural beds and bedding).

- The Cotton Place, P.O. Box 59721H, Dallas, Texas 75229; 214-243-4149 (for natural cotton bedding, clothing, and yarn).

- Granny's Old Fashioned Products, P.O. Box 256, Arcadia, California 91066 (for plant-based shampoos, soaps, and cleaning products; or try your local health-food store).

- Reflections, Route 2 Box 24P40, Trinity, Texas 75862 (for organic cotton clothing).

- Garnet Hill, 262 Main Street, Franconia, New Hampshire 03580; 1-800-622-6216 (for natural-fiber clothing and bedding).

- Janice Corporation, 198 Route 46, Budd Lake, New Jersey 07828; 1-800-526-4237 (for chemical-free clothes, bedding, personal grooming and kitchen products).

- WinterSilks, 2700 Laura Lane, P.O. Box 130, Middleton, Wisconsin; 1-800-648-7455 (for washable silk underwear and outerwear).

- Seventh Generation, Colchester, Vermont 05446-1672; 1-800-456-1139 (for bedding, toys, baby clothes, batteries, paper, and other home and office products).

- Allergy Relief Shop, 2932 Middlebrook Pike, Knoxville, Tennessee 37921; 615-522-2795 (for filters, bedding, clothes, and paints).

- N.E.E.D.S. (National Ecological and Environmental Delivery System), 527 Charles Avenue, Syracuse, New York 13209; 1-800-634-1380 (for appliances, personal grooming products, cleaning materials).

- E.L. Foust Co., Box 105, Elmhurst, Illinois 60126; 1-800-225-9549 (for air purifiers, nontoxic lubricants, masks, books).

- Ceramic Radiant Heater Corp., P.O. Box 60, Greenport, New York 11944; 1-800-331-6408.

- Healthful Hardware, P.O. Box 3217, Prescott, Arizona 86302; 602-445-8225 (for gaussmeters and copies of John Banta's video "Current Switch; How to Identify and Reduce or Eliminate Electromagnetic Fields").

- Bau-biologie Hardware Catalog, 200 Palo Colorado Canyon Road, Carmel, California 93923; 1-800-441-8971.

- The Living Source, 7005 Woodway Drive, Suite 214, Waco, Texas 76712; 817-776-4878 (for untreated fabrics, water filters, personal grooming products, all-cotton pillows, cleaning materials).

- Nontoxic Environments: Products for Aware and Chemically Sensitive Individuals, 9392 S. Gribble Road, Canby, Oregon 97013; 503-266-5244 (105-page catalog of building materials, household furnishings, cleaning products, Ott-Light Systems, books, supplements, personal grooming products, art and pet supplies, appliances).

- Jim Nigra Enterprises, 5699 Kaman Road, Agoura, California 91301; 818-889-6877 (for water and air purifiers).

- Karen's Nontoxic Products, 1839 Dr. Jack Road, Conowingo, Maryland 21918; 1-800-KARENS4 (for cosmetics, personal grooming products, toys, housewares, pet care).

- Natural Chemistry, Inc., 244 Elm Street, New Canaan, Connecticut 06840 (for enzyme-based home, pet, and pool cleaning solutions).

- Enviroclean, 30 Walnut Avenue, Floral Park, New York 11001-9866; 1-800-466-1425 (73-page catalog of all types of cleaning products).

- Earth Care, 966 Mazzoni Street, Ukiah, California 95482-8507; 1-800-347-0070 (for recycled paper products of all kinds).

- Conservatree Paper Company, 10 Lombard Street, Suite 250, San Francisco, California 94111; 415-433-1000 or (outside California) 1-800-522-9200 (for printing and computer paper).

- Colorcon, 415 Moyer Boulevard, West Point, Pennsylvania 19486; 215-699-7733 (for nontoxic printing inks).

- Sinclair & Valentine, 256 E. Marie Avenue, West St. Paul, Minnesota 55118; 612-455-1261 (for soybean ink).

Miscellaneous Resources (Some Free)

- *Everyday Chemicals: 101* Practical Tips for Home and Work, by Beth Richman and Susan Hassol; contact The Windstar Foundation, 2317 Snowmass Creek Road, Snowmass, Colorado 81654; 1-800-669-4777.

- *Toxics: Stepping Lightly on the Earth: Everyone's Guide to Toxics in the Home*; contact Greenpeace, 1436 U Street NW, Washington, D.C. 20009 (or try your local Greenpeace office).

- Household Hazardous Waste Wheel, Recycling Wheel, and Water "Sense" Wheel; contact Environmental Hazards Management Institute, P.O. Box 932, 10 Newmarket Road, Durham, New Hampshire 03824; 603-868-1496 (compact, useful advice on what's toxic, how to dispose of it, and what to use instead).

- "A Home Buyer's Guide to Environmental Hazards"; contact FannieMae, 3900 Wisconsin Avenue NW, Washington, D.C. 20016-2899; 202-752-6527 or 202-752-7124 (forty-page booklet covering radon, asbestos, lead, hazardous wastes, ground water, and formaldehyde).

- "Air Pollution in Your Home?" and "Home Indoor Air Quality Checklist," booklets available from local chapters of the American Lung Association.

- *The Inside Story: A Guide to Indoor Air Quality*; contact the U.S. Environmental Protection Agency, Washington, D.C. 20460 or the U.S. Consumer Product Safety Commission, Washington, D.C. 20207.

- For a 178-page booklet on toxic household products and safer alternatives, contact the Household Hazardous Waste Project, 901 South National Avenue, Box 108, Springfield, Missouri 65804.

- For a list of plants that may combat household toxics, contact the Clean Air Council, 405 N. Washington Street, Suite 104, Falls Church, Virginia 22046.

- For information about seminars, contact the International Institute for Bau-biologie and Ecology, Box 387, Clearwater, Florida 34615; 813-461-4371.

- For a home test kit that tests for carbon monoxide, radon gas, lead, ultraviolet radiation, and microwave oven radiation, contact DSK Safer Home Test Kit, 1609 Bridgeport Drive, Los Angeles, California 90065.

5

In and Under the Rug

O N MAY 3, 1989, with mixed feelings, forty-four-year-old
Steve Shapiro climbed the steps of one of our capital's massive old buildings. He was on his way to testify before the
Subcommittee on Superfund, Ocean, and Water Protection of the
Committee on Environment and Public Works of the U.S. Senate.
Outside, the day was bright and beautiful, the air freshened by recent rains. The cherry blossoms were gone, but other flowers brightened Washington's gray public buildings. Inside, the windows of
the hearing room, which had let in fresh air for many years, were
now sealed shut, thanks to Washington's energy-conscious, "closed
climate" zeal.

At issue was Senate Bill 657, Senator George Mitchell's Indoor
Air Quality Act of 1989. But before the hearing began, several of
Shapiro's co-workers and a few other chemically sensitive people,
who had traveled across the country (one woman was from Oregon) to attend the hearing, left the room. Even though they were
wearing respirators, the perfumes and after-shave lotions of those
assembled had begun to make them sick. After a news photographer
came into the room and laid his camera and camera bag full of film
on the press table, several more of Shapiro's co-workers began to
have severe reactions to the chemicals in the film and had to leave
the room. It was ironic that indoor air quality in the room where the
Senate was conducting a hearing on indoor air quality had become

intolerable to nearly a dozen people who were seeking redress from the U.S. Congress.

Shapiro was the third person to arrive at the hearing room. Soon, others drifted in, including a woman who sat near Shapiro and began marking some papers with a pink highlighter. Shapiro, explaining his own acute chemical sensitivity, immediately asked her to put it away and use a pen instead. But the damage was done. Already somewhat anxious about testifying, Shapiro had been affected by this brief exposure and now had the additional burden of being unable to draw fully upon his mental faculties. As some of his co-workers entered the hearing room fifteen to twenty minutes later, they too reacted to the now-odorless residue of the highlighter.

Despite these exposures, Shapiro managed to testify about an illness that he and many of his co-workers had acquired when their workplace had been carpeted and remodeled (he represented sixteen co-workers who had provided written statements that were not read): "Our health and life have been radically affected by the indoor air," he began. "There are those [of us] who don't know that it is the indoor air . . . that is affecting their health and productivity. Throughout the work week these people pop Sudafeds and go through a box of Kleenex." Some of his colleagues, unable to continue functioning, had simply quit their jobs. Their health improved. Of those who could no longer work in Shapiro's office building—including "people in their prime, in their twenties, ex-joggers, an ex-marathon runner, a karate black belt, and others in good health before they were affected"—most had no history of allergies. They and their doctors were baffled, Shapiro testified, and some of the affected workers got worse whether they were in the building or not.

"We exchange experiences among ourselves about other office buildings, hotels, stores, malls, indoor markets, schools, doctors' offices, hospitals and clinics, restaurants, places of worship, greenhouses, and other places that affect us [in order] to minimize the Russian roulette effect on us of breathing indoor air. This is somewhat helpful, but we all don't react to the same things, to the same degree, or at the same rate.

"Our lives are full of surprises. You walk into a place you

thought safe, only to be caught in fumes from paint, cleaning agents, perfume, nail polish, magic markers, white-out, new furniture, electronic equipment and jet-ink printers, plastic objects, plastic wrapping, glue, mastics—the list never ends.

Volatile Chemicals of the Twentieth Century

"There are individual chemicals or combinations of chemicals found in offices and office buildings [nationwide]—not all necessarily come from carpet and renovation materials—which can apparently produce short- and long-term health effects. . . . I'm speaking of reactions to parts per million, billion, or even trillion of substances or combinations of substances where reactions are normally associated with parts per thousand. . . . Although [my and my colleagues'] illness was preventable, none of us, except for some of those who have become ill this year, was warned.

"In this situation, what does one do?," Shapiro asked. "Is it sensible to ignore the symptoms—you often react in buildings to things you can't even smell or you smell but don't recognize—and endure the physical misery and temporary mental dysfunction? Or is it sensible to drop out of your life and live as a recluse at home or in a remote area to avoid the volatile chemicals of the twentieth century? There are no good answers to this dilemma," he concluded.

Early Warnings

Why were these workers so sick? Where did they work? What is the building that made them so sick? By now you may have guessed the answers to these questions. The building is Waterside Mall, the Washington, D.C., headquarters of the EPA, the agency entrusted with the protection of your environment. But, in one of the most monumental ironies in bureaucratic history, the EPA had been caught with its carpets down. Synthetic, wall-to-wall carpeting, the post-World-War-II darling of the American homeowner, had made hundreds of EPA employees ill and finally alerted that agency to the increasing susceptibility of human beings to the volatile chemicals in indoor air. Sick building syndrome had arrived.

The illness affecting these workers, you may also have guessed, was EI/MCS. This illness was scarcely recognized by anyone until Dr. Randolph first noticed the relationship between certain petroleum-based chemicals and human health in 1951. Since then, thousands of his patients and the patients of other environmentally oriented physicians have learned about it and gotten better by learning how to avoid toxic chemicals. How, in 1989, did the EPA *not* know about it? How could this condition seem so mysterious and puzzling to EPA staff members, their bosses, the physicians they consulted, everyone?

Actually, from its inception in 1970 the EPA had had several warnings about the effect of indoor air quality on human health, warnings it had apparently ignored. Its own medical science advisor, Dr. Lawrence Plumlee, a graduate of Johns Hopkins Medical School, found his health sliding downhill with exposures to auto exhaust, tobacco smoke in his office, and fumigants and cleansers in hotel rooms when his work required travel. Finally, in the late 1970s, his weight down from 135 to 93 pounds, he resigned and left Washington for the purer air of rural Arkansas: "I had become so ill that although I loved my job at EPA, it didn't seem feasible to continue. It's difficult to put a price on health." In 1980 the EPA's own journal published an article, "On the Cutting Edge," about Plumlee's battle with what was then called "environmental overload." In his fight back to health, Plumlee had been helped by a stay in Dr. Rea's Dallas Clinic; at that time Dr. Rea, a former chest surgeon, was a member of EPA's Science Advisory Board. Curiously, neither Dr. Plumlee's publicized illness nor Dr. Rea's presence on its board seems to have tipped off the EPA.

In 1981, seven years before the carpet-related epidemic at EPA, an employee got off the elevator in Waterside Mall into a newly carpeted room and immediately reacted with tearing, burning eyes and burning throat and lungs. She and a second affected worker were sick at home for two and a half weeks. The first worker can no longer tolerate perfume; the second cannot go into a fabric or carpet store without becoming ill. At least two other employees have had long-term effects from this episode. When EPA tested the carpet, the glue holding it together was found to contain pentachlorophenol, believed to cause cancer and birth defects, and other volatile organic chemicals. In July 1987 a group of professional EPA employees newly affiliated with the National Federation of Federal Employees negotiated a clean-air policy specifying nontoxic carpeting in EPA headquarters. Thus by 1988 the EPA was not totally unaware of the dangers from certain modern chemicals. Why then was it caught with its carpets down?

By the time the new carpet was installed in Waterside in 1987–88, EPA's management had largely ignored employees' complaints, according to Bobbie Lively-Diebold, another Waterside employee severely afflicted with EI/MCS. On July 20, 1989, she testified before the House Subcommittee on Natural Resources, Agriculture Research, and Environment of the Committee on Science, Space, and Technology. This subcommittee was considering Massachusetts Representative Joseph Kennedy's H.R. 1530, a companion bill to the Indoor Air Quality Act of 1989 which the Senate had passed. (Four years later, undaunted by House inaction on indoor air, Representative Kennedy introduced H.R. 2919, the Indoor Air Quality Act of 1993. As of this writing, the bill is still in committee.) As Lively-Diebold walked through the building toward the hearing room, a person smoking a cigarette crossed her path, causing a throat spasm that left her unable to speak for a time. After she finally regained her voice, she told the committee that as far back as 1987 some staff of the EPA's internal environmental health and safety division—more irony—had complained of respiratory and other problems associated with carpeting in a satellite EPA headquarters site in Washington. And, unbelievably, after imposing a moratorium in April 1988 on further laying of the carpet that was making people ill in Waterside, the EPA nevertheless announced, in a misguided economy move, that it would install some of the remaining carpet at [its] labs in Edison, New Jersey, and Research Triangle Park, North Carolina." In April 1989, the owner of Waterside allowed another tenant, the General Accounting Office, to install new carpeting. This carpeting was believed to emit the chemical 4-phenylcyclohexene (4-PC), which researchers at the University of Arizona had determined was toxic to animals. Vapors from this carpet go into EPA's hallways, she said, but the EPA considered itself off the hook because the matter was "beyond its jurisdiction."

Another of the multiple ironies in the EPA's story is that in June

1987, a month before the carpet-layers arrived, the EPA itself published the TEAM study (described in Chapter 2), which showed that indoor air pollution was at least three to seventy times greater than outdoor air pollution—even in the smoggiest areas of the country. This report cited one *acute* effect on human health, "sick building syndrome," in what may have been the first written use of this term. Since then, of course, SBS has become familiar to many through their own and media exposures. It refers to an illness acquired by some people who live or work in new, tightly constructed buildings that are inadequately ventilated and that recirculate toxic fumes from construction and cleaning materials, furnishings, office equipment, and personal grooming products. The illness, sporadic at first, can develop into chronic EI/MCS when those affected become "sensitized" to multiple chemicals. The EPA's 1989 indoor air health survey of its headquarters employees concluded that more than 40 percent were suffering from SBS. The TEAM study cited two possible *chronic* health effects: cancer and "chemical sensitivity . . . an ill-defined condition marked by progressively more debilitating severe reactions to various consumer products such as perfumes, soaps, tobacco smoke, and plastics. The incidence of this syndrome is unknown; however, anecdotal accounts indicate that it may be increasing sharply. The effects on productivity of affected persons can be severe." Good work, EPA, but a bit too late to help those soon to be victims.

Terrible and Life-Altering

The "ill-defined condition" was about to become better defined. Says J. William Hirzy, a senior scientist in what is now the EPA's Office of Pollution Prevention and Toxic Substances: "The spate of multiple chemical sensitivity cases appearing during 1988 put a whole new light on our efforts. National media covered our story, and we were then flooded with letters and phone calls from people telling us of similar problems in their homes and offices." Fortunately, the new union of EPA scientists was in place. Its members organized afflicted workers into a Committee of Poisoned Employees (COPE) and used their own expertise to assess the data that were beginning to accumulate. In varying degrees, about 880 employees had reacted to the carpeting and renovation; 40 of them developed multiple chemical sensitivities. Belatedly, the EPA discovered that it had a "serious indoor air pollution problem," Hirzy said in 1990, "one that we have found we share with much of the public. . . . The union believes that the suffering of our fellow workers, terrible and life-altering as multiple chemical sensitivities is, can be used to benefit our fellow citizens by getting action quickly on this problem." Note that "multiple chemical sensitivities" has finally joined EPA's vocabulary.

Right Hirzy was—and compassionate too, but "quickly" was another story. A few in the media noticed the irony of the EPA's own indoor air pollution problem. Though *Time* magazine's January 2, 1989, "Planet of the Year" issue did not mention MCS or much of any other effect that chemicals were having on human health, it did cite the EPA's problem in a 1988 article on sick building syndrome. Another newsmagazine reported that the EPA's emergency response team—usually mobilized for chemical spills and toxic waste dumps—had had to be assigned to its own offices, adding to the mounting list of ironies.

Prompted by the employees' union, the emergency response team tested rolls of the carpet for the chief suspect, 4-PC, which the University of Arizona researchers had already dubbed "essence of new carpet." At the EPA building, tests were planned to see if airing out or steam cleaning the carpet would solve the problem. A notably fatuous EPA administrator observed that if the tests succeeded, "we can proceed [with installing the carpet] and get employees into good, healthy, attractive space so that they can get on with the job of protecting the environment."

Airing out and steam cleaning did not work. In the fall of 1989 workers began ripping out the twenty-seven thousand square yards of carpeting that had already been installed and replacing it with presumably safer carpeting and vinyl tiles. How much did this cost the government, i.e., us taxpayers? No one knows for sure, but one disabled employee has computed the approximate cost to herself and the government for her illness as of 1989: $1,500 for prescription drugs, $2,750 in medical bills, and $580,000 for the government's investment in her education and her employment as a U.S. Navy veteran and five-year EPA worker. The government had paid for three and one-half years of her graduate school and dissertation research; as a good government employee, she included overhead in her calculations. Before the carpet was laid she was healthy. Now even the slightest exposure is disabling: she gets "respiratory tract inflammation from exposure to volatile emissions from [certain] computers and . . . from other plastic products such as the hard, smooth, black plastic used in many [electronic] products." She has "stopped reading newspapers and some other types of printed materials because of a reaction to the inks." Unable to work at either the EPA or the Department of Defense because of their use of computers, she worries about her employment prospects.

Nationwide Health Effects

How many people nationwide have been affected by the hazardous chemicals in new carpeting? No one knows, though in summer 1989 the CPSC issued a press release and sent letters to allergists across the country asking them to refer patients with carpet complaints to a CPSC hotline. During its study of carpet-related health complaints from 1988 to early 1990, the CPSC received complaints from 206 households involving 335 residents with symptoms. (When this writer called CPSC in 1991 for the latest figure, I was first asked, "What company are you with?" As if the EPA dealt only with companies, not people like you and me.) According to the survey, the hazardous carpets were mostly made of synthetics, especially nylon. Most had been applied wall to wall with foam or latex padding, were a light color, and were additionally treated with chemicals to ensure stain resistance. Two-thirds of those with symptoms were women. Most sufferers reported upper respiratory symptoms. More than two-thirds of the complainants saw their doctors. Twenty-five people were hospitalized. Most physicians reportedly treated the symptoms but did not connect them with the carpeting. One hundred and ninety-nine people said that their symptoms did not fade or go away with time. A few had their carpets tested for chemicals; formaldehyde (presumed to cause cancer in humans) and toluene diisocyanate (which the EPA in 1990 added to its TRI list), among others, were found. Most had not removed the carpeting, because of the cost. Unbelievably, the study's chief investigator reported that "the evaluation of these complaints could not establish a cause and effect relationship between the carpet and the health effects experienced." A curious fact is that while the CPSC can, by law, tell manufacturers about the complaints it receives about unsafe products, it can't tell consumers without the manufacturer's approval.

As usual, more studies were called for: the CPSC intends to work with the EPA on the carpet problem. A less sanguine Hirzy: "Given that it took EPA from 1973 until 1989 to regulate asbestos under the Toxic Substances Control Act, there is little reason for optimism that 4-PC will be regulated before the turn of the century by the 'regular' process." In 1993 the CPSC's recorded message (1-800-638-CPSC, extension 129) reported five hundred health complaints associated with new carpeting since 1988 but claimed that it "does not currently have evidence that specific chemical emissions coming from carpeting are responsible for the health complaints associated with carpet installation." The message also said that forty chemicals, including styrene, formaldehyde, vinyl acetate, and propylene glycol, have been identified in new carpeting.

Occasional tales of carpet poisoning have crept into view. In 1988 the *Arizona Republic* reported that employees at a media center in a suburban high school complained of headaches, dizziness, numbness, and a metallic taste almost immediately after new carpeting was installed. At a public hearing on a proposed new library building in northern Illinois, a popular teacher told of acquiring EI/MCS after new carpeting was installed in her high school. Previously healthy, she experienced rashes, disorientation, and respiratory problems shortly after the carpeting was laid. She was permitted to transfer to a different, uncarpeted building, where she finds students willing to accommodate her chemical sensitivities by wearing no perfumes or other scented cosmetics to her classes. On Los Angeles's KNBC-TV, chemical victim Kenneth Pressberg described his adverse health reactions to the carpeting in his office, especially to the formaldehyde it contained. Pressberg's new, chemically-less-contaminated home has nontoxic paint, natural fabrics, and no carpeting: "If you use natural products there's less likelihood you're going to have any outgassing or [to develop] chemical sensitivities. Once you begin to use more synthetic items in the construction or the development or the finishes of a house, you're going to bring in these toxins that are ultimately a part of your home." Of course, few illnesses require the building of a new home as part of the cure. Few sufferers from EI/MCS, or any illness, can afford to build a new house to help cure themselves.

In what was one of the first known cases of carpet poisoning, the entire Glenn Beebe family, in Cincinnati, became severely sensitized in 1981 after installing only seventy-nine square yards of commercial carpeting in work space in their family business. At first their headaches, nausea, and facial burning disappeared on weekends. Later these symptoms and new ones—fatigue, mental confusion, depression, and incoherent speech—became chronic. Sharon Beebe, the formerly healthy wife and mother, developed a "lung disorder, shortness of breath, a severe and persistent sore throat, and itchy skin." Finally suspecting the carpeting and getting no help from their local Board of Health, they hired a private chemist, who found that the carpet had been releasing "several dozen toxic chemicals, including ethylbenzene, formaldehyde, methacrylic acid, toluene, and xylene." (Toluene and xylene—the chemicals in printer's ink— are also found in many household cleaning products.) Expecting to recover their health, the family had the carpeting removed. Eight years later they were still chemically sensitive—and afraid that they would remain so the rest of their lives. Their lawsuit against the carpet manufacturer was dismissed on the grounds that the toxicity of the implicated compounds was not fully known at the time of manufacture and purchase. Though the manufacturer offered them $100,000 to drop the case and remain silent, the family declined, preferring to be in a position to warn others of the dangers from carpeting. The Beebes have since set up a carpet-injury network and published *Toxic Carpet III*, available from Toxic Carpet Information Exchange, P.O. Box 39344, Cincinnati, Ohio 45239. Because of their chemical injuries, they have had to give up their million-dollar business.

In 1985 Linda Sands, her husband Stephen, and their five children became ill after new carpeting was installed in their home in Montpelier, Vermont. Though the family's health improved after they completed a long, expensive detoxification program in Los Angeles in 1991, one son was reafflicted when new carpets were installed in his high school. Sands is suing the carpet maker and the installer. Even if she loses the suit, Sands says, she will continue the fight: "My children have been denied a normal childhood. I won't stop until there are warning labels on carpets and regulation of the industry. I don't want what happened to my family to happen to anyone else."

Carpet cleaning can also have adverse health effects. In 1990 the *Harvard Medical School Health Letter*, reporting research by the New York Hospital-Cornell University Medical Center in New York City, described an association between carpeting and Kawasaki syndrome, a mysterious illness that sickens small children and can cause massive heart attacks: "The only factor clearly differentiating the [affected group and a control group of children] is whether rugs in the home have been shampooed, beaten, or vigorously cleaned within a month before the child became sick." Dust mites, first suspected, were later ruled out. Some symptoms of the condition—conjunctivitis, fever, skin and throat redness, and rash—are remarkably like those experienced by many workers at the EPA just two years before, although this investigating team seemed unaware of the EPA's experience. The U.S. has about three thousand cases of Kawasaki syndrome a year, though many more may go undiagnosed, said Jane Newburger, a cardiologist at Children's Hospital Medical Center in Boston. Adults too: a California woman's doctor confirmed that her half-shut eyes and misshapen face were due to chemicals used to clean her carpeting (a chemical company faxed the doctor a list of the product's ingredients).

Part of the problem may be what the carpet has acquired after being laid. Dust vacuumed from carpets in an EPA study of eight homes contained detectable levels of seven potentially carcinogenic PAHs, including benzo(a)pyrene, chrysene, and benz(a)anthracene, according to a report given by Seattle consulting engineer John W. Roberts at a 1993 Helsinki (Finland) conference on indoor air quality and climate. Total PAH levels inside even the less-contaminated homes "far exceeded the 1 ppm limit requiring cleanup of residential soil at hazardous waste sites in Washington State." For carpet lovers, Roberts recommended using doormats, removing shoes at the door, and vacuuming.

Action at the EPA

Meanwhile, back at the EPA, an action occurred in 1990 that is said to be unprecedented in the history of the United States Civil Service. The union of EPA professional employees petitioned the then head of the EPA, William K. Reilly, to regulate 4-PC, the chemical apparently involved in the infamous incident at the EPA, as well as the possibly associated chemicals produced in the manufacture of carpeting, glues, and other products. Union scientists, including experts in both toxicology and chemical processing, were worried not only about their own and their co-workers' future safety and health, but also about the safety and health of unsuspecting members of the general public who might be looking to the EPA to protect them from dangerous chemicals. Thus were civil service workers formally asking the head of their agency to do what he should have been doing all along.

The union's petition was filed on January 11, 1990, under TSCA's Citizen's Petition section. The petition asked then-Commissioner Reilly to immediately begin regulating 4-PC, "a byproduct in the manufacture of the adhesive used in building most synthetic fiber carpets in the U.S." Basing their results on collected data and risk analysis, these union scientists determined that if 4-PC levels were held to 5 parts per trillion in indoor air, breathers of that air would be protected from acquiring EI/MCS. A level of 17 parts per trillion would protect people against respiratory and eye irritation. No one, however, seemed interested in stopping the production of 4-PC altogether: government agencies regulate on the basis of calculated risk.

The scientists' petition also asked for

- product-content standards for carpet and glue, based on industry testing

- epidemiology and laboratory studies going beyond the CPSC's study

- public notice of the risks associated with 4-PC

- a requirement that industry buy back products that exceed the standards.

The petition made several other points. Carpeting and glues, the scientists warned, might contain other harmful chemicals besides 4-PC, which has been found to cause similar health effects in other products. More immediately, it should not be necessary to wait for scientific discovery of the exact mechanism by which these chemicals are making people ill for action to be taken against their indiscriminate use. (This is especially important because researchers always want to do more research, while clinicians want to go on trying to help the sufferers. "Health hazards do not wait for scientific certainty before they extract their toll," says Earon Davis, a lawyer-advocate for people with EI/MCS.) Perhaps, the petition offered, there may be only a few "bad batches" of carpet reaching the market; in any event it would not cost a lot to remedy the situation. And finally, these EPA scientists pointed out that not all cases of EI/MCS are the result of exposure to 4-PC. At last, the EPA was beginning to be aware of the widespread existence of this condition.

What was Reilly's response, three months later, in April 1990, to the union's petition? Essentially he called for voluntary action and more study. "Because the Agency disagrees with the specific assertions regarding the health risk posed by carpeting and with the remedies sought," it would not set up the new rules the union wanted. Instead, the EPA (1) asked the carpet industry to voluntarily and periodically test all of its products for chemical emissions and to report its findings to the public, (2) planned to do more research, and (3) set up a one-year "public dialogue" group of government experts, industry, and interested citizens. But, the EPA insisted, this group was not to concern itself with anyone's health! What, you may ask, was this entire experience all about, if not health? The EPA was once more sweeping things under the rug.

Frustrated, several EPA employees who had developed EI/MCS filed suit. Also, in the fall of 1990 the union drew up an 104-item list of recommendations for safe alternative workplaces for affected employees and presented it to the EPA's personnel office. By 1991, forty-seven employees made ill by the carpeting had been officially granted alternative workspace. One of these was an EPA scientist who reacts to computers, paper, and mold, among other things. She had become so chemically sensitive that she could not tolerate the paper and inks of certain magazines that came to her house. When asked if the EPA had any information on the toxicity of inks, she replied matter-of-factly, "Oh no, the EPA is a follower, not a leader."

And a distant follower at that. As of March 1990, for example, the EPA's Great Lakes regional office, covering six states, had 213 open cases involving air pollution. The oldest open case in this office had been pending for seven years. A Chicago public interest attorney, Martha Churchill, calculated that "at the rate the agency is making decisions, it will not clear its pending caseload until 2002. And that's if it gets no new requests for variances."

The EPA-initiated carpet policy dialogue group labored for a year, from August 21, 1990, to September 27, 1991, and brought forth a series of sixteen "accomplishments," only one of which had anything to do with informing the public of possible danger—a brochure called "Indoor Air Quality and New Carpet: What You Should Know." The mildly worded brochure said that "indoor air pollution at low levels is difficult to study" and that "limited research to date has found no link between adverse health effects and the levels of chemicals emitted by new carpet." Nevertheless, hedging its bets, the EPA's brochure cited a number of precautions, which included asking the carpet industry for low-emitting adhesives and recommending plenty of ventilation during and after carpet installation. Copies of the brochure may still be available from the EPA's Public Information Office at 202-260-7751, though Representative Bernard Sanders (I-VT) has asked that the EPA stop distributing it because of the inaccuracy of the preceding quotation. The other "accomplishments" were mostly voluntary agreements by carpet, padding, and adhesives companies to do more testing and research and use less-toxic ingredients. One "accomplishment," couched in the usual bureaucratese, was that "the General Services Administration established an initiative to develop requirements to make a low volatile-organic-chemical covering available for use in Government offices." In other words, the government is taking steps to provide less-toxic carpets for itself, while providing minimal warnings for the rest of us.

On October 29, 1992, the carpet controversy burst into public view again with CBS's "Street Stories," which showed white mice dying from exposure to carpet fumes in experiments run by scientists at Anderson Laboratories, in Dedham, Massachusetts. People who had become ill after their wall-to-wall carpeting was installed had sent carpet samples to the laboratory. According to scientist Rosalind Anderson, owner of the laboratory, these results did not implicate any particular chemical, but perhaps more than one "bad guy." Viewers heard Bob Axelrad, head of the EPA's indoor air division, say that because there was no "good science" yet about adverse effects from carpeting and because this was a matter of "public policy" (i.e., would affect a large industry), the EPA was not warning the public. Although the carpet industry had begun a voluntary "green tag" program, CBS reporters did not find them in evidence at a large carpet store. Viewers also heard Bill Hirzy say that "it's a moral outrage that EPA is now buying safe carpet for its own people but not warning the general public."

Worried by this bad publicity, the Carpet and Rug Institute (CRI) hired an independent, highly regarded University of Pittsburgh researcher to duplicate Anderson's tests. When these new results turned out just the same, the CRI decided it didn't like them. Industry researchers, looking for a "smoking gun," then tested 4-PC and found no adverse effects on mice. When the EPA's own researchers tested carpet samples, they found no adverse effects until it was pointed out to them that they had forgotten to hook up a crucial pump. Two Congressional hearings on carpets, in October 1992 and June 1993, were inconclusive. Testifying at the latter hearing, EPA official Victor Kimm said that "we spent hundreds of thousands of dollars trying to figure out what caused the problem ['several' EPA employees becoming ill after the renovation] and we were never able to make a connection. This remains a mystery to us."

Part of the problem is the number of chemicals used in synthetic carpeting—at least a thousand, immunologist Jack Thrasher was told at a 1992 meeting with a major carpet manufacturer. Thrasher and his colleague Dr. Alan Broughton had been asked to tell the company's toxicologist about their studies, which had found abnormal immunologic test results in numerous cases of people exposed to carpeting. While a Canadian Carpet Institute official maintains that three toxic chemicals—formaldehyde, benzene, and toluene—are not used in the manufacture of carpeting, CPSC studies of new carpet samples direct from the mill revealed emissions of all three.

Mystery or not, Representative Sanders in 1992 wrote the EPA that with carpeting "we have a serious health hazard" and asked the agency to ask the CRI to suspend its testing and its new green-label program as incorrectly implying that a carpet is safe. In early 1993, in what may eventually become the first class action of its kind, fourteen plaintiffs in three states filed three separate suits representing as many as a hundred thousand persons. They charge that several carpet manufacturers and distributors and the CRI have known since 1980 that the adhesives and materials used in making carpets pose health hazards and can cause the symptoms, such as headaches and dizziness, they experienced after carpets were installed in their homes, and that the carpeting was falsely advertised as safe.

Feeling the heat, the CRI in November 1993 agreed to begin placing warning labels on all new carpet sold after January 1, 1994, even though it says that there is no scientific evidence to suggest that carpet constitutes a public hazard. (Once again, an industry is trying to hide behind the lack of definitive, controlled, double-blind studies published in prestigious journals like *JAMA* and *NEJM*.) The new label says, in part, "Important health information: Some people experience allergic or flu-like symptoms, headaches, or respiratory problems which they associate with the installation, cleaning, or removal of carpet or other interior renovation materials. If these or other symptoms occur, notify your physician of the symptoms and all materials involved. Sensitive individuals: Persons who are allergy-prone or sensitive to odors or chemicals should avoid the area or leave the premises when these materials are being installed or removed." This label no longer implies that tagged carpets are safer, only that the manufacturer of the carpet bearing the label "participates in a program which seeks to develop ways to reduce emissions by testing samples of carpet."

Also, the CRI is distributing to retailers copies of "A Carpet Owner's Manual," which emphasizes fresh air ventilation of carpet during renovation and redecoration, how to care for carpets, and how to prevent high emission rates. This step is not a bad thing, says Mark Goldman, of Anderson Labs; it's just not enough. The carpet industry "needs to change the carpet chemistry to prevent outgassing." Anderson Labs now suspects the carpet chemical problem may come from a commonly used latex substance called styrene butadiene rubber. Whatever scientists eventually decide is the culprit, you need to protect yourself.

Carpet Caveats

If you are one of those who think that the EPA is busy protecting your environment and your health, you may have found the preceding account disillusioning and depressing. That reaction is rational—but would you rather not know? With carpeting, the EPA's nemesis, your safety lies mostly in your own hands. Here are a few carpet caveats:

- Avoid synthetic carpeting, especially wall-to-wall and glued down.

- Avoid rubber or latex padding; use natural fiber padding or none at all.

- Avoid chemically treated carpets.

- For names of manufacturers of less-toxic carpeting, area rugs, and carpet glue, consult the resources at the end of this chapter.

- If while in a carpet store you have *any* symptoms—a cough, sneeze, head pain, palpitation (heart irregularity), nausea, dizziness, or just a "funny feeling"—beware of that store's carpeting.

- Before you buy wall-to-wall carpeting, try living with a small sample; keep it under your pillow for a night or two to see if you react.

- When you buy any carpeting, ask the carpet dealer to make sure the carpet is aired out before delivery—and follow up by asking just how they will do that.

- If your new carpeting *has* any odor, ventilate, ventilate, ventilate. Keep windows open and air moving through the carpeted area during and after installation, for forty-eight hours or longer— probably much longer. (It is better to buy carpeting in spring or fall, when rooms can be easily aired out.)

- If you already have synthetic wall-to-wall carpeting, you might want to try a product that blocks toxic fumes from outgassing—AFM's Carpet-Guard, available from such distributors as Nontoxic Environments, 9392 South Gribble Road, Canby, Oregon 97013; 503-266-5244.

- Steam cleaning solves the problem of outgassing only temporarily. As soon as the carpet dries, the outgassing continues.

- For use in some home areas and in institutions like schools and libraries, the good news is that, according to a survey of five major city school systems, vinyl composition tile is cheaper to install and maintain than carpeting, as well as less toxic and easier to keep clean.

- Best of all are bare wood floors, waxed with a plant-based wax, or ceramic tile floors. Such floors are the safest and can look beautiful. Using an old-fashioned dry mop to clean bare floors will keep them cleaner than any carpet, which collects and holds dust, dust mites, molds, and toxic chemicals. If you want some floor covering, use accent rugs of wool or washable cotton, heavy enough to stay in place; try to find wool that has not been heavily mothproofed.

* * * *

To Find Out More

- Copies of the CPSC's report "Carpet Related Health Complaints" may be obtained from Carpet Complaints, Room 529, U.S. Consumer Product Safety Commission, Washington, D.C. 20207.

- To network, contact Toxic Carpet, 8441 Livingston Road, Cincinnati, Ohio 45247.

Some Sources for Safer Carpeting

- Bremworth Carpets, 1940 Olivera Road, Suite C, Concord, California 94520; 1-800-227-3408 (woven wool carpet, jute backing).

- Carousel Carpet Mills, 1 Carousel Lane, Ukiah, California 95482; 707-485-0333 (all-wool carpets).

- Desso Carpet, P.O. Box 1351, Wayne, Pennsylvania 19087; 1-800-368-1515 (woven wool carpet, jute backing).

- Eco-Carpet, Eco-Container Corp., 14651 Ventura Boulevard, 3rd floor, Sherman Oaks, California 91403; 818-382-3060 (natural-fiber carpet).

- Foreign Accent, 2825E Broadbent Parkway NE, Albuquerque, New Mexico 97107; 505-344-4833 (woven wool area rugs).

- Gordon T. Sands Ltd., 40 Torbay Road, Markham, Ontario, Canada L3R 1G6; 416-475-6380 (woven wool carpet, felt carpet pad).

- Helios Carpet, P.O. Box 1928, Calhoun, Georgia 30703; 1-800-843-5138 (woven wool carpet).

- Hendricksen Naturlich Flooring Interiors, 6761 Sebastopol Avenue, Suite 7, Sebastopol, California 95472-3805; 707-829-3959 (natural wool carpet, jute padding without glue, Auro adhesive, Envirotec adhesive, true linoleum).

- H & I Carpet Corp., 115 Dupont Street, Toronto, Ontario M5R 1V4; 416-961-6891 (woven wool carpet).

- N.E.E.D.S., 527 Charles Avenue, Syracuse, New York 13209; 1-800-634-1380 (least-toxic carpet adhesive, air filters).

- CYA Products Inc., 211 Robbins Lane, Syosset, New York 11791; 516-681-9394.

6

Why We Are So Well Preserved

FORMALDEHYDE IS A COLORLESS GAS, a simple compound of the chemical elements carbon, hydrogen, and oxygen. It has a pungent, irritating odor that is unmistakable to anyone who has worked in or near a biology or medical laboratory or a funeral home. Actually, whether we can smell it or not, we are all exposed to it every day from many different sources, for it is present in thousands of consumer products, from particleboard in furniture, cabinets, counter tops, and subflooring to lipstick, shampoo, toothpaste, insulation, carpeting, draperies, and most clothing fabrics (for a lengthier inventory, see the list at the end of this chapter). Especially when new, these products emit, or "outgas," formaldehyde; this accounts for its distinctive odor in stores selling furniture, fabric, and clothing.

Since 1868 formaldehyde has been used as a biological preservative; by 1889 it was being commercially produced and marketed as a preservative and bonding agent. Formaldehyde production in the U.S. has gone up from 987 million pounds in 1951 to 6,730 million pounds in 1988—an increase of 581 percent. According to the Formaldehyde Institute, a professional organization of manufacturers using formaldehyde to make their products, U.S. production of formaldehyde-containing products accounts for eight percent of the gross national product. Jobs are provided for more than 1.4 million people employed in some 45,000 U.S. facilities with an annual payroll of nearly $8 billion. Formaldehyde is essential to plant operations in seventeen major industries and is an important basic raw material in seventy other industries. "Restrictions [on its manufacture]," warns the Institute ominously, "would touch consumers deeply and directly."

Cancer and the EPA

But how is it touching consumers' health? And the health of those who work with it? In 1986 the Formaldehyde Institute denied that formaldehyde constitutes any health hazard, claiming that when used properly it may cause only temporary eye and nose irritation or some skin sensitization. (The National Safety Council, on the other hand, says that "contact can cause severe eye and skin burns, leading to permanent damage" and [it] "can cause an asthma-like allergy.") As for cancer, says the Institute, "the scientific evidence available to date fails to show a link between formaldehyde and cancer in humans." A link between formaldehyde and nasal cancer in animals was not confirmed by several epidemiological studies of possible nasal and respiratory cancer in formaldehyde workers, said the Institute. Nevertheless, Institute members have "taken steps voluntarily to reduce the formaldehyde levels significantly in the workplace and in consumer products." Shouldn't one wonder why?

That was 1986. Yet by the early 1980s the CPSC had received over three thousand complaints about formaldehyde gas from construction products, two thousand of them involving urea formaldehyde foam insulation (UFFI). The CPSC is still receiving many complaints about formaldehyde; in 1991 one such complaint stated that a sixty-eight-year-old man died after exposure to formaldehyde vapors from foam insulation in a new mobile home. As early as 1980, the Federal Panel on Formaldehyde (under the NTP) concluded that "formaldehyde should be presumed to pose a risk of cancer to humans." Prompted by a 1983 lawsuit by the NRDC and APHA, the EPA took a closer look at formaldehyde and finally concluded, in 1984, that formaldehyde "is a potential carcinogen in humans." Formal announcement to the media, however, did not come until 1987.

The EPA's slowly-arrived-at conclusion was based primarily on animal studies and on the assumption that a large number of people are at risk, though not at a high level. Five years later the EPA took another look at formaldehyde, when its Science Advisory Board (SAB) reviewed the EPA's Office of Toxic Substances' update on formaldehyde risk assessment—trying to decide, to put it more simply, how much risk you should be subjected to. The SAB affirmed that animal data were "unequivocal" in showing formaldehyde to be a nasal carcinogen and expressed mild surprise that threshold levels for damage to animals were much lower than originally thought. Further, it recommended that the animal data be compared with the "most appropriate" human studies, possibly those done by American Cyanamid. However, the EPA had said in 1984 that "although many epidemiological studies have been made of formaldehyde, the chemical is so prevalent in our environment that it would take an epidemiologic study of immense proportions to detect significant increases in risk in the general population. . . . Occupational studies, where higher exposures occur, are also difficult to interpret because of exposures to other chemicals."

In other words, the EPA does not have the resources to really determine the human health risks from formaldehyde. We humans continue to be the guinea pigs—and in enormous numbers. Most at risk are residents of mobile and "conventional" homes—over one hundred million of us, the EPA estimated in 1984—and almost eight hundred thousand clothing workers. Also exposed are millions of high school and college students, in or near biology laboratories. "When the individual risks are considered with the widespread exposure to these risks, a large number of cancers can be expected in the lifetimes of the populations exposed," said the EPA. Why, then, is the EPA so cautious? One reason is its stated reluctance to "send incorrect signals to the public." It doesn't want to alarm us. Another reason is its desire not to offend or affect industry. In EPA's own words, "The existence of potential harm does not in itself constitute unreasonable risk. If the economic or other adverse impacts of regulatory control outweigh the risk of harm, EPA would not find the risk unreasonable." At least the EPA is saying it straight out: industry is more important than our health. Is the EPA subtly raising the spectre of job loss? If so, it is setting up a false dilemma. The oft-cited equation "health gain means job loss" is an oversimplification. Alternatives usually exist.

Other Health Effects

What of other possible human health effects from this formaldehyde blanketing of our homes and workplaces? The EPA knows little of them; it was looking only for evidence of cancer, gene mutations, and birth defects. The NAS, on the other hand, has estimated that "fewer than 20 percent but perhaps more than 10 percent of the general population may be susceptible to formaldehyde and may react acutely at any concentration." In the *American Review of Respiratory Diseases 1988*, three researchers cautiously concluded that "although the irritant properties of formaldehyde are documented, evidence of health effects at concentrations found in residences and offices is inconclusive."

Curiously, it was one of these three researchers, Dr. John Spengler, professor of environmental health at Harvard University and former chairman of the NAS's Committee on Indoor Pollution, who in the early 1980s noted that "we should in no way expect the Formaldehyde Institute to respond in a completely unbiased way in doing studies." He was referring to the Institute's multi-million-dollar public relations campaign to protect formaldehyde from government regulatory agencies. In 1987 the same Dr. Spengler testified at Senator George Mitchell's hearings on indoor air pollution that "even if only a small percentage of the nation's mortality rate for cancer, which is about 350,000 cancer deaths per year, were attributed to radon, passive cigarette smoke, formaldehyde, or organic vapors, it would exceed the risk from any other single manmade cause including routinely operating nuclear radiation."

In contrast to the respiratory researchers, Ball State University's Thad Godish has demonstrated a "dose-response relationship between the level of formaldehyde present in residential environments such as mobile homes and homes with particleboard subflooring and the severity of sixteen different symptoms . . . eye irritation, dry/sore throat, runny nose, cough, sinus irritation, sinus infection, headaches, unusual fatigue, depression, difficulty sleeping, rashes, bloody nose, nausea, diarrhea, chest pain, and abdominal pain . . .

at an average concentration of 0.09 parts per million." Danish and Canadian studies produced similar results, and several studies have suggested a link between formaldehyde and menstrual disorders, Godish reported in 1989. Also, he says, "studies of residents of mobile homes exposed to formaldehyde above 0.1 parts per million for 10+ years indicate a significantly increased risk of throat cancer [of] approximately two in ten thousand." Among the many published studies of the health effects of formaldehyde is one showing that formaldehyde produced lasting impairment of memory, equilibrium, and dexterity in histology technicians. In another study, the Houston, Texas, Bureau of Occupational Health found that workers in stores with lower-priced clothing experienced more formaldehyde-related health effects than workers in stores with higher-priced clothing, which includes fewer permanent-press (formaldehyde-treated) items.

Perhaps the most significant work on formaldehyde is that done by immunologists Jack Thrasher, PhD, and Alan Broughton, MD, authors of *The Poisoning of Our Homes and Workplaces: The Indoor Formaldehyde Crisis*. For several years these researchers have been studying the immune-system effects of chemicals such as formaldehyde and those in pesticides, solvents, and plastics. They have observed the immune systems of several hundred people ill from chronic inhalation of formaldehyde, many of whom had been told by their exasperated physicians to see a psychiatrist. They have studied aerospace and office workers; occupationally exposed workers (those with more than the usual exposure to formaldehyde); mobile home residents; and people in a community subjected to acute exposure from an overheated tanker car containing urea formaldehyde resin. Their results suggest not only that there are measurable immunological changes associated with such exposures, but that formaldehyde can cause a "subtle but chronic activation of the immune system." The former is important because chemical sensitivity, which rarely shows up on common diagnostic tests, is frequently rejected as a diagnosis. Until now, EI/MCS has usually been diagnosed by symptom/exposure relationships rather than by the existence of antibodies or detectable physiological changes. Headaches and dizziness are not quantifiable; antibodies are. "Activation of the immune system" means that toxic chemicals like formaldehyde can cause an immune-system dysfunction that often starts out with persistent flu-like symptoms and fatigue and ends up with sensitivity to many chemicals.

Referring to Senator Mitchell's 1987 hearings on indoor air pollution, Thrasher and Broughton ask an important question of us all: "If Senator Mitchell, these witnesses [such as Dr. Spengler], and [other] experts have so much concern for your health and welfare, why shouldn't you?" Yes. Indeed. Until Senator Mitchell's indoor air quality bill becomes law (and even after it does), you are well advised to be concerned for your own health.

Common Symptoms

Dizziness, or vertigo, is a common health complaint affecting more than fifteen million people, according to Dr. Vijay Dayal, professor of head and neck surgery at the University of Chicago Medical Center. While technical advances in the diagnosis and treatment of vertigo are being made, doctors do not seem to be looking at causes other than Meniere's disease, which involves the inner ear. Yet people who complain to the CPSC about formaldehyde often report dizziness, as well as headaches, breathing problems, nausea, and other symptoms, from using such products as bubble bath, carbonless paper, paneling, bedsheets, mattresses, carpeting, refrigerators, a baby "bath ring," and sofas and other furniture. The CPSC considers formaldehyde a strong sensitizer and requires warning labels on products containing more than 1 percent formaldehyde; one complainant said that employees of a furniture store were actually told to remove warning labels of formaldehyde from furniture to be sold to consumers.

In New York State, Onondaga County officials refused to pay for 271 new desks after several employees complained of headaches and dizziness attributed to the formaldehyde used in their construction. Though air-quality test results were ambiguous, some officials said that it was really very simple: "People felt ill when the desks were placed in a room with them, and felt better when they were removed."

The National Headache Foundation estimated in the 1980s that forty million Americans suffer from frequent or severe headaches.

The figure now may be as high as seventy million, according to specialists brainstorming at a 1991 headache conference. How many of those headaches are being caused by formaldehyde? One can only guess. How many doctors are asking the right questions of those suffering from dizziness and headache? Not many, probably.

In nursing school, Michele Fox worked on a formaldehyde-preserved cat, sometimes carrying it to and from her home. Soon she noticed that exposures to auto exhaust and gasoline fumes brought on severe headaches, a hearing loss, and temporary blindness. Working as a nurse, she continued mixing medicines and using toxic cleaners but feeling worse and worse. Finally her health broke down completely and she was diagnosed with an extreme case of EI/MCS. After multiple blood transfusions, removal of her spleen, and intravenous replenishments of essential nutrients, Fox is better but lives a very restricted life in order to avoid common twentieth-century products like synthetic perfumes, deodorants, and detergents.

A Pennsylvania mortician had to sell his 114-year-old family-owned funeral home because of ill health from exposure to the formaldehyde used in embalming. Responses from a trade journal article he wrote about his experiences indicated that others in the business were unaware that their similar health problems could be caused by formaldehyde. In 1969 Irene Wilkenfeld became chronically ill while teaching Spanish in a new secondary school in New Jersey, but it was not until 1984 that a letter to the editor of a local newspaper virtually describing her own symptoms gave her the clue she needed. Once she realized that her health problems stemmed from that long-ago exposure to formaldehyde in building materials, she was able to reorganize her life to avoid formaldehyde and the many other chemicals that she now reacts to if inadvertently exposed. Finally diagnosed with EI/MCS, she writes, "There's no such thing as 'itsy-bitsy' amounts of formaldehyde. These days our homes are literally embalmed in it."

Dangerous Insulation

Before the oil crisis of the 1970s, when energy costs were low, most of us paid little attention to how well our homes were insulated or how tightly constructed they were. As costs rose and we were urged to have "energy audits" done, many people "tightened" their homes, caulking and weatherstripping everything in sight, and installing insulation. One popular insulating material was UFFI, composed of urea-formaldehyde resin, a foaming agent, and water. Usually blown into holes in outside walls, UFFI was installed in as many as half a million U.S. homes. Once installed, UFFI continues to outgas formaldehyde as it hardens, with levels of the gas declining rapidly during the first forty weeks after installation, according to the CPSC.

But because it soon became apparent that UFFI was making some people sick, the CPSC in 1982 decided to ban its use in homes and schools. The formaldehyde industry quickly went to work, and after a long court battle the U.S. Court of Appeals overturned the ban in April 1983. Thus you can still use UFFI if you want to, though because of extensive publicity about its health effects, very few people now do.

One who wishes she had never heard of UFFI is Paula Kolodzie's mother. At age twelve, Paula won public-speaking honors at her school in Ontario, Canada, for a speech about her mother, who had always wanted to be an interior decorator. After Mrs. Kolodzie renovated and redecorated their hundred-year-old house in the late 1970s, a success that won her several customers, she thought her dream was coming true. But within a year she gradually progressed from headaches and persistent sore throats to constant feelings of fatigue and sickness, to frequent fainting spells, to convulsions when she smelled dish detergents or auto fumes, and finally to severe weight loss despite eating six to nine meals a day. Her brain and entire nervous system were affected. To breathe normally, she needed an oxygen tank. Finally—from newspapers and television—the family discovered the culprit. It was the UFFI that they had had installed in their previously uninsulated home. Although all the family were affected, she was by far the sickest. In 1981 she entered the Randolph Clinic, where she learned how to alter her lifestyle to avoid all the chemicals and foods that she was reacting to. Paula's mother's new dream, said her daughter, was to create "a safe home for all of us because we were all affected by the gassing-off of the formaldehyde insulation. A safe home for a chemical victim is called an oasis. No perfumed products will be allowed. No smokers can get past the front door. Our air will be filtered through de-pollution units. Heat will be electric. Food will be unsprayed with chemicals, colouring, or preservatives, and the decorating will be very simple." Paula's mother is still an interior decorator, though with quite a different approach.

Hazardous Particleboard

A hundred years ago, or even twenty-five, formaldehyde-laden particleboard and other building materials scarcely existed. Yet now, "economically and chemically, formaldehyde is impossible to replace," according to Gary Gramp, a chemist for the Hardwood-Plywood Manufacturers Association, "and it's not a great problem in my opinion." However, he adds, "If I were adding to my house, I'd look for low-formaldehyde products."

So would Connie Smrecek, who was a healthy Minnesota housewife until she and her husband remodeled their house in the late 1970s using an inexpensive particleboard subflooring that they cut and laid themselves. Soon she began suffering "extreme irritability, nausea, burning eyes, respiratory problems, dizziness, nasal congestion, and other allergy-like symptoms [plus] an overpowering desire to sleep." When she slept during the day, her two little boys would try to rouse her, but she was too sick. "No, shut the door," she would reluctantly respond. After two years of this, with her husband and children having similar symptoms, though not so severe, the Smreceks saw a television program on the health effects of formaldehyde—and recognized themselves. The Minnesota public health department found unusually high formaldehyde levels in their house, prompting the Smreceks to have the flooring ripped out, but for Connie Smrecek it was too late. She was sensitive not only to formaldehyde but to other common chemicals as well. She had acquired EI/MCS: "Her system was so overloaded that she could not even read the day's mail without suffering reactions from synthetic compounds in the ink or in lingering perfume from somebody who had touched the paper." Now living in a specially constructed chemical-free home that she and her husband built, she still has problems in walking, breathing, and thinking. Since much of the outside world, such as fumes from a passing car, is poisonous to her, she remains homebound, a victim of toxic building products containing formaldehyde. She may never fully recover. Despite her disabilities, she formed an organization, Citizens United to Reduce Emissions, or C.U.R.E., to try to prevent others from acquiring her illness.

Unfortunately, her message did not reach Ann Hardacre, in Indiana, who suffered stomach pains, severe headaches, body aches, and flu-like symptoms for four years until Godish discovered the cause. The minute he walked into her house he could smell the formaldehyde coming from the pressed-wood products used in the home's construction. Though none of her doctors had suspected her house as the cause of her symptoms, it was indeed making her ill.

Connecticut architect Paul Bierman-Lytle has identified fifteen hundred hazardous components used in home construction. Formaldehyde, he says, is the most dangerous because "it's in almost everything." Nevertheless, Bierman-Lytle predicts that "if you eat healthy food, and you want safe products to consume, the same thing will become an obvious choice for homes. People are starting to be better shoppers, and they are also starting to ask housing brokers and inspectors about radon, asbestos, lead paint, formaldehyde emissions, and insulation."

The Risks and What to Do About Them

How much formaldehyde does it take to get sick from it, and who is most at risk? Authorities' opinions are confusing and contradictory. The CPSC says that 0.015 parts per million can be considered a safe level in air. Godish reports studies of indoor air indicating that "levels of formaldehyde as low as 0.05 parts per million are sufficient to cause symptoms in sensitive individuals." Home air levels of formaldehyde can range from 0.02 to 2 parts per million, he has found, with the highest levels in mobile homes, especially those manufactured before 1980 (mobile homes now contain less particleboard than previously). The EPA in 1984 estimated an average level of around 0.03 parts per million in nonmobile homes, with newer homes sometimes over 0.1 parts per million. The American Lung Association cautions that "irritation of eyes, nose, and throat can occur at concentrations as low as 0.25 parts per million. However," continues the ALA, "investigations of consumer complaints suggest that peak formaldehyde levels of less than 0.1 parts per million are associated with the irritant symptoms of building-related illness. . . . Conventional particleboard subflooring, measured two to five years after installation, has shown peak levels in the range of 0.2 to 0.3 parts per million"—five times more than enough to cause symptoms, Godish found. According to the Illinois Department of Public Health, most healthy adults would not be expected to experience acute toxic effects from formaldehyde exposure below 0.1 parts per million. Thus the CPSC says that 0.015 parts per million is safe, Godish warns about 0.05 parts per million, the ALA warns about 0.1 or 0.25 parts per million (take your pick), and a state public health department warns about 0.1 parts per million, while home levels from formaldehyde commonly range from 0.02 to 2 parts per million—in other words, from not dangerous to very dangerous.

As might be expected, those considered most at risk are infants, homemakers, and the elderly—persons spending the most time at home. Also at risk are the chemically injured and those with allergies or respiratory problems, whose immune systems may already be impaired. If you want to measure formaldehyde levels in your home, passive air samplers designed for this purpose are readily available; you might consult one of the sources listed at the end of this chapter.

What can you do to avoid dangerous formaldehyde emissions? Don't be floored by the Formaldehyde Institute's eighty-five-item list, which makes it look completely impossible to avoid breathing the stuff. Especially for your home, where you do have some control over your environment, there are many substitute products that contain less or no formaldehyde. Labels, unfortunately, are of little help. Our society has not yet recognized the need to have all ingredients, even minute quantities, listed on all products. But if you learn to recognize the smell of formaldehyde as you gradually rid your home of petrochemical-based products, you will be able to detect some products that contain it. For those you need to find substitutes.

If you or someone in your family is having symptoms that baffle your doctors, you can do some of your own testing before deciding either to buy a test device or to call in a professional to test the air in your home. Try filling one of your rooms with obvious sources of formaldehyde (synthetic clothes, drapes, carpets; foam pillows; pieces of particleboard). Shut the room's door and windows for a week, and then spend some time there watching for symptoms of any kind. Or you can move suspected items out of one room to create a nonchemical "oasis" and see if you feel better there. Or you can spend several hours in a fabric store full of synthetic, treated, permanent-press fabrics to see how you feel.

If formaldehyde seems to be a problem for you, the first step is to make your bedroom, where you spend at least seven or eight hours a day, a safe room, by removing as many formaldehyde sources as possible. Substitute all-cotton, undyed, unprinted, untreated sheets and pillowcases for synthetic, dyed, printed, treated ones (inks and dyes can contain formaldehyde). For pillows and covers, use only untreated cotton, wool, down, or feathers (for more suggestions on safe home furnishings, see Chapter 4). If you are allergic to down and feathers, use cotton pillows or folded cotton blankets. Remove as much particleboard furniture and as many synthetic clothes and furnishings as you can. Remove as many of the products listed at the end of this chapter as possible. Very important: keep the bedroom doors closed and windows open as much as possible. Once your symptoms are relieved, you can begin dealing with the rest of your home.

Basically, there are four approaches to the formaldehyde problem at home:

- Remove the source. When the source is movable, this is the easiest and best solution, though you may find it hard at first to give up some cherished clothes, cosmetics, and cleaning or other products. Later, however, you may be very glad that you did. Alternative products abound.

- Treat the source. If you own your home and have UFFI in your walls, you can reduce your exposure by covering walls with special, relatively nontoxic paints or sealers (see Chapter 4 for sources) and by putting gaskets in electrical outlets. (For advice on removing UFFI insulation, consult "Building Practice Note #23," available from Publication Section, M-20, Division of Building Research, National Research Council of Canada, Ottawa, Ontario, Canada, K1A 0R6; 613-993-2463.) Use aluminum tape (try your local hardware or Sears store) to block any construction gaps. Sealers and tape can also prevent outgassing of formaldehyde from pressed-wood furniture, cabinets, and counter tops; run your fingers along their undersides to detect any telltale rough surfaces. Solid-wood furniture and cabinets are better but are likely to have formaldehyde-emitting finishes, as are hardwood floors. Ammonia fumigation, found effective in reducing mobile home formaldehyde levels, should be applied by only trained operators. (For more information on ammonia fumigation and for a building-related-illness checklist, contact Thad Godish, PhD, Director, Indoor Air Quality Research Laboratory, Ball State University, Muncie, Indiana 47305.)

- Purify the air. Activated-charcoal or other filters will remove some of the formaldehyde and other chemicals from the air in your home (and your car). They can be expensive and they require some maintenance, but are worth it in health-cost savings. Spider plants, highly publicized as formaldehyde removers on the basis of NASA research, are ineffective, according to Godish, because the humidity they create actually increases formaldehyde emissions and thus counterbalances the formaldehyde they absorb.

- Ventilate the air. Because formaldehyde outgasses more into hot or humid air, air conditioning may help in the summer. For the same reason, "baking out" a new house or mobile home by shutting it up, increasing its air temperature, and then airing it out may help reduce formaldehyde emissions. In winter, heat-exchange air-to-air ventilation systems draw in outdoor air while retaining heat. Outdoor air may not be "fresh" or "pure," but the EPA has found indoor air as much as a hundred times more contaminated than outdoor air even in heavily polluted areas. Thus, airing your home out at least once a day will help reduce formaldehyde levels. The trade-off between energy costs and your family's well-being is well worth it.

Is our government setting standards for formaldehyde? In 1992 OSHA reduced the permissible occupational level from 1.0 to 0.1 parts per million—quite a drop. The new level is in striking contrast to the target level of the U.S. Department of Housing and Urban Development (HUD): 0.4 parts per million for new mobile homes. According to Godish, "the HUD target level reflects the ability of wood product manufacturers to make products which do not exceed the target level. . . . Rather than protecting consumers, it provides regulatory sanction for the manufacture of defective products which are a significant threat to public health."

Once again, then, you are pretty much on your own when it comes to protecting your health. If the measures just recommended do not help your symptoms but you still suspect formaldehyde, you may need to consider moving. The decision will depend partly on the severity of your symptoms. Says Godish, "The release of formaldehyde from source materials will never completely stop."

* * * *

To Find Out More

- *The Poisoning of Our Homes and Workplaces: The Indoor Formaldehyde Crisis,* by Jack Thrasher, PhD, and Alan Broughton, MD, Santa Ana, California, Seadora, Inc., 1989; write Seadora, Inc., 1715 E. Wilshire #715, Santa Ana, California 92705.

- "Health Effects of Formaldehyde," by K. Gupta, U.S. Consumer Product Safety Commission, Washington, D.C. 20207, 1983.

- "Health Risk Assessment for Formaldehyde," U.S. Environmental Protection Agency, Washington, D.C. 20460, 1987.

- *The Inside Story: A Guide to Indoor Air Quality,* U.S. Consumer Product Safety Commission and U.S. Environmental Protection Agency, September 1988 (has section on formaldehyde).

- Contact your local American Lung Association office.

- Contact your state's public health department.

Sources for Passive Air Samplers
(for information only, not as a recommendation)

- Advanced Chemical Sensors Co., 350 Oaks Lane, Pompano Beach, Florida 33069; 305-979-0958.

- Air Quality Research, Inc., 901 Grayson, Berkeley, California 94710; 415-644-2097.

- E.I. Du Pont Company, Applied Technical Division, P.O. Box 110, Kennett Square, Pennsylvania 19348; 1-800-344-4900.

- 3M Corporation, Technical Service Department, Building 260-3-2, St. Paul, Minnesota 55144; 1-800-328-1667.

- Assay Technology, Inc., 1070 E. Meadow Circle, Palo Alto, California 94303; 1-800-833-1258.

- Crystal Diagnostics, 30 Commerce Way, Woburn, Massachusetts 01801; 617-933-4114.

- GMD Systems, Inc., Old Route 519, Hendersonville, Pennsylvania 15339; 412-746-3600.

Sources for Sealers
(for information only, not as a recommendation)

- Valspar Corporation, 200 Sayer Street, Rockford, Illinois 61101; 815-987-3775.

- Pace Chem Industries, Inc., 779 S. La Grange Avenue, Newbury Park, California 91320; 1-800-350-2912.

* * * *

A Sampler of Common Products Containing Formaldehyde
(source: the Formaldehyde Institute)

acrylic
aerosol insecticide
air and furnace filters
air fresheners
antihistamines
antiperspirant formulations
antislip agents
antistatic agents
automotive exhaust
barber and beauty shops
binders
binding on paper bag seams
brake drums
carpet and upholstery latex
  backing
cigarette smoke
coated papers used for cartons
  and labels
coatings for appliances
counter and table tops
dental bibs
dental fillings
deodorants
detergents
diaper liners
disinfectants
drapery and upholstery fabric
dyes for textile industry
electrical insulation parts
electronic equipment
embalming agents
examining-table paper rolls
explosives
facial tissues and napkins
fiberboard
fiberglass and mineral wool
  insulation

filter papers (some)
flour preservative
Formica
furniture adhesives
glues
hair-waving preparations
hardware
hospital bed sheets
housings for electric shavers
  and mixers
insecticides
knobs and buttons
lawn and garden equipment
mascara and other cosmetics
melamine tableware
mildew preventatives
milk
nail hardener
nail polish
nitrogen fertilizers
nylon fibers
orthopedic casts and bandages
paint and wood finishes
particleboard
permanent press cotton
pharmaceuticals
plastic/plastic parts for vehicles
plumbing fixtures
plywood
preservatives
pressed wood furniture
primer coat for automobiles
rayon
resins and oil-based paints
Sanforized cotton
shampoo
soap dispensers

softeners and lubricants
sporting goods
stove and refrigerator hardware
synthetic lubricants
textile-treating agents
textile waterproofing
tire rubbers
toilet seats

UF foam insulation
utensil handles
water-softening chemicals
wax and butcher wet strength
  paper
wheat grains and agriculture
  seeds
wool

7

Which Pesticides Are Safe: Fighting the Deadly Dandelion

WHAT YOU NEED TO KNOW about pesticides is really very simple. They are all designed to kill. "Cide" means "kill," whether the word is pesticide, insecticide, herbicide, fungicide, termiticide, miticide, rodenticide, or bacteriocide, or any other "-cide." Pesticides are designed to kill unwanted living things, or pests, whether they are insects, weeds, fungi, termites, mites, rodents, or bacteria. All pesticides are dangerous to living things—and that includes human beings. The few, inorganic (non-carbon-containing) pesticides used before World War II were called "economic poisons" because of their economic benefit to farmers. "Economic poisons" became "pesticides," which became, in some circles, "plant protectants." With each change in terminology, the sense of toxicity became more remote.

Though pesticide applicators speak of "nontarget organisms," pesticides do not discriminate between targeted and nontargeted living things. "If you go into your back yard with a machine gun and blast back and forth, it is not very choosy about whom it will kill. Pesticides . . . are like that too," says Dr. Janette Sherman, author of *Chemical Exposure and Disease*. While human beings are seldom if ever intentionally targeted for lethal pesticide exposures, pesticides have killed some people:

- In 1982, U.S. naval lieutenant George Prior, a healthy thirty-year-old, died an agonizing death after playing golf on a course that had been repeatedly sprayed with the fungicide Daconil, which was pinpointed as the cause of death. (The capital "D" indicates a trade name.)

- For a man who wanted to take a break after burglarizing an empty house that was being fumigated, crime did not pay. He went back into the house to eat a snack and watch television. Neighbors found him writhing naked on the front lawn of the San Fernando, California, home, having torn off his clothes in an attempt to rid himself of their pesticide contamination. He later died in a local hospital.

- In Texas, four suspected illegal aliens were found dead in a boxcar half-filled with boxes of tortilla flour. The car had been fumigated with the pesticide Phostoxin, and the local coroner found evidence of internal bleeding, a typical sign of pesticide poisoning.

- In 1987 *NEJM* reported the deaths of three patients from respiratory failure, the result of organophosphate pesticides affecting nerve connections.

- Worldwide, anywhere from one million to twenty-five million people are estimated to suffer from accidental pesticide poisoning each year, with more than twenty thousand dying, according to the World Health Organization. Between 1975 and 1980 in Sri Lanka, 79,961 patients were hospitalized because of pesticide poisonings and 6,083 of them died. In fact, pesticides have become a drug of choice for committing suicide: WHO estimates that each year two million people in undeveloped countries purposely ingest the pesticides so easily available to them. Many more cases of pesticide poisoning worldwide, it is thought, go unrecognized or unreported.

Obviously, pesticides are not something to fool around with. But most of us do not burglarize houses, work for exterminators or lawn-care companies, or hide in boxcars illegally. Where do we encounter pesticides? The answer is "everywhere," or almost everywhere. According to the GAO, "people are exposed to pesticides in the food they eat, the water they drink and swim in, the air they breathe, and in their homes and workplaces. In the home, pesticides are used in treated fabrics for apparel, diapers, or bedding; in bathroom and kitchen disinfectants such as common household bleach; in insect repellents applied directly to human skin; in pet flea collars and in swimming pool additives." Their major use is on crops, but pesticides are also used "in homes, backyard gardens, stores, schools, restaurants, office buildings, industrial workplaces, sports facilities, hotels, hospitals, and theaters, on lawns and golf courses, and along highway rights-of-way." As if this were not enough, add to the list churches, synagogues, health clubs; florists, paint, carpeting, deodorant soaps, shampoos, lanolin creams, pressure-treated wood; soil, groundwater, and rain and you have an idea of what can expose you to pesticides in twentieth-century America.

Most churches, synagogues, and health clubs hire exterminators for routine spraying, whether needed or not (just ask your church, synagogue, or health club). Pesticides are likely to be on the beautiful plant you bring home from the florist (just ask), in the latex paint you brush on furniture and walls, on the back of wallpaper, and on the brown paper bags you bring home from the supermarket. In 1990 the EPA warned parents against buying "Miraculous Insecticide Chalk," which could cause nausea and flu-like symptoms in children. A 1991 EPA study found pesticide residues in the dust and carpeting of all surveyed houses, making floors potentially hazardous for infants and toddlers. Dust in older houses yielded banned pesticides. Deodorant soaps that kill odor-causing bacteria contain disinfectants and fungicides that *Clinical Toxicology of Commercial Products* characterizes as moderately or slightly toxic. Certain human (not animal) shampoos contain the fungicide Captan, according to Dr. Marion Moses, a California physician who has treated many migrant farm workers with pesticide-related illnesses and who is now head of San Francisco's Pesticide Education Center. Researchers at Oregon State University discovered pesticides in lanolin-based ointments such as those used for sore nipples by nursing mothers; babies could thus start their pesticide exposures at an early age, though many begin *in utero*, for chemicals can pass through the umbilical cord. You see how they all add up.

Green, pressure-treated wood, which contains the pesticide copper-chromated arsenate, has made carpenters sick with respiratory illness, coughing, and general ill health, according to a manufacturer's memo obtained by the National Coalition Against the Misuse of Pesticides (NCAMP). One carpenter, who had coughed up blood after exposure to sawdust from pressure-treated wood, won a settlement of $667,000 from several companies. Connecticut agricultural scientists in 1989 found ethylene dibromide (EDB), a fumigant banned in 1983, in the soil of a former tobacco farm where it had last been applied in the late 1960s. "The soil is acting as a reservoir," explained Joe Pignatello, one of the scientists," not only for EDB, but for herbicides, solvents, and PCBs [another banned chemical]."

One kind of reservoir leads to another: by 1989 eight states had discovered unsafe levels of EDB in their groundwater. And by 1988, according to Lawrie Mott, an NRDC scientist, forty-six pesticides from agricultural runoff had been found in water in twenty-six states. In North Carolina, for example, groundwater testing had by 1992 found pesticides in eight of forty-nine randomly-selected wells selected for sampling. A 1991 EPA study found that "perhaps" 750 community water supply wells and 60,900 rural domestic water supply wells nationwide are expected to contain pesticides at "levels of health concern." This estimate reflects increasing groundwater contamination, especially in rural states like Iowa. Agricultural runoff—mainly pesticides—now contaminates 55 percent of river miles and 58 percent of lake acres surveyed by the EPA, as reported by Water Quality 2000, a coalition of environmental, business, and governmental groups. In 1993 the GAO put out another of its clearly titled reports: "Drinking Water: Stronger Efforts Needed to Protect Areas Around Public Wells." And rain—heaven's gentle dew—now contains pesticides, in some Midwestern states in concentrations above the EPA's standard for drinking water. Scientists don't know what health effects the contaminated rain may have. (Be sure to carry your umbrella.)

"What gets into the soil, what gets into the water, what gets into the air, eventually gets into us," warned U.S. Senator Paul Simon in a speech to constituents. The senator may have had in mind the EPA's ongoing survey of foreign chemicals in Americans' fatty tissues. In 1982, for example, the study found each of thirteen different pesticides in at least 53 percent of the body fat samples tested.

One pesticide was in all samples. By 1993, 177 organochlorines (persistent pesticides) had been found in the tissues and fluids of people in North America. Over the period 1970 to 1983, the study found oxychlordane, breakdown product of chlordane, a commonly used termiticide, in over 90 percent of fat samples tested, according to the Freshwater Foundation. In April 1988, chlordane, thought to promote the growth of tumors in animals, was taken off the market. Acute exposures to chlordane, the EPA believes, can disrupt the nervous system and even cause death. While an expert in preventive health asserts that since thirty million U.S. homes had been treated with chlordane, "if there were an epidemic out there, we'd know it," a pathologist thinks that "the consequences of chlordane exposure to human health can't be clearly defined yet." True to scientific form, the latter recommended more research. But can we wait? Does it shock you to know that pesticides and other toxic chemicals have taken up lodgings in your body fat? What might they be doing to your health?

Pesticides and Your Health

Next to AIDS, cancer is arguably the most feared modern disease. Yet the NTP by 1990 had identified only thirty agents or processes as definitely causing cancers in human beings. Of these, almost all also cause cancer in animals. Among them is only one pesticide—arsenic and certain of its compounds. However, several hundred other chemicals, including at least seventy of the four hundred pesticides used on food crops, cause cancer in animals. Should we wait to find out whether they also cause cancer in humans? Cancer has a long lead time—as long as forty years. No sane person is advocating controlled double-blind cancer tests on human beings, with one group unknowingly exposed to suspected carcinogens and another group—the lucky ones—carefully selected to be controls.

Several epidemiological studies (of voluntary though probably unknowing exposure to carcinogens) have shown a possible connection between pesticides and cancer. The NCI found that Kansas farmers who used the weed killer 2,4-D (a common herbicide) had a higher-than-average risk of contracting malignant cancer of lymph tissues (known as lymphoma), and an Iowa study found that people living in areas with high herbicide use were 60 percent more likely to die of leukemia. A carefully done study reported in the *Journal of Rural Studies* found that "for three of the five categories of cancer [studied], agricultural chemical use was the best predictor of cancer mortality." A 1987 study by the NCI found that children in households where home and garden pesticides were used are up to nine times more likely to develop some form of leukemia than in households where pesticides were not used.

Of 238 Missouri families studied in 1992 for their use of pesticides, 98 percent used pesticides in home or garden at least once a year and 64 percent used them more than five times a year; half of the families used insecticides to control fleas and ticks on pets. A 1993 controlled study of Missouri children showed "statistically significant associations between childhood brain cancer and several types of pesticide use in the home, including no-pest strips and flea and tick collars on pets." According to the NCI, the years 1973–1988 saw a "dramatic rise" in brain cancers among children as well as older people.

Children are especially at risk from pesticides. In 1989 the NRDC estimated that "at least 17 percent of the preschool population [3 million children out of a total of 17.6 million] are exposed to neurotoxic organophosphate insecticides above safe levels just from eating raw fruit alone." ("Safe" refers to government-set levels based on risk assessments.) Children have a long lifetime of ingesting pesticides ahead of them, and their developing bodies are more susceptible to poisoning. Since a fourth of the American public are now contracting cancer by various means, there could be about 4.5 million cancer cases among present preschoolers during their lifetimes. And, estimated Dr. Richard Jackson, chairman of the American Academy of Pediatrics environmental hazards committee, pesticides may cause five thousand of those cancers.

Actually, the NAS has estimated that as many as twenty thousand Americans a year will develop cancer because of pesticide residues on produce that they eat. And according to the *Wall Street Journal*, the EPA itself has ranked pesticide residues as the nation's number three cancer risk. Yet for one pesticide alone, alachlor, a pesticide widely used on many crops, the EPA has said that the risk of getting cancer "at current levels in the food or drinking water supply was generally one in a million from such exposure over a seventy-year period and added that the dietary risk posed by the substance was reasonable." Reasonable for whom? Is it "reasonable" for just one pesticide to cause cancer to one-in-a-million seventy-year-olds a few years down the road? Not if you're that one. And what about all the other pesticides? The other routes of exposure? Toxicologist Marvin Legator believes that "the EPA is grossly underestimating the risk to the public" when it sets pesticide tolerances.

Animals get cancer too. Unwittingly, mankind has not been kind to its best friend; dogs whose owners use 2,4-D on their lawns are twice as likely to develop lymphoma as those whose owners don't use it, again according to the NCI. Malignant cancer in dogs is similar to non-Hodgkin's lymphoma in humans, the incidence of which in Americans increased by about 50 percent between 1973 and 1991.

Another cancer whose incidence has increased in the human population is breast cancer, which in the U.S. went up from one in twenty in 1950 to one in nine in the 1990s, up 8 percent between 1973 and 1980 among women younger than fifty and up 32 percent among women over fifty. The latter are those most exposed to DDT between 1945 and 1972, the years it was in common use. In 1992 a controlled study of forty women examined at Hartford Hospital, in Hartford, Connecticut, by a team led by Dr. Frank Falck Jr., of the University of Michigan, revealed that the breast tissues of those with breast cancer contained "elevated levels of DDT, DDE, and PCBs, compared with the breast tissues of women with benign breast disease." (DDT is a persistent organochlorine pesticide banned in the U.S. in 1972 for most uses; DDT breaks down in the body to DDE.) In 1993 a team led by Dr. Mary S. Wolff, of the Mount Sinai School of Medicine, in New York, found a fourfold increase in the relative risk of breast cancer in 58 women with high blood levels of DDE, compared with the blood levels in 171 matched control women without cancer, over a six-year period. Said Dr. Wolff, "Given the widespread dissemination of organochlorine insecticides in the environment and the food chain, the implications are far-reaching for public health intervention world-wide." In Israel, after consumer pressure forced the government to ban several pesticides found in dairy products, researchers noted a dramatic drop in breast cancer mortality rates.

In the June 17, 1993, *New Yorker*, Paul Brodeur ended his article "Legacy" with a paragraph on the possible connection between pesticides and breast cancer and the words "Rachel Carson lives." (Carson died of cancer in 1964.) For years the *New Yorker* has kept a wary eye on twentieth-century technology; in the late 1940s it devoted almost an entire issue to John Hersey's article on Hiroshima, and in the early 1960s it published portions of Carson's *Silent Spring*, its title referring to the pesticide-caused deaths of songbirds then occurring across the country. On the publication of this beautifully written and meticulously researched book, Supreme Court Justice William O.Douglas called it "the most important chronicle of this century for the human race."

In January 1988 the *New Yorker* published "The Fumigation Chamber," one of Berton Roueché's always fascinating "Annals of Medicine." This one is the story of a woman doctor in Pennsylvania who gradually developed a series of mysterious symptoms—nausea, abdominal cramps, diarrhea, heart irregularities, double vision, muscle weakness, chest tightness, twitching in her legs, and a prickling sensation in the soles of her feet. After visiting several specialists without any improvement, she and her doctor husband finally deduced that her symptoms were caused by the routine spraying of organophosphate pesticides in their summer cabin. Later she suffered similar symptoms from insecticide spraying at an indoor tennis court and a flower show. The article ended with the doctor's statement: "I'm just beginning to realize that the world is a very dangerous place. It's something nobody really wants to think about. I mean the thousands and thousands of toxic chemicals that have become so much a part of modern living. I mean the people who use them without really knowing what they can do. I mean the where and how and why they use them. It's frightening. I think I'm prety much recovered now. I haven't had any trouble for over a year. But you never know. The only thing I'm sure of is that I'm going to have to be very careful for the rest of my life."

Other Health Effects

Yes, cancer is not the only danger from pesticides. Much suffering reflects damage to the nervous system—not surprisingly, for many of the most widely used modern pesticides trace their origins to the nerve gases sarin, soman, and tabun developed in Germany during World War II. These pesticides are known as the organophosphates because all are "organic" (i.e., carbon-containing) and are derived from phosphoric acid. The organophosphates are less chemically stable than organochlorines (containing carbon and chlorine) like DDT, which persist in the environment and, as their derivatives, in our body fat. Organophosphates like chlorpyrifos, mevinphos, diazinon, malathion, and parathion have largely replaced the organochlorines for home and garden use. The organophosphates (and the carbamates, another common class of pesticides) affect the nervous system by inhibiting an enzyme called cholinesterase. The resulting interference with nerve function can cause twitching, paralysis, tremors, convulsions, and death from respiratory failure, according to Professor George Ware, of the University of Arizona. Moreover, according to biochemist Bambi Batts Young, they can produce such varied effects as nausea, vomiting, and diarrhea; heart irregularities; excessive sweating, salivation, and watering of the eyes; chest discomfort; headaches; and abnormal brain function and behavior. And according to EPA Region VI, in Texas, they can mimic brain hemorrhage, heat exhaustion, heat stroke, gastroenteritis, asthma, and pneumonia. Designed to zap insects' nerves, they can also affect the nerves of "nontarget organisms" like you or me.

That is exactly what happened to unsuspecting workers in a Nevada casino sprayed with a pesticide containing a carbamate as well as the "carriers" 1,1,1-trichloroethane, methylene chloride, and xylene. Twelve out of 113 workers reporting symptoms such as dizziness, racing heartbeats, trembling, nausea, and weakness developed an intolerance to perfumes, gasoline, newsprint, cleaners, and other solvent-containing materials (they now had EI/MCS). Even the OSHA industrial hygienist investigating the occurrence became ill, with cramps, chills, nausea, and headache. Cholinesterase inhibitors can also produce "significant aggressive and violent behavior," including murder, according to Dr. Orrin Devinsky, of New York University School of Medicine, and his associates, who reported on four cases in the *Journal of Neuropsychiatry*. Three had come in contact with organophosphate lawn chemicals; two of these had committed brutal murders. The fourth was a professor of medicine who had sprayed a carbamate powder on his cat. The violent behavior included verbal and physical abuse of friends, family, strangers, or themselves. All four held responsible jobs and had no history of fighting, arrest, or psychiatric diagnoses. All returned to normal after the pesticide exposure and their violent behavior. The two murderers are both in prison, feeling long-lasting, overwhelming guilt.

As if these dramatic health effects were not enough, pesticides also have subtle, long-term effects. In 1984 researchers found that when as little as 0.1 parts per billion of organochlorines, which are also neurotoxic, were removed from the blood of chemically sensitive patients in an environmentally controlled hospital unit, the patients' IQs went up between 5 and 15 points. More recent research by toxicologist Warren P. Porter at the University of Wisconsin found that rats became both aggressive and learning-disabled after being given low-level pesticide mixtures. Concerned about the implications of his research, Dr. Porter warns that "we will not be able to maintain a highly ordered technological society if we raise a generation of children who are learning-disabled and hyperaggressive." Reports such as these have caught the attention of psychologists, one of whom, Professor David Overstreet of the University of North Carolina, says, "The basic take-home message is that we have to be extremely careful about exposure to these compounds everywhere."

Pesticides affect not only our nervous systems, but our immune systems. "About five million Americans . . . risk severe immune reactions ranging from runny eyes and itchy skin to shock and death when they are exposed to [pesticides]. Another eleven million have moderate reactions to pesticides ranging from tearing and dripping noses to hives and muscle and joint pain," according to Dr. Russell Jaffe, principal scientist at Serammune Physicians Lab, a biotechnology laboratory in Reston, Virginia. The lab's five-year study of more than eight thousand patients is "the first to clearly link pesticides with immune recognition responses," claims Dr. Jaffe. "It is no longer a matter of guesswork. Now we can determine for an individual his or her sensitivity to pesticides." The Serammune Physicians Lab has developed ELISA/ACT, which tests blood samples for immune system reactions to 235 foods, pesticides, and other environmental chemicals.

San Francisco immunologist Alan Levin sees patients whose immune systems have been wrecked by pesticides. "The most common symptom we see is a gradual intolerance developing to environmental chemicals of all types, including vehicle exhaust, fumes at the gas station, perfumes, alcohol, some foods. We ask them if they have to hold their breath when they walk by the detergent shelves in the supermarket. They almost always say 'yes.' They feel like they have the flu all the time." Such patients often have skin problems, food and mold allergies, and lowered counts of infection-fighting white blood cells. Toxicologist L. John Olson of the Wisconsin Department of Health agrees: "Research has demonstrated that subtle immune system defects can have serious, even fatal consequences to both animals and humans." Wildlife included: the National Wildlife Federation says that pesticides used in the U.S. jeopardize about 250 endangered and threatened species.

Yet pesticide use in the U.S. is on the increase, though accurate figures are hard to come by; most states do not mandate reporting of pesticide use or sales, and definitions of the word "pesticide" differ widely. *Public Citizen* in 1988 estimated an increase in pesticides (broadly defined) going from 120 *million* pounds in 1950 to more than 2.6 *billion* pounds in 1988. In 1991 Greenpeace said that our use of pesticides has gone up 3,000 percent since 1940, with an increase in pesticide potency of 1,000 percent. For 1991 the EPA estimated U.S. pesticide use at about 2.2 billion pounds, including wood preservatives, sulfur, and some disinfectants, but not chlorine products registered with the EPA for disinfectant or drinking water treatment uses. U.S. pesticide sales in 1991 were $8.3 billion. Pesticide sales worldwide went from $3 billion in 1970 to $19 billion by 1990.

Thus these poisons now cover the earth. Where are you most likely to encounter them, how effective and how necessary are they, and how have they been affecting people who are most exposed?

Farm Use

In 1991 U.S. farmers applied about 76 percent of all pesticides sold in this country (more than one billion pounds, as narrowly defined), over half of them herbicides. But astonishingly, according to the National Toxics Campaign, less than than 0.1 percent of these chemicals reach the intended pest. The rest, 99.9 percent, contaminate our soil, water, and food. And the pesticides that do reach the pests are losing their effectiveness. Between 1940 and 1984, crop losses to insects almost doubled even with a twelve-fold increase in the use of insecticides. "Corn losses to insects more than tripled . . . between 1945 and 1985 despite a thousand-fold increase in insecticides used on corn crops," according to the textbook *Environmental Science*. Over a twenty-five-year period, according to a 1993 report, *Agrichemicals in America: Farmers' Reliance on Pesticides and Fertilizers*, there was a 125 percent increase in pounds per acre of pesticides applied to U.S. cropland, with fruit and vegetable farms using more than livestock and dairy farms.

One reason that farmers are using more pesticides is that the number of insect species resistant to one or more pesticides grew from 185 in 1965 to 447 in 1984. By 1992 more than 500 species were resistant to pesticides. Insects reproduce very quickly, and because of natural selection, "chemical insecticides are great at suppressing bug populations in the short run, but over time they are just a particularly efficient method of breeding tougher, hardier insects."

Can we get by with fewer pesticides on crops? If American farmers stopped using half the chemical pesticides they now spray on crops, it would cause only a slight rise in food prices and would bestow major environmental and public health benefits, according to a 1991 Cornell University study. Several farmers agree. The late Robert Rodale, publisher of *Prevention* and *Organic Gardening* magazines, maintained that techniques developed on his experimental farm proved that "farmers can get the same yield with much less use of fertilizers and pesticides. And sometimes in a dry year we've even had better yields." Biochemist-turned-farmer John B. Clark has farmed his eighteen hundred acres in southwestern Michigan without pesticides since 1978 and without soluble chemical fertilizers since 1985. The results on his farm and all over the world, Clark says, are almost always the same: "Yields get better as organic practices are continued, *and pest problems virtually disappear* [italics his]. Natural pest controls, which are suppressed in chemical farming, get healthier and more effective every year. Plant and livestock health improves; soil tilth improves every year, and so does soil moisture retention. . . . The sad truth . . . is that all the risks associated with pesticides are *unnecessary* risks."

The chemical companies "have convinced a lot of people that we can't farm without chemicals, and I don't believe that's true," argues Iowa farmer Tom Furlong. Progressive Iowa was in 1993 the only state to tax pesticides and then pay farmers to find better alternatives, like crop rotation; these farmers find that crop yields increase. Dick Harter, a California rice farmer, says that government agencies and the land-grant colleges (those with influential agriculture departments) have been slow to take alternative farming seriously. Hence alternative farmers must do their own research, for the bulk of agricultural research is "subsidized by the government and the companies that make pesticides and fertilizers. They're big supporters of the land-grant universities."

What is the chemical industry saying in response to such criticisms? Here's a sample, from the president (in 1987) of the National Agricultural Chemicals Association. "[Groundwater] contamination is not unique to my industry." "Any time you're dealing in the biological sciences like this, there's no black and white. . . . Having peer review by the appropriate scientists doesn't allow the process to move quite as fast as some people would like for it to move." "What I would like to see is the EPA become a more credible, scientifically oriented organization." "Some of the scientists are too quick to have their papers appear in the popular print, without peer review." In other words, the best defense is offense—blame everyone else but your own industry.

The power of the agricultural chemical industry is reflected in the fact that in 1991, according to the head of the Organic Foods Production Association of North America, only about one in four hundred farmers was farming organically, that is, controlling disease and weeds without using chemicals. (What a change from a hundred or even sixty years ago, when such chemicals did not even exist and everyone farmed without them!) However, you can take some comfort in knowing that the United States Department of Agriculture's (USDA's) National Organic Standards Board has been holding public hearings in order to set national standards for organic farming, with a target date of October 1994. If the resulting standards are not too watered down, they should clarify the previously unreliable use of the word. Another sign of change is that at least one land-grant college, the University of Iowa, now has a center, the Aldo Leopold Center for Sustainable Agriculture, to investigate alternative farming methods. (Aldo Leopold was an early-twentieth-century ecologist and conservationist.) Residents of that highly agricultural state are increasingly aware of the groundwater studies and the leukemia studies.

Also heavily exposed to unnecessary risks from farm chemicals are migrant farm workers. In the fall of 1979 farm worker Minnie Cox was sprayed with Paraquat by a California crop duster. The following December she died of pneumonia. The California Department of Food and Agriculture's investigating doctor said that she died of "atypical viral pneumonia, not pesticide related." An OSHA doctor said that she died of Paraquat poisoning. In Florida in 1989 more than seventy-five migrant farm workers, sent into a cauliflower field without sufficient protective clothing and too soon after it had been sprayed with the pesticide Phosdrin, fell ill with headaches, dizziness, nausea, vomiting, and breathing problems. Some workers were hospitalized, one victim in intensive care. Four years later, all the way across the country, Washington State halted the use of Phosdrin on apple orchards, an action said to be the first time a pesticide was banned because of its harmful effect on farm workers rather than consumers.

Even farm neighbors are at risk. On a windy summer day in 1971 a Wisconsin farm couple, the Freedlunds, and their six children watched with fascination the aerial spraying of a neighboring farm with the brushkiller 2,4,5-T, one of the components of Agent Orange, the defoliant used in Vietnam to clear jungles. The next day the entire family was sick, with "intense bellyaches, headache, fever, nauseous feeling, sleeplessness, children rising up in their sleep to yell, groan, mutter, and sleepwalk. Many trips to the bathroom with diarrhea. Baby screamed in pain and fear. Convulsions."

.

Gradually the symptoms eased, though they can recur when family members are exposed to any herbicide. "It's never going to be over for us," said Ruth, one of the daughters. Ridiculed by some for their belief that the symptoms were caused by the spraying, the Freedlunds fought for recognition of the dangers of pesticides, and in 1983 were present when Wisconsin's governor signed a bill banning 2,4,5-T in Wisconsin. Earlier, in 1979, the federal EPA had banned most uses of 2,4,5-T after it had been linked to a dramatic increase in miscarriages in Oregon. Nettie Freedlund, the mother, had two miscarriages in the 1970s, and one of her daughters has had a miscarriage. Joseph Prince, an EPA toxicologist who studied the Freedlunds, was compassionate but unconvinced until in 1979 a group of forty-seven railroad workers cleaned up a tank car spill of 2,4,5-T without protective clothing. Prince found serious defects in their immune systems. "These chemicals compromise the immune system," said Nettie Freedlund. "For years, if [any illness] went around, we caught it."

Commercial and Government Use

In 1991 government and business used 18 percent of the pesticides sold in this country. Government buildings, including those in our capital, are usually sprayed with pesticides. Corporations and businesses, especially those in the food industry, hire exterminators as well as lawn-care companies. Railroads spray their yards and their rights-of-way. Park districts, forest preserve districts, municipalities, and county boards have "weed control" programs using herbicides. Schools routinely spray both inside and outside their buildings.

Many governmental bodies spray residential areas and their residents from the air for such insects as mosquitoes, gypsy moths, and Mediterranean fruit flies (medflies). Yet for mosquitoes, most mosquito abatement experts consider larviciding (spot spraying of mosquito larvae in standing water or other breeding grounds) safer and more effective than adulticiding (blanket spraying of adult mosquitoes in residential areas). "Spraying up and down the street is totally ineffective," according to Khian Liem, a medical entomologist in the South Cook County (Illinois) Mosquito Abatement District, which abandoned residential spraying in 1978. The spray trucks are sent out, he said, "basically as window dressing, just to show the public they are doing something." Some Illinois districts still adulticide, forcing one resident, Beth Horner, a musician and professional storyteller, to leave town to avoid an asthma attack. A Lake County (Illinois) resident told his village board that his two daughters began vomiting and got fevers after a spraying. Dr. Samuel Epstein argues that there is no public health justification for adulticiding unless there is clear evidence of an infectious disease danger to humans, and then the decision to spray should be made by a state's governor or public health department, and only a pesticide uncontaminated by toxic solvents and so-called "inert" ingredients should be used. A sensible, health-oriented approach.

Instead of a synthetic chemical, some districts use a natural substance called *Bacillus thuringiensis (B.t.) israelenis*, considered toxic only to mosquitoes and black flies. Another form of *B.t.* (*B.t. kurstaki*) has been widely used to control gypsy-moth infestations, mainly in the northeastern U.S., despite indications that widespread use quickly creates *B.t.*-resistant insects. Though proclaimed nontoxic, some *B.t.* preparations can contain as much as 97.1 percent unidentified "inert" ingredients. When asked to identify such ingredients, manufacturers refuse, claiming "trade secrets." (No informed consent there.)

Malathion is the pesticide sprayed over much of Southern California in an attempt to control the Mediterranean fruit fly. Yet, according to Dr. Epstein, there are at least twenty-six studies showing that malathion has carcinogenic, reproductive, and neurotoxic effects. As if that were not enough, the malathion is killing off the area's natural predators, like the ladybugs, lacewings, and small wasps that eat aphids. In 1990, to save their orange trees California homeowners were spending $4 each for tubes of ladybugs to replace those killed by the pesticide, which also killed the honeybees that pollinate fruit trees.

Since California's repeated aerial malathion sprayings for medflies began in 1989, numerous Los Angeles families have reported suffering from rashes, colds, stomach upsets, flu-like symptoms, eye problems, rashes, diarrhea, headaches, and earaches, according to an article in *Woman's Day*. Parents fear for their children, whose immature organ systems make them more susceptible to toxic chemicals. One mother, concerned about the effect of the malathion on her already chemically sensitive five-year-old daughter, started a newsletter, *Mother to Mother*, protesting the spraying. After the helicopters go over, the little girl becomes hyperactive: "I act nasty," she says. "I don't feel wonderful. I hit and kick." Another mother, a lawyer with a four-year-old daughter who developed conjunctivitis and a permanent rash, apparently from the spraying, fears that malathion is "an experiment in which one million people are being made into guinea pigs." As for the spraying's effectiveness, she says "If you start spraying in August and you're still finding flies in April, doesn't logic tell you that the spray isn't working?" At least she and her daughter can go indoors when the helicopters buzz overhead: the Legal Aid Society of Orange County has filed a federal suit on behalf of homeless people, who have little protection against the poison from the skies.

In World War II our government hailed the synthesis of DDT and used it widely to prevent disease in the South Pacific. Marketed between 1943 and 1972, DDT was banned for most uses in the U.S. after it was found to be both carcinogenic and a prolific producer of pesticide-resistant bugs. However, it is still with us in our soils and the produce grown in them; as a metabolite, DDE, in our body fat; and as an "inert" ingredient in some pesticide formulations. DDT continues to be manufactured here and can come back to us on imported produce (DDT use is still legal in many countries) in what has been called a "circle of poison." About DDT and other persistent pesticides, food writer Patrick Quillin has said, "Daniel Webster made a deal with the devil for a limited period of prosperity in return for his soul. Pesticides have been like a deal with the devil. Hopefully, we can extract ourselves from this deal, as Daniel Webster did."

A Los Angeles nurse recalls that as the child of a soldier stationed on Guam after World War II, she and other children used to run after trucks spraying the streets, shouting "DDT! DDT!" The first word her baby brother uttered was "DDT." In New Jersey, Bernie Jorgensen was exposed to DDT as a child, when she and a friend were lying on the beach behind a sand dune. A truck went by on the other side of the dune, and a "cloud of pesticide drifted over the top of the dune and washed down upon our bodies." She recognized the smell of DDT from previous sprayings for mosquitoes on the beach.

Now diagnosed with EI/MCS, having experienced symptoms such as nausea, numbness, partial paralysis, and severe chest pains from later exposures to toxic substances, she must avoid many fumes, foods, and fibers by living in a trailer in the Arizona desert, away from husband, children, and friends. Before they visit her, they must wash with special soaps and shampoos and dress in cotton, but their visits still leave her exhausted and ill from the small amounts of chemicals they cannot completely rid themselves of. Bernie hopes eventually to live with her family in a safe home built where the trailer sits, after her body has cleansed itself enough in the fresh air of the desert for her to be able to tolerate daily assaults of pollutants. "Someday soon," she says, "the twentieth century will welcome me back." In the meantime, this century may be affecting as many as twenty-four million Americans who have symptoms similar to hers but don't know the cause, says her physician, William Rea.

Another common governmental use of pesticides is in our schools. Surveys done in 1987 found that ten out of eleven Southern school districts used pesticides and that in two California counties, all but one school district regularly applied pesticides. A 1992 Sierra Club survey found that 91 percent of 128 Chicago-area schools spray routinely, usually monthly, a third of them immediately before or during school hours. What are we doing to our children! Fortunately, a few school districts nationwide have changed to integrated pest management (IPM) policies, which use pesticides only as a last resort after nontoxic methods have been tried (better still would be no pesticides at all). In a wise move, the Berkeley, California, school district requires clearance from the city's department of health before any pesticide can be applied. The worst policy, in schools especially, is routine application when children are present; the best policy would be a move to alternative, nontoxic methods of pest control.

Home, Garden, and Lawn Use

Though only about 6 percent of the nation's pesticides are used in homes, gardens, and lawns, that may be where you are most likely to use or encounter them. An estimated 85 percent of American households have at least one pesticide in storage (again narrowly defined). Most American families, not realizing the dangers or unaware of the least-toxic alternatives, buy and use pesticides to kill weeds and insects, sometimes carelessly. Or they hire exterminators for indoors and lawn-care companies for outdoors. And very few people realize that their deodorant soaps are really pesticide soaps (broadly defined).

Another unsuspected risk is from the use of termiticides, required by some localities. Actress Kirstie Alley and her husband, living in a home in the Los Angeles area, both became very ill and went to many doctors for help, to no avail. It took a toxicologist to discover that the spraying of their house with the termiticide methyl bromide had caused their illness. Methyl bromide is commonly used in California when houses are sold, Alley said. According to the OTA's *Neurotoxicity*, methyl bromide has caused severe neurotoxic effects and death in fumigators, applicators, and structural pest control workers. (Methyl bromide is also effective at destroying the ozone layer—about forty times more so than chlorine, according to scientists reporting the 1992 Montreal Protocol, an international agreement aimed at reducing damage to the ozone layer.)

If you live in apartment, you have less control than in a house. After exposure to a gas leak, Annie Berthold-Bond felt tired and depressed for an entire winter, but things got much worse after the New Haven, Connecticut, apartment in which she and her husband, a Yale graduate student, lived was sprayed with pesticides. Her symptoms—severe headaches, inability to concentrate, lack of strength, extreme anxiety—led her doctor to send her to a mental health clinic. Diagnosed as an "atypical manic depressive," she was hospitalized and put on antidepressants. Finally, the true source of her problems was discovered through testing: the gas and pesticide exposures had made her sensitive to many modern chemicals in her environment. Her immune system was "wildly over-reactive." As described by Donella Meadows, adjunct professor of environmental studies at Dartmouth College, Berthold-Bond reacted to any of the thousands of traps the modern world sets for the chemically sensitive: from chemicals in a campus bulletin board to pesticides in fruit, from poorly tuned car engines to fungicide-soaked swabs in telephone receivers. Now chemically injured, she and her husband cannot live near orchards, farms, power lines, train tracks, golf courses, major highways, or many kinds of businesses. They can't use synthetic fibers or cosmetics. They clean with baking soda and unperfumed soaps. Living in a carefully planned, chemical-free home, Berthold-Bond has become well enough to have a baby, to publish a book, *Clean & Green: The Complete Guide to Nontoxic and Environmentally Safe Housekeeping*, and to publish a magazine, *Green Alternatives*. Like many with EI/MCS, she has a strong urge to warn and help others.

Your pesticide exposures may come through use on lawns—your apartment building's, your neighbor's, or your own. According to the Professional Lawn Care Association, fifty-three million homeowners maintain their own lawns, while nine million hire a lawn-care service. About 40 percent of the nation's lawns are treated with pesticides, with owners using about four to eight times as many chemical pesticides an acre as farmers, in a widening disparity, according to the NAS. The risks of common lawn chemicals have been spelled out by NCAMP: nine of them may be carcinogenic, ten may cause birth defects, three can affect reproduction, nine can damage the liver or kidneys, twenty attack the nervous system, and twenty-nine cause rashes or skin disease. Pesticides, said NCAMP's head Jay Feldman, are defined as "acceptable poisons. But nothing out there is safe," as some have discovered:

- In Florida a two-year-old girl ran barefoot onto grass that had been sprayed an hour before. Within a week she had developed respiratory problems, a rash, and a high temperature. Later her hands and feet swelled, blistered, and peeled. She suffered bad headaches and muscle aches and lost both weight and appetite. "Lawn-care companies have perpetrated a massive con job on the American people. Let's fight the deadly dandelion, they say, even if it means using deadly toxins," says Dr. Epstein.

- One summer night in 1985, a minute or two after Elyse Roberts opened the bedroom window of her northern Illinois home, she shivered and became nauseated and chilled, with sharp shooting pains in her joints and hips. Later, in the hospital, doctors saw her pupils contract to tiny points and monitored her blood-pressure increase, irregular heartbeat, high fever, and decrease in white blood cell count. Fortunately for her, these doctors recognized the symptoms of pesticide poisoning: both that day and that night she had been exposed to nearby lawn spraying with an organophosphate pesticide used for crabgrass control. In intensive care, she was put on an ice mattress and given atropine, the same antidote provided soldiers in the Persian Gulf war six years later. Roberts was lucky. Not only do some doctors not recognize pesticide poisoning, too often "patients aren't told they've been poisoned—but that they're suffering pesticide 'allergies,'" says Lorens Tronêt, board member of NCAMP. Allergies, no. Poisons, yes.

- In a classic case of EI/MCS developing after one acute exposure to 2,4-D, a Midwest suburban woman pushed her children indoors and stood in the doorway of her home on a sunny, breezy spring day in 1989, watching a lawn-care applicator spray her neighbor's property just a few feet away. An hour later she became violently ill, with mental confusion, uncontrollable weeping, acute stomach pains, severe headache, numbness in the left half of her body, muscle twitches, nausea, extreme fatigue, and partial vision. Both the Poison Control Center that she called and her internist said that it sounded like a case of pesticide poisoning but that there was nothing they could do. Advised by her internist to move out of the house for a couple of days, she stayed in a friend's house, but found herself "overpowered" by the smells of fabric softener and printed matter, which she had never before noticed. Back home, she could not tolerate the smell of her leather purse or other familiar objects. In her health club, smells from deodorants and hair sprays left her too weak to work out. As the days went on with little or no improvement, she knew something was radically wrong. When she told her supervisor, he said, "Could this be environmental illness?" He remembered reading about EI in a local paper. Terrified and depressed by her illness, she got the article and called the local EI/MCS support group mentioned in it—a move that she says saved her life.

Sadly, the radical impairment suffered by this last victim is not uncommon to those struck by EI/MCS. At age thirty-three, with a devoted family and ambitious career plans, she saw her life virtually come to a stop. Previously outgoing, healthy, and active with her children and in the community, she was forced to curtail most of her activities. "All was wiped away in ten minutes," she says, with some bitterness. Having been environmentally aware for many years, she found it particularly galling that someone who knew the dangers from formaldehyde in particleboard and who ate additive-free, sugar-free food and avoided caffeine, alcohol, and tobacco would become so sick from her environment. Now, as each day wore on, she got sick and sicker, until by evening, in terrible pain, she could only lie on her sofa, in a fetal position, crying. She had so little energy that she could either take a shower or make dinner, but not both. The household chores—shopping, cleaning, errands—fell to her husband. When he and their children returned home from almost anywhere, they had to shower and change clothes so as to not make her worse.

Life in their community of lovely, green, flat, weed-free lawns and scented fabric softeners became such a nightmare that her husband took a new job and they moved to a mountainside—a spot with few lawns. Somewhat better, she still suffers from residual scents in their rented house. Her husband continues doing laundry and errands, for most laundry products and stores make her sick. He usually cooks dinner and puts their children to bed, for the children's toys and books increase her symptoms. Except for short hikes high up in the mountains, where she regains some of her energy, she is a virtual recluse, with few visitors. The couple's efforts to find a safer house have so far led to nothing.

What do the lawn-care people say about their industry? "The environmental importance of lawns outweighs the very low risk of the products we use," said Barry Troutman, director of education for the Atlanta-based Professional Lawn Care Association, which represents more than a thousand companies. But it's all in how you look at it. "Few humans or animals have become sick or died as a result of weeds," says Dr. Sherman, speaking of the $2.2-billion lawn-care industry that grew 20 percent in a recent decade. The same cannot be said for lawn chemicals. Why expose yourself, your children, your pets? Why take the risk?

Regulation and Testing

The EPA will protect us from unsafe pesticides, right? Contrary to what you may think, EPA registration of a pesticide *does not mean that it is safe*. According to New York Attorney General Robert Abrams, "EPA registration is not a consumer product safety program. It is not intended to determine the safety of the pesticide, but rather indicates that, in EPA's judgment, the benefits justify the risks of use." Benefits to whom? Risks to whom?

In 1972 Congress, concerned that 90 percent of pesticides in use had not been adequately tested for adverse health effects, directed the EPA to reassess the safety of about fifty thousand pesticide products—broken down into six hundred "active" ingredients—registered with the EPA. Incredibly, by 1987 the EPA had completed the reassessment and reregistration of only two active ingredients, according to Congressional testimony reported in "A License to Kill: How the EPA Fails to Protect the Public from Dangerous Pesticides," by *Public Citizen*.

Fortunately for all of us and for our representatives in Washington, Congress's GAO is busy checking up on what the administrative branch of our government is doing or not doing. For some time it has published a series of reports on pesticides with marvelously explicit titles: "Pesticides: EPA's Formidable Task to Assess and Regulate Their Risks "(1986); "Lawn Care Pesticides: Risks Remain Uncertain While Prohibited Safety Claims Continue" (March 1990); "Pesticides: 30 Years Since Silent Spring—Many Longstanding Concerns Remain" (July 1992); "Pesticides: Information Systems Improvements Essential for EPA's Reregistration Efforts" (November 1992); "Lawn-Care Pesticides: Reregistration Falls Further Behind and Exposure Effects Are Uncertain" (April 1993); "Pesticides: Pesticide Reregistration May Not Be Completed Until 2006 (May 1993)." Together, these reports document the continuing failure of the EPA to achieve any comprehensive assessment, much less protection, for Americans at risk. The May 1993 report said that by the end of 1992 EPA had reregistered thirty-one pesticide products out of about twenty thousand such products. (Some companies have withdrawn products because of reluctance to undertake extensive testing.)

In 1990, according to NCAMP, the EPA failed to meet yet another critical deadline in the long process of reassessment, one requiring chemical manufacturers to begin a process of generating health and safety studies. Yet testing by manufacturers, says Dr. Sherman, is in some instances "akin to having Dracula guard the blood bank." As for the toxicity testing that the EPA has already required of pesticide manufacturers, four main things are wrong, says toxicologist Warren Porter: (1) only one pesticide is tested at a time—no mixtures, (2) cancer takes too long to show up, even in rats, (3) neurological, hormonal, and immunological effects are omitted, and (4) the additive effects of multiple exposure routes— skin, food, water, and air—are not considered. Two World Wildlife Fund scientists, Coralie Clement and Theo Colborn, concur. In their 1992 survey of the literature on human exposure to herbicides and fungicides, they say, "We were not able to find daily intake estimates that considered multiple exposure to a number of herbicides and fungicides at one time, as well as information that considered simultaneous exposure via a number of pathways, such as dermal, inhalation, and dietary exposure." Their chief concern: "There must be an assurance that a single low- or/high-dose exposure 'hit' during a critical window of time throughout embryo and fetal development will have no effect on the quality of life and future potential of *in utero* exposed offspring."

Obviously, we do not have that assurance now. And it looks like we'll just have to wait. In the meantime, you are entitled to one free copy of each of the GAO reports: write the GAO at P.O. Box 6015, Gaithersburg, Maryland 20884.

On top of all this delay and inefficiency, in 1978 a leading toxicity testing laboratory, Industrial Bio-Test Laboratories, Inc., was closed after disclosures that thousands of its tests of "high-use" pesticides (and drugs, food additives, soaps, and cosmetics) were faked or improperly conducted. In 1983 three IBT executives were convicted of fraud. The EPA required manufacturers to repeat the invalid IBT tests, which caused part of EPA's delay in reregistering pesticides. One pesticide for which new tests showed tumor-causing potential (while the flawed tests had not) was alachlor, the active ingredient in Lasso, in 1987 the largest selling agricultural pesticide in the U.S., according to the *Hartford Courant*.

No wonder "the general public receives limited and misleading information on pesticide hazards"—the title of a chapter in the GAO's 1986 report on nonagricultural pesticides. According to the Federal Insecticide, Fungicide, and Rodenticide Act (FIFRA), all pesticides sold in interstate commerce must be registered with the EPA (as you have seen, mere registration does not mean that a pesticide is safe). Under FIFRA it is illegal for pesticide manufacturers and distributors to make label claims that are "false or misleading." This includes any statement that a pesticide is "safe" or "nonpoisonous" or "harmless," with or without a qualifying phrase such as "when used as directed." As a matter of fact, EPA's repeatedly stated position is that "no pesticide is 'safe' because pesticides are, by their very nature, designed to be biologically active and kill various kinds of organisms." Yet in a 1992 audit of the EPA's pesticide labeling practices, the agency's own inspector general said that the "EPA cannot provide the public with assurance that precautionary statements on many pesticide labels are adequate to protect humans and the environment from unreasonable adverse effects." It could hardly be put any plainer.

But why, if it is illegal, do you sometimes see claims of pesticide safety on labels or in advertising? One reason is that the EPA seldom acts on false claims by manufacturers or sellers, including those for pesticides. Another reason is that the Federal Trade Commission (FTC), which is empowered to protect consumers against false and deceptive advertising, also rarely acts on false pesticide claims. A third reason is that FIFRA, as amended, does not authorize EPA to control professional applicator safety claims. Hence, when GAO investigators called lawn-care companies to find out what safety information they were giving out, they heard comments like "Our products are practically nontoxic; no one gets sick" and "All [of] our products are legal and registered at EPA as practically nontoxic." In New York, State Attorney General Abrams has taken up some of the slack. He has asked New York State consumers with complaints about fraudulent safety claims to contact his office's Consumer Frauds Bureau or Environmental Protection Bureau.

More statistics on pesticide health effects—or more use of the statistics that are available—are also needed. In his audit, the EPA's inspector general discovered that though adverse health incident reports that the EPA's Office of Pesticide Programs received contained valuable information, the OPP accorded them "little importance." Yet the audit shows that from 1984 to 1991 the EPA received a total of 14,433 incident reports from the National Pesticide Telecommunications Network (1-800-858-7378), a 24-hour hotline that the OPP pays Texas Tech University, in Lubbock, about $825,000 a year to operate. The products causing the most problems are some of the most common home-use pesticides, such as chlorpyrifos, chlordane, diazinon, and malathion. "This may be only a small fraction of the pesticide incidents that occur," said the inspector general.

So-Called Inerts

"Inert" ingredients of pesticides—sometimes more than 99 percent of the pesticide formulation—offer an even murkier story. Though "inerts" may not damage the target organism, they can include such "well-known toxic chemicals as benzene, pentachlorophenol, carbon tetrachloride, asbestos, DDT, formaldehyde, xylene, and hexachlorophene (which contains TCDD, also known as dioxin). . . . Of the [more than] 1,200 chemicals registered as inert, EPA knows 55 to be 'toxicologically significant,' does not know the toxicity of 870, and regards 275 as innocuous." according to chemist Louis Marchi.

"Inerts" do not have to be listed on pesticide labels. Under an obsolete regulation, the identity of such "inerts" in any pesticide product can be kept from the public as "trade secrets" even though manufacturers can now easily find out the inert ingredients in competitors' products. It took four years and a freedom-of-information lawsuit for the Northwest Coalition for Alternatives to Pesticides (NCAP) to get the names of 296 "inerts" that were blacked out on the EPA's list of about 1,450 secret "inert" ingredients. Said Mary O'Brien, a scientist then with NCAP, "You have simply got a basic conflict here, between the chemical industry wanting to keep their pesticide chemicals secret, and the public wanting to know what's in the pesticides that they are exposed to on their food, in their drinking water, on their skin, and in the air."

Yet we do have some general information. Toxic petroleum distillates, like xylene, are used in 10 to 20 percent of all pesticides. Xylene, according to Dr. Marion Moses, helps the skin absorb the active ingredient in the pesticide malathion. Also, unbelievably, hazardous wastes can legally make their way into the inert ingredients in some pesticides, says Peter Montague of the Environmental Research Foundation.

Some have died from the "inerts." In California, Michael London, a twenty-nine-year-old employee of an exterminating company, died suddenly while spraying pesticides in a poorly ventilated crawl space. The coroner ruled that methylene chloride—an "inert" ingredient of the formulation London was using—was the cause of death.

Legal and Political Action

A few municipalities across the country have passed strict pesticide laws. In a landmark decision announced on June 21, 1991, the U.S. Supreme Court said that federal law does not block municipal regulations on the use of pesticides in cases where they are stricter than laws of higher governing bodies. "Local action is warranted because state and federal laws are inadequate," commented NCAMP's Jay Feldman. The "Casey" decision, so-called because it came in a case involving a pesticide ordinance in Casey, a small town in northwestern Wisconsin, was at first thought to open the door to strong local pesticide ordinances, but it is now being undermined by state legislatures "convinced" by pesticide companies to pass laws preempting local control. Legislators easily succumb to the argument that "patchwork" laws are inefficient; yet little is done to promote strong statewide laws.

Strong laws might have prevented several tragic incidents. In 1990 eleven-year-old Kevin Ryan courageously testified before a Senate subcommittee about how neighbors' lawn chemicals made him ill and drastically affected his life. When one of the senators asked, "We wouldn't want to scare people, would we?" Kevin said "No." Later he told an interviewer that after thinking about it, he wished he had said "But we do want to scare people." Kevin and his mother are proceeding with their lawsuit against ChemLawn after it was reinstated in 1991 by a federal appeals court. Though the Ryan family has moved to escape neighbors' lawn spraying, both mother and son can still suffer severe reactions if exposed to pesticides in stores or on playing fields. The court reinstated the suit after the Ryans dropped their request for a federal ban on lawn chemicals, which another judge had considered to be a matter for the EPA, not the courts. In 1988 ChemLawn, the nation's largest lawn care company, lost a $1 million lawsuit to Karen James, a Michigan postal worker who suffered eye and other health damage after she was doused with pesticides from a ChemLawn truck while walking across a lawn.

In a pesticide-related court case, four hundred farmers and growers in twenty states sued Du Pont in 1993, charging that it "knowingly sold a contaminated fungicide that destroyed millions of dollars worth" of fruits, vegetables, and nurseries' flowering bushes. In Georgia, Du Pont settled one such suit out of court for $11.25 million, and in Florida a jury awarded an orchid grower $3 million. Such settlements do little to promote faith in the agricultural chemical industry.

Workplace spraying is a problem for many. In a 1993 case involving four state workers exposed to extensive treatments of their workplace with the pesticide Dursban, the Iowa Supreme Court ruled that a trial court erred in finding "insufficient causation evidence to establish a jury issue simply because there was no epidemiological evidence." The high court relied instead on evidence from doctors who treated the four workers for respiratory and immune problems, brain damage, and fecal and urine incontinence. Said the court, "The best that can be said for epidemiology is that it can prove the risk but cannot prove individual causation. . . . If we were to require epidemiological evidence in all cases of toxic tort injury, we would automatically deny recovery to all claimants who are injured by a toxic substance that is relatively new and as to which a statistical track record has not yet been fully established." In this case, clinical evidence, rather than strict science, prevailed—a definite step forward for the chemically injured. In the words of Dr. Allen Levin, "People who publish papers in medical journals don't see patients, and people who see patients don't publish papers in medical journals."

Minimizing Your Exposure

Yep. "There's no choice: You drink water. You breathe air. You eat food—there's no way to avoid pesticides," said Fumio Matsumura, a toxicologist at Michigan State University's Pesticide Research Center. But you *can* minimize your exposure, and here are some ways to do so.

- Buy a water filter that removes pesticides, preferably from your entire water supply.

- To the extent possible, buy or grow organic (chemically less contaminated) food. What you spend now you'll save later in lowered health-care costs.

- Practice integrated pest management (IPM) in your own home: never use insecticides routinely, only as needed, and then only the least toxic, such as boric acid (try your local health food store or suppliers such as those listed at the end of this chapter)—and after trying all physical methods such as swatting (remember swatting?), practicing better sanitation, and blocking access points. Your health and your children's health are at stake.

- Practice IPM in your yard and garden: use pesticides only as absolutely needed and then only natural, plant-based products (such as Safer or Ringer products or a solution of ordinary dishwashing soap—not detergent) or biological controls—and after trying physical methods like weeding (remember weeding? it's good exercise and gets you outdoors in natural light) and picking off diseased leaves. A healthy soil and well-chosen plants are the best defense against disease and infestation. If you feel that you must have a lawn-care service, beware of "the contract that never expires." Be sure there's a time limit, or you'll be surprised by the sound of motors on your lawn every March, if not earlier.

- If you are chemically sensitive or don't want to be, don't fly to

Antigua, Argentina, Australia, Barbados, Belize, Bolivia, Brazil, Chile, Colombia, Costa Rica, El Salvador, Guam, Guatemala, Jamaica, the Marianas, Mexico, Nicaragua, Panama, Peru, St. Maarten, St. Lucia, or Venezuela. These countries often require cabin spraying with pesticides *before* passengers disembark. Unless you have a letter from your doctor and manage to escape from the cabin, you will be doused while still retained by your seatbelt, according to former flight attendant Diana Fairechild, who wrote *Jet Smart* after she became so chemically sensitive she could no longer fly.

- Especially avoid "deodorant" or "antibacterial" or "antifungal" body soaps or foot powders. They and many underarm deodorants contain pesticides (as broadly defined). Realize that pesticides have silently and subtly been included in many seemingly safe products, often without adequate labeling.

- Whatever commercial product you may decide to use, take the directions seriously. Realize that they don't go far enough. Remember that unnamed "inert" ingredients can be very toxic. And know that a four-year University of Illinois study found that no amount of washing will clean clothes on which undiluted pesticide has been spilled.

- Some states or municipalities have laws requiring lawn-care companies to notify concerned residents before they spray or treat nearby property. If you live in such a state or town, usually you must call the company yourself to request prior notification. Even if you don't, try asking the lawn-care company anyway. If your community sprays routinely for mosquitoes, ask the sprayer to notify you in advance and not to spray your residence and neighboring residences.

- Consider turning all or part of your lawn into a prairie where summer blooms attract butterflies and hummingbirds. Because prairie plants send roots deep into the soil, they need little watering. Or, depending on your climate, consider a rock or cactus garden.

- Realize that most insects are beneficial; resist entomophobia (fear of bugs). Be more frightened of bug-killers. Almost all insects are essential to our survival, says Canadian entomology professor Stuart B. Hill. Only 0.1 percent are "pests." The rest are important to us as pollinators, decomposers, regulators of pests, and food for other beneficial animals like fish and birds.

- Modern lawn care is a recent phenomenon: what did people do before "economic poisons" were invented? Mostly they enjoyed their lawns as is—dandelions and all, ground ivy and all, crabgrass and all. Children and pets could safely roll around on the grass. The "perfect lawn obsession" did not exist; it's a creation of modern lawn-care companies.

To Find Out More

- *Since Silent Spring*, by Frank Graham Jr., Boston, Houghton Mifflin, 1970.

- *Altered Harvest: Agriculture, Genetics, and the Fate of the World's Food Supply*, by Jack Doyle, New York, Viking, 1985.

- *Alternative Agriculture*, by the National Research Council's Committee on the Role of Alternative Farming Methods in Modern Production Agriculture, Washington, D.C., National Academy Press, 1989.

- *Recognition and Management of Pesticide Poisonings*, by Donald P. Morgan, U.S. Environmental Protection Agency, fourth edition (EPA-540/9-88-001), March 1989.

- *Pesticides and Human Health*, by W.H. Hallenbeck and K.M. Cunningham-Burns, New York, Springer-Verlag, 1985.

- *How to Survive in America the Poisoned*, by Lewis Regenstein, revised edition, Washington, D.C., Acropolis Books, 1986.

- *Toxics: Stepping Lightly on the Earth: Everyone's Guide to Toxics in the Home*, Greenpeace, undated booklet with section on pesticides.

- *A Bitter Fog: Herbicides and Human Health*, by Carol Van Strum, San Francisco, Sierra Club Books, 1983.

- *Jet Smart*, by Diana Fairechild, Flyana Rhyme (P.O. Box 300, Makawao, Maui, Hawaii 96768), 1992.

Less-Toxic Pest Control

- *Common-Sense Pest Control: Least-Toxic Solutions for Your Home, Garden, Pets, and Community*, by William Olkowski, Sheila Daar, and Helga Olkowski, Taunton Press (63 S. Main Street, Box 5506, Newtown, Connecticut 06740-5506), 1991.

- *Pest Control for Home and Garden: The Safest and Most Effective Methods for You and the Environment*, by Michael Hansen and the editors of Consumer Reports Books, Yonkers, New York, Consumers Union, 1993.

- *Pest Control You Can Live With: Safe and Effective Ways to Get Rid of Common Household Pests*, by Debra Graff, Earth Stewardship Press (P.O. Box 1316, Sterling, Virginia 22170), 1990.

- *How to Control Garden Pests Without Killing Almost Everything Else*, by Helga and William Olkowski, Rachel Carson Trust for the Living Environment (8940 Jones Mill Road, Chevy Chase, Maryland 20815; 301-652-1877), 1977.

- *Pesticides in Contract Lawn Maintenance*, by Ellen M. Rainer and Cynthia T. French, Rachel Carson Council (8940 Jones Mill Road, Chevy Chase, Maryland 20815; 301-652-1877), 1985.

- *Gardening with Nature: Our Role in a Quality Environment*, by Marjorie J. Smigel and Claire Pike Smith, available from the Rachel Carson Council, 1991.

- *A Chemical-Free Lawn*, by Warren Schultz, Rodale Press (33 E. Minor Street, Emmaus, Pennsylvania 18049; 215-967-5171), 1989.

- *Building a Healthy Lawn*, by Stuart Franklin, Garden Way Publishing (Schoolhouse Road, Pownal, Vermont 05261; 802-823-5811), 1989.

- *Establishing Integrated Pest Management Policies and Programs: A Guide for Public Agencies*, by Mary Louise Flint, Sheila Daar, and Richard Molinar, University of California Statewide Integrated Pest Management Project, 1991; order from IPM Education and Publications, University of California, Davis, California, 95616-8620; 916-752-4162.

Organizations and Publications

- Northwest Coalition for Alternatives to Pesticides (NCAP), P.O. Box 1393, Eugene, Oregon 97440; 503-344-5044; publishes the *Journal of Pesticide Reform.*

- National Coalition Against the Misuse of Pesticides (NCAMP), 701 E Street, SE, Suite 200, Washington, D.C. 20003; 202-543-5450; publishes *Pesticides and You.*

- New York Coalition for Alternatives to Pesticides (NYCAP), P.O. Box 6005, Albany, New York 12206; 518-426-8246 or 9331; publishes *NYCAP News.*

- Rachel Carson Council, 8940 Jones Mill Road, Chevy Chase, Maryland 20815; 301-652-1877; publishes various newsletter and brochures. Also at this address is the Audubon Naturalist Society of the Central Atlantic States, which has published a folder called "Have a healthy lawn without using toxics."

- Agricultural Resources Center/PESTicide EDucation project, 115 West Main Street, Carrboro, North Carolina 27510; 919-967-1886; publishes *PESTed NEWS.*

- Bio-Integral Resource Center (BIRC), P.O. Box 7414, Berkeley, California 94707; 510-524-2567; publishes *The IPM Practitioner*, the *Common Sense Pest Control Quarterly*, and a catalog called "Least-Toxic Pest Management."

- The American Defender Network, Box 911, Lake Zurich, Illinois 60047; 708-381-1975; publishes fact sheets on lawn chemicals, mosquito control, and pyrethrums.

- Environmental Health Coalition, 1844 Third Avenue, San Diego, California 92101; 619-235-0281; publishes *Toxinformer* and fact sheets and sponsors a project called School Pesticide Use Reduction (SPUR).

- International Institute of Research for Chemical Hypersensitivity, 6200 #C, Topia Drive, Malibu, California, 90265; publishes *Informed Consent*, whose Jan/Feb 1994 issue has a long article on the airplane spraying problem.

Catalogs and Suppliers

- Gardens Alive! Natural Gardening and Research Center, Box 149, Sunman, Indiana 47041; 812-623-4201.

- Safer Natural Plant and Pet Care Products, Oakmont, 44 Oak Street, Newton Upper Falls, Massachusetts 02164; 1-800-447-2229.

- Ringer Natural Lawn & Garden Products, 9959 Valley View Road, Eden Prairie, Minnesota 55344-3585; 1-800-654-1047 (ask for information about a natural pesticide from the neem tree).

- EcoSafe Products, Inc., P.O. Box 1177, St. Augustine, Florida 32085; 1-800-274-7387.

- Bio-Control, Box 337, Berry Creek, California 95916.

- Biological Control, Route 5, Jackson, New Jersey 08527.

- Unique Insect Control, 5504 Sperry Drive, Citrus Heights, California 95621.

- TRIK-O, Box 170, Canutillo, Texas 70853 (specializing in the trichogramma wasp, a microscopic parasite that eats certain plant-eating pests).

- Biological Urban Gardening Services (BUGS), P.O. Box 76, Citrus Heights, California 95611; 916-726-5377; publishes a newsletter and a catalog for the organic landscape industry.

Useful Phone Numbers

- U.S. Environmental Protection Agency's Office of Pesticide Programs: 703-305-5805.

- National Pesticide Telecommunications Network: 1-800-858-7378 (or 800-858-PEST) is a toll-free telephone service at Texas Tech University Health Sciences Center, School of Medicine, Department of Preventive Medicine and Community Health, Lubbock, Texas 79430. Funded by the EPA and Texas Tech, the service provides information on pesticide products, toxicology, and health effects; on recognition and management of pesticide poisonings; on clean-up and disposal; and on emergency treatment.

1-800-858-PEST: keep this number handy.

* * * *

A Pesticide Postscript

The following is taken (with permission) from "Why No One Can Say 'Pesticides Are Safe'," by Mary H. O'Brien, *former editor of the* Journal of Pesticide Reform. *Data documentation is available from NCAP, P.O. Box 1393, Eugene, Oregon 97440.*

A pesticide may kill more than the pest. Less than one out of a thousand kinds of insects are pests, yet most insecticides kill many kinds of insects, including those that help control the pest species. Soil organisms account for half by weight of all living matter on earth, yet the effects of pesticides on soil organisms may be the least-researched area of pest control.

A pesticide may remain a long time in the environment. Pesticides can accumulate over the years in soil or pond bottoms, to be taken up later by plants or released by soil organisms to poison further. The half-life of the organochlorine pesticide toxaphene is fifteen years in soil, meaning that fifteen years after it is applied, one-half of the pesticide will remain in the soil.

A pesticide may travel far. Pesticides may travel via air, soil, water, dust, or organisms, coming down in rain or snow. Organochlorine pesticides are stored in the fat of animals and then accumulate in the bodies of other animals or humans who eat them.

A pesticide may turn into another poison. Parathion becomes another compound four times more toxic when it contacts oxygen.

A pesticide may become more poisonous in the presence of other chemicals. This effect is called "synergism." Nonpesticide chemicals can also interact with pesticides. The toxicity of malathion is greatly increased by a common industrial plasticizer, TOTP, even when malathion exposure occurs two weeks following the use of TOTP.

A pesticide may poison by methods entirely different from those intended. Since most pesticides are designed to kill pests quickly, their long-term effects on humans, such as cancer, genetic damage, and birth defects, are all unintended side effects.

Pesticide damage may show up long after the pesticide has left the body. For example, the phenoxy herbicide 2,4-D is rapidly eliminated from the body, but cases are known in which individuals briefly exposed to 2,4-D on their skin developed nerve damage in their arms and legs several weeks later.

A pesticide may be dangerous even if all label directions are followed. For this reason, in the U.S it is illegal to print a label that claims a pesticide is "safe" or "harmless." With pesticides manufactured by, formulated by, or exported into developing countries, the uncertainities multiply. And even if accurately labeled when shipped, a pesticide may be repackaged later in a way that fails to protect handlers and users.

A pesticide may cause damage that was never investigated before it was registered or was not discovered during toxicological testing. In the U.S., almost all pesticides are conditionally registered, which means that not all required tests have been completed and reviewed before the products are allowed on the market. In addition, studies of certain pesticide effects, such as those on children and other especially vulnerable groups, or effects on the body's immune system, are not required and are almost never done. Thus countries whose pesticide regulatory schemes have relied on U.S. data also have inadequately-tested pesticides on the market.

8

Factory Food

WHAT DO CHEMICALS have to do with food? A lot, apart from the fact that everything we eat is composed of chemicals. The tidal wave of new chemicals—most petrochemically based—that washed across the United States in the twentieth century did not bypass food. Since World War II hundreds, if not thousands, of new chemicals have been added to our food, intentionally and unintentionally. Here are just a few, taken from labels of a seasoning mix, a carbonated beverage, and salt: hydrolyzed soy protein extract, sodium stearoyl-2-lactylate, aspartame, sodium silico-aluminate. You can be sure that none of these was put into food a hundred years ago. Some, like the hydrolyzed soy protein, are benign, unless you are sensitive to soy products or monosodium glutamate (MSG). To these add pesticides, dyes, flavorings, preservatives, fluoride in drinking water, sulfites in wine and beer, chemicals leached from packaging, even industrial chemicals contaminating tanker trucks that carry food. Now we hear about fat substitutes, irradiated produce, and "designer" (genetically engineered) food.

What has happened to the pure, natural, unadulterated food our parents and grandparents enjoyed? In nineteenth-century rural America, people grew their own food or walked, market basket on arm, to the local grocery store, where pickles were in barrels, flour was in bins, and the butcher cut up chickens while shoppers watched. Unsanitary? Maybe, though perhaps not more than now, when foodborne illnesses, some caused by bacteria such as salmonella in carelessly handled meat, are on the rise. With the twentieth-century migration to the cities, away from family farms and gardens, and with the speeding up of our lives has come a reliance on prepared, processed foods. Our marvelous, envied, gleaming supermarkets are bulging with brightly packaged edibles. We pride ourselves on having, year round, an abundant variety of convenient, presumably sanitized products.

In recent decades, more and more women have entered the workforce but remained the main food preparers. Those of us who are harried wives or single mothers often find ourselves rushing to crowded supermarkets on the way home from work to buy the box that says "only ten minutes to fix." Or on Saturdays we stock up on stacks of TV and Kraft dinners, anticipating the busy week to come. Convenience, cost, and new taste thrills have become all-important; as for nutrition, the vibrant colors of the foods on the boxes and in the ads must mean lots of vitamins and minerals. Sensing our wishes, if not our real needs, manufacturers have eagerly stepped in to give us food that is easier to fix, less likely to spoil, available whenever we want it, more highly processed, and obviously further removed from its natural source.

But what unfortunate trade-off have we made? All these conveniences have come with a chemical price tag. If you feel exhausted, or headachy, or "spacy" after an hour or so in a huge supermarket, you may be reacting to poorly ventilated indoor air, filled with outgassed chemical molecules from pesticides, from printer's ink on packages, from chicken broiler combustion products, from bakery products that activate your grain sensitivities, and from the VOCs in the cleaning products that produce those gleaming floors. To discover that modern packaging is not airtight, you need only walk down a supermarket detergent aisle to realize that potent invisible particles are escaping from detergent and fabric-softener packages. What does that imply for the packaged food lining the shelves, to say nothing of the disposal of all those packages?

More important, what has happened to the nutrients in, say, the produce in the supermarket bins? A 1993 comparison of nutrient levels found that, ounce for ounce, organic pears, apples, potatoes, wheat, and sweet corn had more than twice the amount of twenty-two essential nutrients found in comparable commercial produce. The fruits and vegetables in health food stores may not look as uniform and shiny and may cost more, but they are likely to give you more nutrition for your money.

What to Avoid

Writers daring to step into the thickets of modern nutritional theories take the risk of being accused of "nutribabble," as writer Anne Mendelson so aptly put it. "I see dozens of cookbooks and hundreds of articles a year purporting to tackle nutritional issues, and the amount of just plain bunk is staggering," she says. The average person ends up totally confused: oat bran is great; then oat bran isn't so great. Coffee is bad for the heart; coffee is OK after all. Don't eat eggs; but a leading heart surgeon eats eggs. Avoid cholesterol; yet the body needs cholesterol and makes it. Switch to margarine for your heart; avoid margarine because of the trans fatty acids it contains. Alcoholic beverages in moderation are good for the heart and help prevent colds; but don't drink if you are pregnant. "Every day I read something different about food," you say. "Why can't scientists make up their minds?"

Actually, ever since World War II, scientists, particularly biochemists, have been discovering a great deal about the body, how it functions, and what it needs. Much is confusing and much remains to be learned. Still, a few things are becoming clear, and there are a few answers to the question we face every day, What to eat? One answer has to do with what should be subtracted from your diet, the other with what should be added to your diet. Subtraction means avoidance—of as many toxic chemicals as possible. Most are synthetic, devised by chemists in laboratories. Let's follow the production trail of our modern food supply.

On the Farm

On U.S. farms, animals are heavily treated with antibiotics, hormones, and veterinary medicines, in 1987 totaling about two thousand active ingredients, according to Americans for Safe Food (ASF), a branch of the nonprofit, consumer-oriented Center for Science in the Public Interest (CSPI). The government, says ASF, lacks "adequate methods to detect residues of 70 percent of the twenty thousand to thirty thousand animal drugs [many containing identical active ingredients] in use today—residues that can appear in meat, milk, or eggs."

Many of these drugs are used illegally. In 1984, 95 percent of the veterinarians surveyed by an animal health magazine admitted using chloramphenicol, an antibiotic banned for meat animals in 1968 because it had been found capable of causing a fatal blood disorder in humans. Some milk and pigs tested in 1986 had illegal levels of residues of permitted sulfa drugs. Cattle in feedlots often are implanted with legal growth-inducing hormone pellets but at illegal places on the animal's body or at double the recommended dose, according to ASF. By 1992 things were no better: the GAO stated that "although FDA intended that extra-label uses under its policy would be rare, several veterinarians who treat dairy cows told GAO that 40 to 85 percent of their dairy cow prescriptions are for extra-label uses."

Almost half of all antibiotics produced in the U.S. are used on animals. And this practice has caused problems in people. Several well-conducted studies have traced human salmonellosis to resistant bacteria in meat from antibiotic-treated animals, according to Beatrice Trum Hunter, food editor of *Consumers' Research*. Also, consumers can "unwittingly develop resistance to antibiotics in the milk they drink, on top of the antibiotics they're ingesting with beef and poultry," warns a 1989 *Wall Street Journal* article headlined "Milk Is Found Tainted with a Range of Drugs Farmers Give Cattle." Suspecting that milk processors and regulators were not testing milk thoroughly enough, both the *WSJ* and CSPI did their own surveys in 1989, with screening for drug residues conducted by Rutgers University scientists. CSPI found that 20 percent of twenty off-the-shelf, randomly selected samples were tainted with sulfa drugs, including sulfamethazine, legal at that time but suspected of causing cancer. The *WSJ* found 38 percent of its fifty retail samples contaminated with illegal residues of sulfamethazine, other sulfa drugs, or antibiotics.

Penicillin, found in these surveys, can cause allergic reactions in wary or unwary milk drinkers. What has happened to pure, wholesome milk, long considered safe and long promoted as essential for all ages? Predictably, a lobbyist for the milk and ice cream industries attempted to rebut the surveys: "I still think milk is the safest product we have." (What does this say for all other foods?)

Also predictably, the FDA, the agency responsible for protecting the interstate food supply and public health, could still assert that the American food supply is the safest in the world, though at least one of its employees disagrees. According to Joseph Settepani, an FDA scientist, the currently narrow scope of testing leaves much milk contaminated with unknown levels of animal drug residues that have not been shown to be safe. Nor, according to Alexander Apostolou, director of toxicology for the Center for Veterinary Medicine, does the FDA always look out for the public health: "Deference to the drug sponsor sometimes results in uncritical acceptance of sponsor claims."

Meanwhile, more and more stores stock beef and other meat from producers like Melvin Coleman, of southern Colorado, Mary Lou Bradley, of Childress, Texas, Barbara MacArthur, of north central Illinois, and John and Merrill Clark, of southwestern Michigan, all of whom produce drug-free beef called, respectively, "Coleman Natural Beef," "B3R Beef," "Strathmore Farms" beef, and "Roseland Farms" beef (the latter two farms do not use pesticides). According to the *Wall Street Journal*, sales of Coleman Natural Beef rose about 20 percent after the publicizing of a European Community ban on the importation of hormone-treated beef.

Crops on U.S. farms are heavily sprayed with pesticides, the most feared and most publicized food contaminant. Pesticides are, after all, biocidal poisons, designed to kill living organisms. More than a billion pounds a year, containing over six hundred active ingredients registered with the EPA (which does not mean they are safe), are sprayed on U.S. crops. Yet FDA scientists in their 1989 annual survey of pesticide contamination found "no pesticide residues at all, or residues well within safe limits, in 99 percent of the domestic foods and 96 percent of the imported foods," according to *Chemecology*, a Chemical Manufacturers Association magazine. Similar assurances have been given in subsequent annual surveys. Another FDA study, called the Total Diet Study, found pesticide and other chemical contaminants "well within standards set by the

United Nations Food and Agriculture Organization, the World Health Organization, and the U.S. EPA," also according to *Chemecology*.

No need to worry, right? Wrong. Consider these statements:

- "Between 1982 and 1985, the FDA detected pesticide residues in 48 percent of more than two dozen frequently consumed fruits and vegetables. However, [the] FDA's analytical methods detect only about one-half of the pesticides that contaminate fruits and vegetables," according to the OTA's 1990 book on neurotoxicity.

- "Sixty-nine different pesticides linked to cancer are legally allowed on food, thirty-two of these are not detectable by FDA's routine monitoring methods, and thirty carcinogens are among 118 pesticides found in food by the FDA in their 1988 food monitoring," warned the U.S. Public Interest Research Group (US-PIRG).

- "Only about 1 percent of all food shipments are tested for illegal residues. In about half the cases in which food is found to contain illegal residues, the food has been sold before the results are back from the lab," according to ASF.

- "Placing your trust in the FDA's monitoring of (pesticide) residues is a lot like standing in a downpour holding a teacup over your head; you have no way of capturing all that's coming at you," says Dr. Richard Jackson, California's chief of communicable disease control and a member of the NAS's pesticides panel.

- California investigators found, under that state's Birth Defects Prevention Act, that "EPA has reached wrong safety conclusions on as many as 58 of 99 pesticides reviewed," according to epidemiologist Samuel Epstein and NCAMP's Jay Feldman.

- David Steinman, reviewing the FDA's Total Diet Studies for 1983 to 1986 in his 1990 book *Diet for a Poisoned Planet*, found that "common lettuce, for instance, had thirty-six [pesticide] residues in sixteen samples. This means that, on the average, each of the sixteen samples of lettuce analyzed had between two and three pesticide residues in it. The study also listed the

different kinds of pesticides found. In lettuce there were nine."
Says Steinman, "I'm not trying to alarm people. I'm trying to inform them to make healthful choices."

Healthful choices are hard to come by in our supermarkets, particularly in winter. According to the OTA, much produce "has been
imported from developing countries where farmers use pesticides
manufactured in the U.S. that have been banned, severely restricted,
or never registered for use here." Such pesticides now account for
about 25 percent of all U.S. pesticide exports and provide approximately one-half of the pesticides imported in most Latin American
countries. One organization, OTA reports, estimates that 70 percent of the pesticides exported to developing countries are used on
crops grown for export to industrialized countries. Also, "the FDA
is not sure which countries are using which chemicals, so they don't
know what to test for," said ASF in its discussion of this "circle of
poison." Government action has been equivocal: a few days before
the end of his term, President Jimmy Carter issued an executive
order which put controls on exports of substances that were banned
or severely restricted in the U.S. Several days after Ronald Reagan
became President, however, he revoked the order.

Thus current federal law permits the circle of poison, and because of inadequate FDA and USDA staffing and limited detection
technology, the extent of such poisoning of our food is largely unknown. At least one case, however, has been well documented.
Chlordane, a pesticide, was banned in the U.S. after it was established as causing cancer and affecting the nervous system. At least
twice in 1988 chlordane-contaminated Honduran beef was imported and eaten by people in Florida, Kentucky, and Minnesota
before the beef was analyzed. In one such instance, the chlordane
residue was reported to be eight times the approved tolerance. Apparently the pesticide got on the cattle from the spraying of nearby
sugarcane. Crop spraying, both abroad and in the U.S., is often
done by poorly trained or illiterate workers who are uninformed
about procedures and hazards and who thus unwittingly endanger
their own health as well as the health of those who eat the sprayed
food.

Consumers have suffered also. In 1985 more than a thousand

people from California to Canada developed twitching muscles or blurred vision or went into shock after eating watermelons laced with aldicarb, a pesticide not approved for such fruits. Just a little slip-up.

How can pesticides affect our nervous systems? In the mid-1970s workers at a Virginia plant manufacturing a chlorinated hydrocarbon insecticide marketed as Kepone developed "disabling neurological symptoms . . . characterized by tremors, muscle weakness, slurred speech, [and] lack of coordination." Biochemical similarities exist between the insect and human nervous systems. What is bad for bugs can be bad for us as well. Yet at present, only one class of pesticides—the organophosphates, accounting in 1984–1989 for only three out of fifty-four new active ingredients—is mandated to be tested for neurotoxic effects.

Finally, many pesticides are applied merely to improve the appearance of fruits and vegetables—an overuse causing increasing concern among public health officials worldwide. Those beautiful, uniform pyramids of produce in your supermarket may be blemish-free but they are not pesticide-free.

In the Food Factories

Most farm-grown foods, except for those sold at roadside stands and increasingly popular farmers' markets, are trucked to factories, where they are subjected to as many as three thousand direct additives (including preservatives, waxes, emulsifiers, and thickening, leavening, bleaching, and anti-caking agents) and many times that number in indirect additives such as solvents, resins, and other processing aids and packaging components. Animals go to packinghouses, to be subject to some of the same contaminants. Some additives are introduced to make food products look and taste better, some to make food products behave better. Most have nothing to do with nutritional value, but are used for other purposes, says Ruth Winter, author of *A Consumer's Dictionary of Food Additives*: namely, to feed our illusions. Lemon-flavored candy is dyed yellow to evoke the idea of a real (but absent) lemon; milkshakes are artificially thickened to heighten our feeling of richness and satisfaction; meat sauces come with "smoke flavoring," to provide the illusion that our dinner is fresh off the fire.

Three kinds of additives appear routinely in our food, just to entice us: sweeteners, colors, and flavors and flavor enhancers. Today, an estimated hundred million Americans regularly ingest aspartame, marketed under the trade names NutraSweet and Equal. Used extensively in diet soft drinks, this low-calorie sweetener is also in thousands of food products, from cocoa mix to cereal, chewing gum to chewable vitamins. It is available in bulk packs for institutional use. In this country, aspartame has largely replaced saccharin, another artificial sweetener whose widespread presence in food generated such health concerns that it is used only rarely today. The manufacturer, in petitioning for approval of aspartame, submitted extensive toxicological studies of both animals and humans. The FDA's protracted review, punctuated by legal actions, took so long that the company threatened to sue the FDA. In 1981, after eight and one-half years, the FDA finally approved aspartame, but with the provision for a review of consumer complaints. Since then the agency has been inundated with more complaints against this additive than about any other in its history. As a result, in 1985 the FDA began its Adverse Reaction Monitoring System: health professionals are requested to report adverse reactions to any food or food additive.

Not all experts agree on the safety of aspartame. The August 1, 1985, *Congressional Record* contains a statement by former FDA toxicologist M. Adrian Gross that the aspartame manufacturer's studies "to establish the safety of aspartame are to a large extent unreliable . . . at least one of those studies has established beyond any reasonable doubt that aspartame is capable of inducing brain tumors in experimental animals and that this predisposition . . . is of extremely high significance." In 1987, at a Senate hearing on aspartame, Jacqueline Verrett, another former FDA toxicologist and author of *Eating May Be Hazardous to Your Health*, called the original aspartame studies "flawed" and said that they "should have been thrown out from day one."

Despite its own assurances, the FDA in 1990 reported a total of 5,338 aspartame-related complaints. The most common complaint was headaches. There were 276 reports of vision problems (including four cases of blindness), 250 of seizures and convulsions, and a host of other reactions, including hearing loss, tinnitus, coma, depression, mood swings, difficulty breathing, anxiety attacks, loss of limb control, numbness of extremities, slurred speech, insomnia, muscle spasms, gastrointestinal and bladder disorders, nausea, loss of taste, rashes, hives, and menstrual problems. Five deaths were attributed to aspartame use. In St. Louis, Anthony Kulczycki, associate professor of medicine at Washington University School of Medicine, in one year heard from 173 people who alleged adverse reactions to aspartame: "Of 75 cases who suspected that their chronic hives might be related to NutraSweet, two-thirds ended their symptoms by avoiding NutraSweet."

Many more incidents have probably gone unreported, says psychiatrist Theodore E. TePas, "either because the patients never reported the symptoms to their doctors or because the doctors were informed but did not bother to file a complaint." Indeed, aspartame complaints have been declining, from six hundred to seven hundred per year in the early 1980s to about three hundred in 1992. Nevertheless, having connected his own earaches to his consumption of a popular diet soft drink, Dr. TePas thinks that aspartame should now be tested as a new drug, not as just a food additive.

Dyes add attractive color to much of our food. Under FD&C (food, drug, and cosmetic) designations, you can find synthetic dyes in many processed foods, as well as in drugs and cosmetics; just read the labels. In 1976 the FDA reported that "95 to 99 percent of children eat some food containing coal-tar (petroleum-derived) food dyes; over four million children will have consumed a total of more than one pound of coal-tar-based food dyes by the time they are twelve years old, and the maximum consumption of food dyes by children is as high as three pounds by age twelve." Yet the consumer-oriented PCHRG views these figures as quite conservative since there has been a 50 percent increase in the total use of food dyes in the past ten years.

Fortunately, of twenty-four food dyes once allowed in our food, seventeen are now banned. But progress has been slow. Here's the story of a single dye, FD&C Red no. 3. In 1977, eight years after studies showed that FD&C Red no. 3 causes thyroid cancer in rats, Ralph Nader's group, Public Citizen, filed the first of four lawsuits to get the FDA to take the dye off the market. In January 1990—thirteen years later—the FDA finally banned this dye as an additive in products where the color is mixed chemically with another additive—as in such products as cake mixes, lipsticks, hand lotions, shampoos, chewing gum, cough drops, and some processed fruits and juices.

Inexplicably, however, FD&C Red no. 3 can still be added to meat, nut products, candy, breakfast cereals, ingested drugs, and some fruit and fruit juices. The rationale, according to Dr. Louis Sullivan, the Bush administration's secretary of the Department of Health and Human Services (HHS), is that "the actual risk posed by FD&C Red no. 3 is extremely small." And according to the FDA, the risk of cancer from a lifetime of consuming the dye is no larger than one in a hundred thousand. Though the FDA compares this risk favorably with the risks from natural disasters and car or plane accidents, it is yet another risk to be added to your total of risks from pesticides and other toxic chemicals in your environment. And cancer is not the only risk from dyes: FD&C Red no. 3 (erythrosine) can cause chromosome damage, and FD&C Yellow no. 6 (tartrazine) can cause severe allergic reactions, according to PCHRG. Natural disasters usually cannot be avoided, but FD&C Red no. 3? Under the risk/benefit safety-evaluation system used by the FDA and EPA, who is getting the benefits? Who is bearing the risks?

Synthetic flavors raise similar questions. Virtually all processed foods are artificially flavored, according to Bill Wasz, principal flavor chemist at Fries & Fries, one of the nation's largest flavor producers. "Canned green beans contain flavorings. And cigarettes are one to two and one-half percent flavor," he says.

The reason? "In processing food to get it into the form people want or to make it safe, flavor is processed out," says Bob Pellegrino, general manager of the same flavoring company. Thus a $750-million-a-year industry was created to put flavor back in. When you buy processed food—the food in cans, bottles, and boxes—in the supermarket, then, you are paying to have the flavor taken out of your food and paying to have it put back in. Yet, ironically, in a topsy-turvy world, unadulterated food often costs more than adulterated. Or companies charge more for foods with reduced fat and calories. And you won't know what flavoring chemicals you are eating or giving your children, for synthetic flavorings may be listed on labels simply as "flavorings" without identifying their chemical compositions. There are too many flavor ingredients, say the flavor producers, to list each one.

The FDA regulates flavorings as food additives, according to Ruth Weisheit, supervisor of consumer affairs at the FDA's Cincinnati office: "Any new flavorings or new uses of a flavoring agent would require FDA testing to make sure [they are] safe." But how safe is the flavor enhancer MSG, monosodium glutamate? This ubiquitous food additive became notorious for what was erroneously dubbed "Chinese restaurant syndrome," a misleading term since MSG is hardly limited to Chinese food. Developed in its modern form in 1908 by a Japanese chemist, MSG was eagerly adopted as a "miracle substance" by U.S. food producers in the late 1940s. In the 1990s it is difficult to find a processed food without MSG, which is "a poison to many people who are sensitive to its effects," says Dr. George R. Schwartz, specialist in emergency medicine and author of *In Bad Taste: the MSG Syndrome.*

A study done by a Harvard medical school researcher found that almost 30 percent of 1,529 surveyed people reacted to MSG, with such symptoms as headache, dizziness, diarrhea, nausea, abdominal pain, visual disturbances, fatigue, shortness of breath, and weakness: "Many people had emotional reactions ranging from depression or insomnia to feeling 'tense.' " Severe, life-threatening asthma attacks after ingestion of MSG have also been reported. "Many asthma sufferers are seen in emergency rooms," says Dr. Schwartz. "How many of these cases are precipitated by MSG has never been analyzed. Rarely are patients with asthma told to avoid MSG or change their diet."

Avoiding MSG is not easy. About a hundred million pounds a year are used by the $280 billion-a-year food industry, in such products as canned soups, bouillons, potato chips, canned meats and tuna, salad dressings, frozen and microwave meals, diet foods, and pizzas, according to the November 3, 1991, "60 Minutes" segment on MSG. (Before the show was aired, the food industry launched an extensive public-relations campaign to try to blunt its effect on sales.) When MSG is only a percentage of a processed-food ingredient, it may or may not be listed on the product label as MSG. Hence it can be hidden in processed foods under other words. If you buy any processed foods, look for these names on the label (they may indicate the presence of MSG): hydrolyzed vegetable protein (HVP), hydrolyzed plant protein (HPP), textured protein, sodium caseinate, calcium caseinate, autolyzed yeast, yeast extract, yeast nutrient, malt extract, barley malt, bouillon, broth, stock, flavoring, natural flavorings, and natural beef/chicken/pork flavoring, gourmet powder, Chinese seasoning, Kombu extract, and PL-50. If you suffer any of the symptoms of MSG syndrome, try to avoid this hidden danger.

The FDA estimates that less than 2 percent of the population suffers MSG's adverse health effects, but that translates to almost five million people. And food producers continue to use it. After all, "the addition of MSG allows [them] to use less product to get the desired taste," says Jack Samuels, an MSG sufferer who has worked since 1988 to get the FDA to require more accurate labeling of MSG. In 1993 he was still trying, while the FDA continued to drag its heels. At least the FDA spokesperson on "60 Minutes" promised that MSG will be some day be listed on labels whenever it is present in another food ingredient in a "significant and functioning level as a flavor enhancer." And enhancing flavor, by stimulating our taste buds and nerves, is all that it does; MSG has no food value whatsoever.

To further enhance the shelf appeal of their products, food processors rely on externals like waxes and colorful, elaborate packaging. Waxes are applied to fruits and vegetables to make them look better as well as retain moisture. Whether derived from petroleum, plants, or insects, the waxes can contain added dyes and fungicides and can trap pesticides applied to the produce. Among these fungicides, considered safe by the FDA at the levels used, are Benomyl and sodium orthophenyl phenate, both suspected to be human carcinogens, and orthophenyl phenol, considered an immune-system suppressant. Though federal law requires retailers to notify customers if produce has been waxed, most do not, citing confusion over labeling requirements. Until the law is enforced or clarified, avoid waxed produce by buying organic or shopping at roadside stands or farmers' markets.

As many as ten thousand components go into modern packaging. Most of these components, such as plastics, were unknown a hundred years ago. Today their health effects are mostly unknown, despite warning signals such as illness resulting from, for example, heated polyvinyl chloride film used by supermarket workers to wrap meat. Plastics, like PVC, are made from gases, some of which get trapped in the plastic and outgas gradually into air and food. Styrene, for instance, known to affect the skin, eyes, and respiratory and nervous systems, has been found carcinogenic to laboratory animals. Also known to affect the earth's ozone layer, styrene is still in common use in fast-food restaurants, for supermarket meats, and as a cushioning filler to protect packaged objects. When used as a container for acid drinks, such as hot tea with lemon, it can disintegrate and leach into the liquid. Once again, old-fashioned, time-tested products, like glass (which is inert), cellophane, and plain, unprinted paper or parchment, are the safest. Whenever possible, avoid packaging that is derived from petroleum, like plastic wrap. Transfer foods into safer containers and wraps.

Alcoholic beverages can be sources of unwanted chemicals, not all of them strictly "additives." In 1985 the Canadian government found possibly dangerous levels of urethane in sixty brands of wine and liquor, some imported from the U.S. Urethane, a colorless, odorless substance, forms naturally during the manufacture of certain alcoholic beverages. It causes cancer in animals. In 1987 the FDA negotiated an agreement with U.S. whiskey manufacturers to reduce urethane levels in their products to below 125 parts per billion by 1989; but the CSPI criticized the FDA for moving too slowly and settling for a dangerously high level. CSPI argues that, as with so many substances, "science has not proved that urethane *does not* cause cancer in humans. In a typical standoff, the FDA and the beverage industry maintain that no one has proved that it does."

You, the consumer, may wish to make informed choices. It is of interest to know that studies conducted before 1988 found that brandies, sherries, bourbons, liqueurs, and port—in that order—had the highest levels of urethane; and beer, vodka, gin, rum, and blended whiskeys the lowest. Wines are also low in urethane, though many wines sold in the U.S. contain lead in quantities far above the amount allowed for drinking water. Imported wines generally contain more lead than domestic wines, with the impurity coming in part from lead foil capsules covering corks. Thanks to CSPI's lobbying efforts, wine bottle labels now state the presence of added sulfites. However, no wine, even organic wine, is completely free of sulfites, since some occur naturally during processing, according to French-born Veronique Raskin, organizer of a group called the California Organic Wine Alliance, which sets standards for organic wines.

En Route

Once food leaves the factory, it is transported to distributors, to grocery stores, and finally to you. Is it safe en route? Not on your life! Many food-grade liquids, for example, are transported in trucks and tanker ships that previously carried toxic chemicals, often without adequate cleaning procedures between trips. This practice is known as back-loading, and it is one more way to increase our own chemical burden.

In 1987 the FDA's Center for Food Safety and Applied Nutrition met with a Canadian tanker company to discuss the contamination of coconut and palm oils with styrene aboard the company's tankers. The company said that the practice of using the same onboard tanks for edible oils following their use for styrene and other industrial chemicals began about twenty-five years earlier and was widespread and expanding. In 1989, three truck drivers from Washington State went to the federal office of the FDA to complain about lax hauling and inspection procedures for tanker trucks. The drivers said that they "crisscrossed the country for two years hauling juices, kosher oils, and bulk food-grade liquids in tankers that also carried chemicals." These drivers blame some food companies, for poor tank inspection; some trucking companies, for lying about what was previously carried in their tanks; and some drivers, who, they say, "will lie, cheat, do just about anything for a few more hours of work."

Other drivers carry contaminated liquids unknowingly. One couple, Jim and Rikki Pomerenke, of Yakima, Washington, after emptying their tanker trailer of what they had been told was a water-based resin, carried fourteen food loads—including kosher canola, soya, and palm oils; whiskey; apple, cranberry, and grape juices; orange and grape concentrates; and non-food-grade molasses destined for cattle feed—before discovering that their earlier load was really a synthetic resin used to develop images on carbonless copy paper. The resin, a toxic substance known as alkylphenol novolac, coated the inside of their tanker with a hardened, non-water-soluble film that eventually had to be scraped out with razor blades. No one knows how much of it got into the foods. Says Rikki Pomerenke of their experience, "I thought that with the testing food shippers did, if the load was contaminated they would be able to tell. That's not true. All they are testing for is a bacteria count. And it only takes one person who might have been allergic to that resin or whatever it was. . . ."

Transport by truck can present another hidden trap for people with food allergies: even if the tank carries only foods, one load may contaminate another with food allergens. If corn oil is still present in a tank as a residue, for example, it can get into a new shipment of soy oil. The corn-sensitive person may then react to the soy oil without knowing why. Thus do still more chemicals or other unwanted contaminants get into our food supply as it makes its way from the farm through the factories to your kitchen.

Overextended, Underfunded, and Shackled

What *is* the FDA doing about these chemicals? Is it protecting us?

Under the Amended Federal Food, Drug, and Cosmetic Act, only drugs are required to be tested on humans. Food, including additives, and cosmetics are not, though some experts feel they should be subject to the same scrutiny as drugs—the additives especially, as the average American consumes about five pounds of food additives a year. Instead, usually based on animal testing only (or sometimes on absent or inadequate testing), additives approved by the FDA appear on its GRAS (Generally Recognized As Safe) list. Though the FDA annually reviews the safety data of about eighty food additives, it does little neurotoxicity testing. As with pesticides, the burden of proof of additive safety rests with the producer, subject to review by the FDA. Once marketed, food additives, unlike drugs, have, until recently, rarely been tracked for adverse consumer reactions—until deaths have resulted, as they have with sulfiting agents.

For food additives the FDA has instituted a concept known as the *de minimus* rule: a known carcinogenic additive is all right if it inflicts cancer on only one person in a million. This stratagem bypasses the only "zero tolerance" standard for carcinogens in U.S. law, the Delaney Clause, a 1958 amendment to the Federal Food, Drug, and Cosmetic Act that prohibited the use of any additive in processed foods that, after appropriate tests, was shown to cause cancer in animals or humans. It's not hard to imagine what companies favored the new standard, which was also accepted by the EPA. Part of the EPA's problem is that it has had two conflicting rules: Delaney and FIFRA. FIFRA permits farmers to use carcinogenic compounds that do not pose an "unreasonable risk" to consumers (but who is doing the reasoning?).

This dilemma appeared resolved, at least for the moment, in late 1992, when an appeals court ruled that the EPA must ban any cancer-causing pesticides that leave residues in food (pesticides are the additives that most people worry about). After the U.S. Supreme Court upheld that decision in 1993, EPA Administrator Carol Browner released a list of thirty-five pesticides that would potentially be banned under Delaney's requirements. The three agencies that regulate food pesticide levels—the FDA, the EPA, and the U.S. Department of Agriculture (USDA)—pledged to work together to reduce the use of pesticides. It was a good start. Perhaps these three agencies had got wind of the about-to-be-publicized five-year NAS study, released in July 1993, which found that infants and children might be "uniquely sensitive" to pesticides on food. Though the report recommended that children go on eating fruits and vegetables for their food value, it also recommended changes in the three agencies' policies.

Did the regulatory agencies know about a report released by the Washington, D.C.-based Environmental Working Group just a month earlier? That group analyzed pesticide data from two different sources: 14,595 produce samples taken by the FDA, plus 4,500 taken by a private testing laboratory hired by supermarkets. The former data revealed 108 different pesticides on just twenty-two fruits and vegetables: 42 different pesticides on tomatoes, 38 different pesticides on strawberries, and 34 different pesticides on apples. The latter data revealed two or more pesticides on 62 percent of the oranges tested, 44 percent of the apples, and from one-quarter to one-third of cherry, peach, strawberry, celery, pear, and grape samples. The group's startling conclusion: when cancer risks from just eight pesticides on twenty fruits and vegetables are added together, the average child exceeds the EPA lifetime one-in-a-million risk standard by his or her first birthday.

In September 1993 the Clinton administration presented Congress with a plan to reduce the use of the most dangerous pesticides and to encourage organic farming, but at the expense of the Delaney Clause—an unfortunate trade-off. If health is really the most important concern, why not retain Delaney, expand it to include nonprocessed food such as produce, and ban weed-killers like atrazine, the nation's largest selling herbicide, one known to cause cancer in animals and to contaminate groundwater?

Another reason for retaining Delaney is the FDA's inability to regulate properly. In 1991 a blue-ribbon advisory panel convened by Dr. Sullivan reported that the FDA is too swamped to do its job right, with problems so severe that they pose a potential threat to public health. The FDA is "overextended, underfunded, and shackled by bureaucratic constraints." Its Washington-area facilities, termed "pathetic" by the panel, are scattered among thirty-two buildings, including a converted chicken coop and converted bathrooms and freezers. While about twenty-five cents of every dollar you spend goes for items regulated by the FDA, the FDA is apparently not getting enough dollars to do the regulating it should be doing—a good reason to do your own grocery-aisle research. If it turns out that Delaney is not retained, then, according to epidemiologist Samuel Epstein, we must try to get pesticides content added to labels. We know how much cholesterol we are getting, why not pesticides?

Another of the FDA's major responsibilities is labeling. In October 1990 Congress passed a new labeling law, the Nutrition Labeling and Education Act, requiring the FDA to clarify labels and give more information to the public. The NLEA requires comprehensive nutrition labeling on most packaged foods and in point-of-purchase displays for the most commonly consumed fruits, vegetables, and raw fish. It restricts health claims on labels to those commonly accepted by scientists and requires the FDA to define such terms as "light" (or "lite"), "low sodium," and "low fat." Products regulated by the USDA—meat, poultry, and eggs—will undergo similar changes. Also, according to the CSPI, this law does not cover food advertising, which is regulated by the FTC. "Only about one-third of all food advertisements contain nutrition or health information," said a CSPI spokesperson, "and practically all of this information is incomplete or misleading." This, too, is to be tightened, by the FTC.

President Bush's 1990 appointee to head the FDA, Dr. David A. Kessler, who was retained by President Clinton, vowed in 1991 to crack down on label violations. Early in his tenure he tackled misleading claims of "no cholesterol" on foods containing high levels of fat, and "fresh" on processed foods. "A fresh product is not a commercially processed product," said Dr. Kessler. "My grandmother knows that, the food industry knows that, the FDA knows that."

In November 1991 the FDA unveiled its proposed new labeling rules, designed to implement Congress's intent: "misleading stuff is going off the label," proclaimed Dr. Kessler. Subject to revision after consumer and industry groups presented their objections, the changes required to be in effect by May 1994 on an estimated three hundred thousand food labels are intended to help consumers tell at a glance the level of fat, sodium, calories, cholesterol, sugars, protein, and fiber in more than eighty thousand types of food on supermarket shelves. Labels can include only nine terms—"free," "less," "more," "low," "high," "fresh," "light (or lite)," "source of," and "reduced"—and they must be well defined. Only four health claims—those based on what the FDA deems sufficient scientific evidence—are allowed: claims for relationships between calcium and osteoporosis, sodium and hypertension, fat and cardiovascular disease, and fat and cancer. Also, if a product makes a health claim but has an unhealthful quality, that quality has to be noted on the label. While most label changes are mandatory, labeling is to be at first voluntary on produce, fish, and meat. At first all uncooked products were to have new safety labels (with handling and cooking instructions) by October 15, 1993. But after losing a lawsuit claiming "not enough time," the USDA in March 1994 extended the deadlines and announced new rules.

Some commentators foresee interesting consequences from this "truth-in-packaging." "It's very hard to describe a product fairly and accurately and still make it saleable," says Tom Pirko, a Los Angeles food and beverage consultant. And from Bob Messenger, editor-in-chief of *Food Business* magazine, "With a lot of these products, when the shingle of health and nutrition is taken off, there's nothing there. It's a nothing product. A lot of these products aren't going to qualify for any health claims under the new rules. And they don't have any taste." Indirect pressure may thus force manufacturers to upgrade the quality of food products. The emperor needs some clothes.

Interestingly, no such industry crisis ensued when California voters approved Proposition 65, which required labels to warn of cancer or reproductive dangers. Despite industry's dire predictions of labeling chaos, "manufacturers are quietly complying with the law by either reducing or eliminating toxic chemicals," according to Illinois state representative Jan Schakowsky. For example, ten days before Proposition 65 went into effect, "all food cans containing lead solder disappeared from grocery shelves," she says. "These cans are the single largest source of dietary lead, a known reproductive toxin." Industry, it would seem, does respond to the subtle pressures of better labeling, in this case by phasing out lead soldering of food cans.

Meanwhile, the FDA has *phased in*, without mandatory labelling, a genetically engineered, "recombinant" growth hormone—bovine growth hormone (rBGH), also known as bovine somatotropin (BST). In 1988 the European Economic Community banned the use of hormones to promote livestock growth and in the following year banned imports of hormone-treated beef. Following the opposite path, the FDA in 1991 tentatively concluded that rBGH can safely be used to increase milk production in cows, with no ill effects to humans—an economic boon to some large milk producers, perhaps, though not to small family farms, especially marginal ones trying to survive in an already milk-glutted market.

However, veterinarian Richard Burroughs, formerly in charge of the FDA's review of rBGH, claims that he was fired (in 1989) because he "pointed to important flaws in the [producing] companies' safety studies that his superiors had overlooked in their eagerness to approve rBGH. 'It used to be that we had a review process at the FDA,' he said. 'Now we have an approval process.'" In 1991 Burroughs was ordered reinstated by the Agency's Merit Protection Board—a small victory for scientific objectivity.

In 1993 enterprising freshman Senator Russell Feingold (D-WI) inserted a ban on rBGH into the Senate version of President Clinton's first budget bill, on the basis that boosting milk production would force the government to spend more money on milk price supports. When the bill became law, a temporary ban on the sale of rBGH went into effect. In November 1993, however, the FDA pronounced rBGH safe for cows and people, opening the way for its commercial use, unlabeled, in milk. Environmentalists fear human health effects; an end result of using rBGH could be premature growth and breast stimulation in infants and breast cancer in adults, according to Dr. Epstein. Another predicted result is increased mastitis in cows, necessitating increased use of antibiotics, which are in turn passed on to consumers in milk. Opposition to rBGH centers on the lack of labels, and rightly so: why can't our consent to this latest additive at least be informed?

Once again, powerful forces are trying to rush us into a techfix without fully considering its far-reaching effects—on human and animal health and on people's livelihoods. The same is true of irradiation. Dr. George Tritsch, a cancer researcher at Roswell Park Memorial Institute in New York, thinks the evidence shows that irradiation causes the formation of mutagens and carcinogens in food. "It's much too short a time to start seeing the effects now. People who started smoking in their teens may not get lung cancer for thirty or forty years," he says. But while you wait for the possible health effects of modern technology to show up, you can learn to avoid *some* of the modern chemicals in our food—primarily by avoiding processed foods as much as possible and by reading the fine print on available labels.

Where to Turn

When it comes to choosing healthy food, how confidently can we rely on the government to tell us what to eat? For decades the USDA has been advising us about diet. Yet a 1993 GAO report says that the government information on food is flawed and unreliable, with most data provided by industry on a voluntary basis. Long beholden to the food industry, the USDA is overseen by Congressional agriculture committees. Of these committees, former Assistant Secretary of Agriculture Carol Foreman, who served under former President Jimmy Carter, said, "When it comes to food safety and nutrition, the agriculture committees are country lanes down which public-health provisions are lured and quietly strangled."

By now almost everyone over the age of six has heard of the four basic food groups, long touted by the USDA: meat and meat substitutes; dairy products; grains; and fruits and vegetables (the latter now separated by the USDA, to make five). For decades, this oversimplified approach has been mainstream nutrition's standard recommendation. Nationwide, conscientious meal planners built countless menus around the four food groups. If you didn't include all four in each meal, you weren't doing right by your family, your customers, or those dependent on your dietary acuity.

Then, with all the hue and cry over the need to reduce fat, cholesterol, and sugar, in 1991 the USDA devised its "Eating Right Pyramid," which gave greater emphasis to grains, fruits, and vegetables than to meat and dairy products, and even less to fat and sweets. Shortly after the pyramid was announced, however, then-USDA-Secretary Edward Madigan withdrew it from distribution, a decision, according to *Consumer Reports*, that was influenced by affected segments of the food industry. A year later, after spending $855,000 to survey the eating public, Madigan unveiled a remarkably similar pyramid, renamed the "Food Guide Pyramid." How could the average consumer be anything but confused?

Government dietary advice, then, is flawed, politically influenced, and simplistic. There's far more to good nutrition than four, five, or a whole pyramid of food groups. Can you turn to your doctor for advice on diet? Doctors are taught little about nutrition in medical school. Out of 125 medical schools in the U.S., only 30 have a required nutrition course. The average physician receives less than three hours of nutrition training in medical schools. At a meeting of the American Medical Women's Association, one doctor drew "knowing laughs" when she commented on her lack of medical training in nutrition: "They had one lecture—on a Saturday morning—and it wasn't compulsory. I don't remember what was in the lecture, because I didn't go." But awareness is finally creeping in. Early in 1994 the Food and Nutrition Board of the NAS's Institute of Medicine said that nutrition, even though it is largely ignored, is the most effective way to prevent and treat chronic diseases.

Fortunately, some doctors have educated themselves about nutrition and its relationship to health. Psychiatrist Melvyn R. Werbach has published three books reviewing clinical research on the relationship of nutrition to health—*Nutritional Influences on Illness; Supplemental Chapters: Nutritional Influences on Illness;* and *Nutritional Influences on Mental Illness.* These books are intended primarily for health professionals, to acquaint them with the latest research in nutrition and health. Ask your doctors if they know about them.

Another progressive physician, Leo Galland, author of *Superimmunity for Kids,* believes that "children have a remarkable ability to heal themselves; doctors and medication do not prevent or cure disease. When a child is given an antibiotic for an infection, you may think it is the antibiotic that cures the infection. It isn't. It is the child's immune system. . . . *The key to a strong, healthy immune system is optimal nutrition.*" Unfortunately, he says, American children today get most of their calories from sugar, processed cereal grains such as wheat and corn, processed oils, dairy products, and fatty meats. Several of these foods—sugar and the hydrogenated oils in margarine—he considers "antinutrients," together with excessive salt and phosphates; pesticides; and "free radicals." Free radicals, compounds formed in the body when cells use oxygen, damage cell membranes and destroy essential nutrients. To combat them, we need adequate supplies of vitamins A, C, E, B-2, and B-3 (antioxidants), as well as the minerals zinc, copper, manganese, and sulfur, says Galland.

In *The Kellogg Report: The Impact of Nutrition, Environment & Lifestyle on the Health of Americans,* Joseph Beasley, MD, and Jerry Swift point out that to date, fifty essential nutrients for human beings are known. We need some, like the five major nutrients—protein, carbohydrate, fat, water, and fiber—in relatively large amounts. Others—minerals and vitamins—we need in smaller amounts, though for optimal nutrition we need more of these micronutrients than the recommended dietary allowances (RDAs). (With the new food labeling terminology, "RDAs" will probably be replaced by "RDIs"—Reference Daily Intakes—and "DRVs"—Daily Reference Values.) Often the recommended amounts merely prevent deficiency diseases like scurvy.

What relationship is there between food and health? "The chronic diseases—both social and medical—are really symptoms of a much more vast underlying problem," say Beasley and Swift. "They are the final culmination of years of inadequate nutrition, a toxic environment, sedentary lifestyles, familial and social disruptions, and dependence on artificial agents (from cigarettes to cocaine) for happiness. Every cell in our bodies—from the brain to immune system—is affected by these abuses. The effects are particularly devastating in developing children—both in and out of the womb." With food, the stakes are high. In addition to the links between diet and chronic illnesses, nutrition can affect human behavior and personality. Animal studies have found that eating causes characteristic changes in brain composition, and studies of humans have found ample evidence of hypochondriasis, depression, and hysteria following deprivation of certain vitamins.

About chemical exposures, Beasley and Swift argue that "the more contaminated one's environment or the more reactive one is, the better one's nourishment should be to head off potential chronic illness down the road." To these observers, most of us are suffering from both toxicity *and* malnutrition—results of the vast technological changes of the nineteenth and twentieth centuries that have put toxins in our air, water, soil, and food, while at the same time removing nutrients by means of the practices used in growing, transporting, storing, cooking, and refining our foods.

Sugar is a good example. In *A Diet for Living*, Dr. Jean Mayer wrote that sugar is a new food: "It didn't exist in the West until the seventeenth century. And the argument that sugar is an essential food is a lot of nonsense." In fact, refining of raw cane sugar into white sugar removes most (93 percent) of the ash, and with it go the trace elements necessary for the metabolism of the sugar: 93 percent of the chromium, 89 percent of the manganese, 98 percent of the cobalt, 83 percent of the copper, 98 percent of the zinc, and 98 percent of the magnesium. These essential elements are in the residue molasses, which is fed to cattle. No wonder the USDA puts sweets at the top of the food pyramid—meaning that they should be eaten sparingly.

Yet by 1977, the average American was eating 137.8 pounds of sugar and other sweeteners every year—a 33 percent rise in per capita consumption since the beginning of the century. By 1989 more than half of that total had been replaced by corn sweeteners (labeled under such names as high-fructose corn syrup, dextrose, dextrin, glucose, polydextrose, mannitol, and sorbitol). But even these "alternative" sweeteners present another health trap for many: corn allergy—or sensitivity, depending on your definition—is one of the most common food allergies in the U.S. today.

What to Eat

That is the question—the one we all face every day. You've seen what to avoid. But what should you choose? What should you eat in order to be as healthy as possible? The answer is not easy: ideas change, fads are rampant, diet books come and go, and myths abound. Mainstream nutrition advises first one thing, and then another.

The myths are mostly oversimplifications, whereas nutrition is a "complex, evolving science, with many areas that are still poorly understood," according to Beatrice Trum Hunter. Wholesale generalizations linking diet to health must certainly be viewed with skepticism: the U.S. Surgeon General said in 1988, "Definitive proof that specific dietary factors are responsible for specific chronic disease conditions is difficult—and may not be possible—to obtain, given the available technology." Adds Hunter, "It is time for Americans to challenge both the official dietary recommendations as well as the advertising claims about various components of food. . . . At stake is not only one's pocketbook, but also one's health." And the bottom line for health is nutrients. In all the hype about new taste thrills, exciting cuisines, low-calorie sweeteners, and bright colorings, we forget the self-evident truth that we eat for one reason only—to obtain the nutrients we need to nourish our cells, to sustain ourselves, to survive. But beyond mere survival, we need *opti-*

mal nutrition—the maximum amount of the essential nutrients required to maintain good health.

Views of health professionals like Drs. Werbach, Galland, and Beasley form the basis for the Nutrition for Optimal Health Association (NOHA), an unusual, nonprofit Chicago-area organization devoted to sound nutrition education. Founded in 1972, the group was originally inspired by biochemist Roger J. Williams's *Nutrition Against Disease*. NOHA presents its dietary recommendations in a handy one-page "bull's-eye," which places foods in five rings based solely on nutrient density. In the center are the most nutrient-dense foods: naturally raised poultry; fresh fish; wild game; fresh fruit and vegetables; raw nuts and seeds; dried beans and legumes; plain yogurt; whole grains as well as nutritious nongrains like buckwheat, amaranth, and quinoa. Around the outside are the foods with the fewest nutrients (some of these may directly cause specific health problems, says NOHA): most sweeteners, including brown sugar and honey; chocolate and cocoa; coffee; hydrogenated fats and tropical oils; foods containing synthetic sweeteners, colors, or flavors; dairy substitutes; fried snack foods such as potato chips; and most "commercial" (processed, or factory-made) cereals, cookies, cakes, pies, sausages, bacon, hot dogs, and luncheon meats. For a copy of this convenient chart, send $2 to NOHA, P.O. Box 380, Winnetka, Illinois 60093.

One specific health problem that both physicians and patients have found to be related to food is migraine and other headaches. In England, Dr. Jean Monro has conducted several studies of headache patients. "Without exception," she says, "if we investigated long enough, and extensively enough, we found foods that triggered symptoms." These were not the foods traditionally thought to cause headaches—chocolate, alcohol, and cheeses—but common, frequently eaten foods like wheat and dairy products, and also tea, oranges, apples, onions, pork, and beef. Her patients were usually able to reduce their reactivity by avoiding suspect foods, by ridding their environment of molds, house plants, tobacco smoke, petroleum-based products, gas appliances, and other triggering factors; and by following a rotation diet (rotating means not repeating any food until your body has gotten rid of it, usually for four days).

The rotation diet, because it provides nutrient variety as well as nutrient density, can be healthful for everyone, including people with food allergies. Dr. Alan R. Gaby, research director of Baltimore-based Consumers for Nutrition Action, believes that "millions of Americans suffer from unrecognized food allergies, which can cause [or worsen] a wide range of physical and emotional disorders," from infantile colic, Crohn's disease, and depression to arthritis. Another health benefit, cited by the *New York Times*: "A more varied diet lessens the risk of a buildup of any single pesticide." And because cravings for particular foods tend to disappear on the rotation diet, it is a good way to lose weight and to maintain weight loss. Katy Lebbing, of Villa Park, Illinois, was never able to keep her weight down until she was diagnosed with wheat allergy. Then, on a wheat-free diet, she lost fifty-one pounds in six months and has kept them off. Both of Lebbing's parents had had alcoholic tendencies; with wheat, she had satisfied her addictive needs with a socially acceptable food, wheat. In fact, Dr. Randolph, who recommends the rotation diet to his patients with food sensitivities, believes that alcoholism is really a form of grain addiction and that alcoholics need to stay off whatever grain they are allergic/addicted to in addition to staying off alcohol.

Ours is a grain-based society. Living without grains—and that means not just wheat, but oats, barley, rye, rice, millet, and corn—is unthinkable to most of us (imagine breakfast without any grains!). Yet our ancestors did, and they were healthy. Dr. S. Boyd Eaton, a Harvard Medical School graduate now practicing medicine and teaching anthropology at Emory University in Atlanta, reminds us that our genetic makeup hasn't changed much since the first modern humans. Our Stone Age ancestors did not suffer from the "chronic degenerative diseases, such as heart disease and strokes, and cancer of the lung or colon, [that] kill 75 percent of Americans today," he says. Also, the hunter-gatherers (mostly before the development of modern agriculture, though some exist today in primitive societies) were tall, relatively healthy, and good athletes. With the coming of grain-centered agriculture, people ate less protein and average heights dropped, to rise again with the reinstatement of animal proteins in the modern diet, which, however, lacks the vitamin and mineral content of our ancestors' diet.

Similarly, English scientists Michael and Sheilagh Crawford concluded, after extensive research in Africa, that our modern diets have become highly deficient in structural fats, which are needed *inside* every cell in our bodies, especially in our brains and arteries. "Invisible" structural fats are made in animals' bodies from polyunsaturated fatty acids in soft, liquid vegetable oils. The chemically different fats that plague many of us today are the storage fats that lodge visibly in our bodies, making them bulge and adding to our weight. Storage fats are made from visible animal fats and from sugar, starch, and protein eaten in excess. Hence the maxim "eat as close to nature as possible": avoid processed and obviously fatty foods in favor of the kinds of fibrous, naturally oil-rich plant foods that African wild game eat—and the lean wild game itself. A tip: in evaluating processed foods in their laboratories, the Crawfords found that homemade chicken soup contained "ten times the amount of structural fats as [the] chicken soup from a packet or a tin." Grandma was on the right track, after all.

What to eat? Buy and use NOHA's bulls-eye, rotate as many of your foods as you can, make your own chicken soup . . . and consider adding supplements to your diet.

Supplements

On the question of whether to add vitamin, mineral, and other supplements to our food intake, research psychologist Bernard Rimland has some persuasive arguments favoring them. He warns that essential nutrients are often missing in modern food. Soils have become depleted, he reports; some oranges grown on such soils contain zero vitamin C. Prescription drugs can damage nutrients, and pesticides compete in the body for valuable vitamins and minerals. A study of Californians revealed that one-third of them eat no vegetables and two-thirds no salad, with only a half eating one serving of fruit a day. So much for the conventional advice, which says "get your vitamins and minerals from food, not supplements."

Are vitamins safe? For the years 1983 to 1990, Poison Control Center data reveal this contrast: deaths from prescription drugs, 2,556; deaths from vitamins, 0. Rimland's advice: the RDAs for minerals are "adequate" for healthy people; but for vitamins, the RDAs are "absurd." It has been demonstrated that "generous amounts" of vitamins may help prevent certain conditions. After all, Rimland says, "many people have been exposed to Legionnaires' disease and AIDS, yet only a few exposed get these illnesses. The immune system depends on adequate amounts of vitamins and minerals." Supporting this assertion, a long-term University of California at Berkeley study found that a daily multivitamin and a good diet may delay the onset of AIDS in people infected with the HIV virus. A house-to-house vitamin distribution program in Cuba halted a mysterious epidemic that sickened more than fifty thousand people in 1993. Interestingly, Rimland cites a report by the research division of the NAS revealing that the more courses nutritionists and physicians take, the more likely they are to use supplements. Doesn't this tell us something? We would all be well-advised to take supplements, particularly vitamins—in addition to, not instead of, a healthy diet, of course.

Are vitamins and other supplements effective? Here are several of the scientific studies that suggest a "yes" answer. In 1991 Harvard University researchers found a significant reduction in heart attacks associated with both beta carotene from fruits and vegetables and vitamin E taken as a food supplement. A study of 120,000 men and women reported in *NEJM* found that those who consumed 100 international units of vitamin E a day developed coronary heart disease at a rate 40 percent less than those consuming low levels of vitamin E. A five-year study by American researchers in China found that daily doses of beta carotene, vitamin E, and selenium reduced cancer deaths by 13 percent.

Taking supplements is becoming mainstream. In January 1992 the magazine *Consumer Reports*, relied on by millions, said that many scientists have "jumped ship" from the medical and health establishment's position that supplements are unnecessary. "Popping pills has become part of [the scientists'] own daily routine" as they become aware of the "mounting evidence that certain vitamins and other nutrients may offer protection against cancer, cataracts, Parkinson's disease and other disorders." Said one scientist who takes a daily regimen of vitamins C and E, beta-carotene, and a multivitamin tablet, "I'm not sure it does any good, but I'm certainly not sure that it doesn't." On April 6, 1992, that bellwether of American culture, the *Time* magazine cover, blazoned the words "The

Real Power of Vitamins: New research shows they may help fight cancer, heart disease, and the ravages of aging." The April 25, 1993, *New York Times Magazine* "Good Health" issue, riding off in both directions, cautioned against easy solutions, such as antioxidant vitamins A, C, and E, for the cellular damage caused by free radicals, but recommended eating lots of leafy green and yellow vegetables to get those vitamins and other protective nutrients.

The Alliance for Aging Research says that every day healthy adults should take 250–1,000 milligrams of vitamin C (the equivalent of fifteen oranges or twenty-five green peppers); 100–400 international units of vitamin E (vs. one half to two cups of sunflower oil or six to twenty-four cups of almonds); 17,000–50,000 international units of beta carotene, a precursor of vitamin A (vs. five carrots or six cups of butternut squash). Though experts differ, Jeffrey Blumberg, chief of the antioxidant research laboratory at the USDA Human Nutrition Research Center on Aging, in Boston, says "We have the confidence that these things really do work."

Yet despite increasing evidence of the benefits of supplements, in 1992 Kessler's FDA—alarmed by their increasing use and skeptical as the FDA has always been about them—launched a campaign of harassment of health food stores and even some alternative doctors who use injections of vitamins, minerals, and amino acids to build up patients' immune systems. In Texas, state health inspectors raided health food stores and removed such products as vitamin C, aloe vera, and herbal teas. In Kent, Washington, FDA agents accompanied by local police pointing guns kicked down the door of Dr. Jonathan Wright's alternative medicine clinic and seized equipment as well as many nutritional supplements. The FDA appears ready to re-classify as drugs all vitamins and minerals in dosages over the RDA—subjecting natural, unpatentable products to prohibitively expensive testing, which will result in expensive, prescription-only products that many patients will be unable to afford. And in December 1993, attempting to curb what it considers label abuses, the FDA announced new regulations that will force dietary supplements to live up to the same standards as foods. Prior approval will be required for health claims on supplement bottles, in catalogs, or implied by a product's name.

Label accuracy is desirable, but so is freedom of choice. In response to the FDA's implied and real threats to that freedom, Jon Carroll, of the *San Francisco Chronicle*, writes: "In these tight budgetary times, it seems to me that people who believe claims that the aging process can be reversed and eternal life is a possibility should be allowed to spend their money any way they want, particularly when they're spending it on stuff that might actually do them some good. . . . People are taking vitamins and remaining alive. Perhaps they are spending their money foolishly, but spending money foolishly is the backbone of our nation's economy. Cosmetics! Car phones! Chewing tobacco! Running shoes! Vitamins are actually good for you, which is more than you can say for anything made by Estee Lauder."

Eating Wisely

What, then, are you to make of this complex, vital, controversial, emotionally loaded subject called "food"? What should you eat and how should you prepare it? How can you work toward your own personal optimal health? Tired of conflicting advice, many Americans have retreated from the better eating habits they adopted in the 1980s, according to a Harris poll cited by Dr. Todd Davis, of the American Medical Association. But if you are one who wants your diet to improve your health, here are a few suggestions:

- Avoid processed foods whenever possible. Eating "close to nature" doesn't mean you have to live in a cave; it only means choosing more of such foods as, for example, nuts and seeds— plain, undyed, untreated, without coatings or seasonings to make them "taste better." It means making your own chicken soup in large batches from unsprayed ingredients, and freezing leftovers in glass jars. If you're musing "I don't have time," think instead of how important your health is to you. You'll find time if you have a strong incentive.

- Seek out organic food. Shop at health food stores or at the new chains, such as Whole Foods Market and Fresh Fields, popping up around the country, selling organic and exotic produce and unusual grains like spelt and kamut. If their food costs more than that in supermarkets, remember that it probably contains more nutrients.

- Be sure to ask whether such stores spray their stores with pesticides.

- Grow your own produce. Unfortunately, in a world so pervaded by pesticides, "organic" really means only "chemically less contaminated."

- Beware of supermarkets. Shop the walls, with their fresh, refrigerated, and frozen basics—not the aisles, with their rows of enticingly packaged, long-shelf-life, factory-produced food. Remember that you want a long life instead.

- Read labels carefully. Check the fine print in the ingredients list. Avoid foods you think you are allergic to (often those you crave most!). Watch out for disguised ingredients; even with the new food labeling law, you may still find "casein" instead of milk, or "dextrose" instead of corn. Avoid foods containing synthetic sweeteners, colorings, and flavorings; and any chemical, like propylene glycol, that sounds as if it belongs in your car's radiator. Even common preservatives like the synthetic antioxidants BHT, BHA, and TBHQ are petrochemically based. If it doesn't sound like food, it probably isn't.

- Never buy irradiated or genetically engineered food. Realize that you are being treated as a guinea pig.

- Vary your foods. Even if you don't follow a strict rotation diet, you'll have a better chance of obtaining essential trace elements, and you may discover new taste treats. Try unusual, delicious foods now becoming available, like starfruit; Asian pears; taro; daikon; jicama; amaranth and buckwheat (alternatives to grain); spelt and teff (rare grains). Put lovely, edible nasturtium flowers in your next salad.

- Read as much as you can. Much has been written on the subject of safe, healthful nutrition; one source leads to another, and soon you'll become familiar with what to avoid and what to eat. Also, you will learn to separate the reliable from the unreliable.

- Cook foods simply. Some, such as fruits, need not be cooked at all.

- Experience or re-experience the wonderful taste of raw, natural, unprocessed food. Is there anything more delicious than an unsprayed, unsweetened, sun-ripened, juicy red strawberry in June? Or a crisp, aromatic apple fresh from an unsprayed tree in the fall? Or plain, organic almonds—toasted or untoasted? Don't worry: your taste buds are not yet too jaded for such treats.

* * * *

To Find Out More

- *The Driving Force: Food, Evolution, and the Future*, by Michael Crawford and David Marsh, New York, Harper & Row, 1989.

- *Dr. Wright's Guide to Healing with Nutrition*, by Jonathan V. Wright, MD, Emmaus, Pennsylvania, Rodale Press, 1984.

- *Superimmunity for Kids*, by Leo Galland, MD, New York, E. P. Dutton, 1988.

- *Prescription for Nutritional Healing*, by James F. Balch, MD, and Phyllis A. Balch, CNC, Garden City Park, New York, Avery Publishing Group, 1990.

- *Nutritional Influences on Illness: A Sourcebook of Clinical Research*, by Melvyn R. Werbach, MD, New Caanan, Connecticut, Keats Publishing, 1988.

- *Supplemental Chapters: Nutritional Influences on Illness*, by Melvyn R. Werbach, MD, Tarzana, California, Third-Line Press, 1993.

- *Nutritional Influences on Mental Illness: A Sourcebook of Clinical Research*, by Melvyn R. Werbach, MD, Tarzana, California, Third-Line Press, 1991.

- *Food—Your Miracle Medicine*, by Jean Carper, New York, Harper Collins, 1993.

- *The Balanced Body Secret: Nutrition and a Woman's Chemistry*, by Nancy Appleton, Cambridge, Massachusetts, Rudra Press, 1991 (four audio tapes and a workbook).

- *Super Nutrition for Women*, by Ann Louise Gittleman, New York, Bantam, 1991.

- *Sugar and Sweeteners: Making Safe and Healthy Choices*, by Beatrice Trum Hunter (completely revised and updated), Pownal, Vermont, Storey Communications, 1989.

- *Fats and Oils*, by Udo Erasmus, Vancouver, Canada, Alive Books, 1986.

- *A Consumer's Dictionary of Food Additives: Definitions for the Layman of Ingredients Harmful and Desirable Found in Packaged Foods, with Complete Information for the Consumer*, third revised edition, by Ruth Winter, New York, Crown Publishers, 1989.

- *Aspartame (NutraSweet): Is It Safe?*, by H.J. Roberts, MD, Philadelphia, The Charles Press, 1990.

- *Bittersweet Aspartame: A Diet Delusion*, by Barbara Alexander Mullarkey, Oak Park, Illinois, NutriVoice, 1992.

- *Diet for a Poisoned Planet*, by David Steinman, New York, Harmony Books, 1990.

- *Pesticide Alert: A Guide to Pesticides on Fruits and Vegetables*, by Lawrie Mott and Karen Snyder, San Francisco, Sierra Club, 1987.

- *Environmental Poisons in Our Food*, by J. Gordon Millichap, MD, Chicago, PNB Publishers, 1993.

- *Safe Food: Eating Wisely in a Risky World*, by Michael Jacobson, Lisa Lefferts, and Anne Witte Garland, Washington, D.C., Center for Science in the Public Interest, 1991.

- *How to Grow More Vegetables Than You Ever Thought Possible on Less Land Than You Can Imagine*, by John Jeavons, Ten Speed Press, Berkeley, California, 1991 (revised edition).

- *The New Organic Grower*, by Eliot Coleman, Post Mills, Vermont, Chelsea Green, 1989.

- *Rodale's All-New Encyclopedia of Organic Gardening*, Emmaus, Pennsylvania, Rodale Press, 1992.

- *The Allergy Self-help Cookbook*, by Marjorie Hurt Jones, RN, Emmaus, Pennsylvania, Rodale Press, 1984.

- *Dr. Mandell's Allergy-Free Cookbook*, by Fran Gare Mandell, New York, Pocket Books, 1981.

- *The Yeast Connection Cookbook: A Guide to Good Nutrition and Better Health*, by William G. Crook, MD, and Marjorie Hurt Jones, RN, Jackson, Tennessee, Professional Books, 1989.

- "Enjoy Nutritious Variety: The Rotation Diet," by Marjorie Fisher, Winnetka, Illinois, Nutrition for Optimal Health Association, 1980.

Some Organizations and Newsletters

- Mothers and Others/Parents and Others for Pesticide Limits, Natural Resources Defense Council, Box 96641, Washington, D.C. 20090.

- Americans for Safe Food, Center for Science in the Public Interest, 1875 Connecticut Avenue, N.W., Suite 300, Washington, D.C. 20009; 202–332-9110 (can supply list of organic food mail-order suppliers).

- Food & Water, Inc., Depot Hill Road, R.R. 1, Box 114, Marshfield, Vermont 05658; 1–800-EAT-SAFE; publishes *Safe Food News*.

- MSG Sensitivity Institute, P.O. Box 961, Concord, New Hampshire 03302–0961; publishes *The MSG Healthline*.

- The Feingold Association, P.O. Box 6550, Alexandria, Virginia 22306; 703–768-FAUS; publishes a newsletter, *Pure Facts*, about the relationship of diet to learning disabilities and hyperactivity.

- Natural Food Associates, P.O. Box 210, Atlanta, Texas 75551; 903–796-3612; publishes a magazine, *Natural Food & Farming*.

- *Mastering Food Allergies*, published by Marjorie Hurt Jones, RN, 2615 N. Fourth Street, #616, Coeur D'Alene, Idaho 83814.

- *The Felix Letter: a commentary on nutrition*, published by Clara Felix, P.O. Box 7094, Berkeley, California 94707.

- Nutrition for Optimal Health Association, P.O. Box 380, Winnetka, Illinois 60093; publishes a newsletter, *NOHA NEWS*.

9

Skunk Mail and Other Invasions of Personal Airspace

POISON: A POTION OF PASSION. That object of your desire emerges from Europe. Poison. Its powers have yet to be charted. An intoxication. A bewitchment. And another prolific chapter in the legacy Dior. A fragrance so new, so different, so long lasting you've never worn anything like it.

THESE ODDLY FLAMBOYANT WORDS, a perfume ad in a December 1986 major urban newspaper, are an attempt to capitalize on the holiday market and the prevalent craze to be sexy at all costs. In all likelihood, this new perfume is derived not from beautiful flower petals, but from smelly petrochemicals. And in all likelihood, this perfume is a poison to some people.

Scented intrusions, from skunk (scented) mail to air "freshener," are becoming more and more common as artificial fragrance makes its way into virtually everything—deodorants, detergents, fabric softeners, lotions, marking pens, baby oil, soap pads, shower caps, and the air in some buildings, to name but a few sources. As with pesticides, you can hardly escape artificial scents. Manufacturers seem to think that a product won't sell unless it is scented. And many Americans have become active participants in this smelly game: the *Los Angeles Times* reports that the average person applies twelve aroma products a day.

But scent, whether called "perfume" or "cologne" or just "fragrance," is only part of a widespread problem: untested cosmetics and other personal-care products. According to the FDA in 1988, approximately four thousand different chemicals were being used in cosmetics, another four thousand in fragrances. Manufacturers mix these chemicals to form the forty thousand combinations used in a wide variety of products. And according to the CPSC, during 1987 alone hospital emergency rooms treated forty-seven thousand cosmetic-related injuries, from a wide range of sources—soaps, creams, lotions, facial masks, nail preparations, shampoos, permanents, hair dyes and straighteners, and other common products.

Scented or not, these personal-care products were toxic to many. How many have been tested for health effects? When the NAS reviewed existing toxicity testing for cosmetic ingredients in 1984, it found that only 16 percent permitted either a complete or partial health hazard assessment—less than for pesticides, drugs, and food additives. In other words, while the FDA knows little about the toxicity of food and drugs, it knows even less about the toxicity of cosmetics—yet these are the three things it is supposed to regulate.

Government Investigations

The NAS's startling results led to several Congressional hearings on cosmetic products, including perfumes. In 1985, the Subcommittee on Investigations and Oversight of the House Science and Technology Committee held hearings on neurotoxins at home and in the workplace. Estimating that millions of people are exposed every day to neurotoxic industrial chemicals, including solvents, pesticides, drugs, food additives, and cosmetics, the subcommittee reported that "very little neurotoxicity testing is *actually* being done." Instead, much of the current knowledge about the effects of neurotoxins has come about "through painful human experience."

In 1988 some of those painful human experiences were revealed in testimony at hearings by the Subcommittee on Regulation and Business Opportunities of the House Committee on Small Business, chaired by Representative Ron Wyden (D-OR). Concerned mainly about potential health hazards of cosmetic products used in small businesses, this subcommittee heard testimony from cosmetologists Kristie Smith, who developed chronic, irreversible asthma while in beauty college, and Edith Khatami, who, together with a co-worker, developed dizziness, nausea, vision problems, disorientation, chest pains, and difficulty breathing while spraying wigs in a poorly ventilated back room of a wig shop.

Beth Shulman, of the United Food and Commercial Workers International Union, testified about the health problems that professionals nationwide have experienced from inhaling the cosmetic products they are using. "The tools of the hair care profession are chemicals—chemicals like formaldehyde, methylene chloride, and ethyl methacrylate," she said, "that are causing problems in terms of neurological damage, asthma, long-term effects that we do not even know today." Of these chemicals, methylene chloride in particular can afford hazardous exposure below the level at which people smell its odor, so the nose cannot be used as an early-warning device. (Skeptics often trivialize chemically sensitive people as "odor sensitive," as if they were reacting merely to unpleasant odors, not to molecules of toxic substances. A chemical doesn't have to have a smell in order to be toxic!) Shulman asked not that chemical cosmetics should be banned, but that "workers and consumers alike should not be human guinea pigs when it comes to cosmetics." The final goal should be to keep all toxic ingredients out of all cosmetics and to use only nontoxic ingredients.

Perhaps the most startling fact to emerge from these hearings came when Representative Wyden gave NIOSH an industry-provided list of 2,983 chemicals used by the cosmetics industry. When NIOSH compared those chemicals with their registry of chemicals with toxic effects, it found that *884 cosmetic ingredients had been reported to the government as toxic substances.* The inescapable fact is that almost a third of the ingredients in cosmetics have had some toxic effect on human beings. Who knows how many toxic effects have gone unreported?

At the 1985 Congressional hearings on neurotoxins, British-born neurotoxicologist Peter Spencer, director of the Center for Research on Occupational and Environmental Toxicology at the Oregon Health Sciences University, described his research on two commonly used aroma chemicals. One was musk ambrette, an aroma chemical that was introduced in the 1920s and is commonly used in "fine fragrances." Spencer and his co-workers reported in 1984 that musk ambrette applied to the unbroken skin of rats produced nervous system damage that weakened their hind limbs. Research reported in 1979 had shown musk ambrette to cause "marked loss in weight, progressive weakness of the hind quarters, leading to complete loss of the use of the legs . . . muscular atrophy, and blood changes" in laboratory animals. Yet at the time of the hearings, the FDA had not removed musk ambrette from the market.

The other aroma chemical that Spencer studied was musk tetralin, also called AETT. "In 1955," he testified, "AETT was introduced into fragrance preparations without testing for chronic toxicity and, in 1977, voluntarily withdrawn by the fragrance industry after repeated exposure to the unbroken skin of rats had demonstrated degeneration of brain neurons and structural changes in spinal cord and in nerves supplying the limbs. An unusual early sign was increased irritability," said Spencer, "a behavioral change I remember well because the rats had a tendency to bite!" Between 1955 and 1976, AETT was "widely used as a significant ingredient of colognes, creams, after-shave lotions, and perfumes, and was often used to mask product odor in so-called unscented preparations." Though industry quite rightly stopped using AETT *and* took the evidence of ill effects to the FDA, that agency "chose not to regulate on that particular compound, so it can be introduced at any future time," Spencer cautioned in his testimony. He also cautioned that nerve damage can be irreversible: the nerve cell is "unable to divide like a liver cell or a blood cell . . . if one loses a nerve cell, that's it. As one depletes these nerve cells, it is suspected [that] throughout a lifetime of chemical exposure eventually the result . . . is expressed either by subtle behavioral changes . . . or more frank neurological deficits."

Other testifying experts agreed. Dr. Bernard Weiss, director of the Environmental Health Sciences Center of the University of Rochester School of Medicine and Dentistry, explaining why some people are affected by aroma chemicals and others not, said that we may not "be aware of destruction within the nervous system until we reach the limits of [its] reserve capacity." Rodney D. Wolford, director of the Department of Health and Safety of the International Brotherhood of Painters and Allied Trades, said that "highly exposed persons may stop having symptoms after the natural defense mechanisms of the body are overcome. They think they are conditioned to the substance when, in fact, they are still being harmed." Donald E. McMillan, chairman of the Department of Pharmacology at the University of Arkansas, said that "virtually no neurobehavioral toxicity testing whatsoever is done of the thousands of chemicals routinely used in cosmetics." In the 1989 report of its 1985 hearings, "Neurotoxins: At Home and the Workplace," the oversight committee agreed: "Countless . . . substances applied daily to the skin of consumers in the form of soaps, perfumes, aftershaves, and detergents have yet to be tested for their chronic neurotoxic effects." An oversight indeed.

In 1991 the EPA analyzed the VOCs given off by thirty-one "fragranced" products and sampled the air in fifteen different commercial and residential environments for VOCs. Fragrances are especially volatile; their whole purpose is to get as many scent molecules into the air as possible. The results: 150 chemicals—highly toxic linalool was one of the most common—were identified in these everyday products; and a total of one hundred chemicals—including toluene, xylene, methylene chloride, and 1,1,1-trichloroethane, all known to be toxic to animals—were found in these locations. Some chemicals, such as ethanol and limonene, were found emitted both by the products tested and in the indoor air sampled. The air in department and clothing stores, shopping malls, potpourri shops, and craft/hobby stores was found to have *more* chemicals than the air in the auto part shop, tire shop, carpet store, detergent and pet food departments, health club, room with air "freshener," and closet with cedar chips, and near the new shower curtain tested. Toluene was most abundant in auto parts stores and in department stores' perfume sections. Romantic?

Neurotoxicity

What little private neurotoxicity research does exist is not reassuring. In addition to musk ambrette and AETT, other aroma chemicals that have been toxic to laboratory animals are cyclohexanol (lethargy, spasms, "depressive action on the central nervous system"), linalool (lethargy, depression, "respiratory disturbances leading to death"), methyl ethyl ketone ("narcosis, emphysema of the lungs, and congestion of the liver and kidneys"), eugenol (intoxication), and musk ketone (blood and liver disorders). According to International Flavors & Fragrances' 1989 figures, linalool occurred more often in perfumes, household products, and soaps than any other aroma chemical and was fifth in average concentration in perfumes, with eugenol the twenty-fifth, and musk ketone the fifteenth. With the perfume industry constantly looking for new marketable scents, the use of aroma chemicals is probably on the increase. Yet unless laws are changed, you are not likely to see any of these names on perfume labels. Only recently have the mass media paid any attention to the possible neurotoxicity of fragrance chemicals. Most sources, such as Ruth Winter's *Consumer's Dictionary of Cosmetic Ingredients*, have concentrated on "allergic contact dermatitis." This is perhaps understandable, as cosmetics are intended to be applied to the skin, as they were in the experiments with rats. It is also understandable—but not fully understood—that cosmetics applied to the skin move through the skin into the bloodstream. "Skin absorption is so good that more and more prescription medicines are being manufactured in a patch form. . . . People who slather creams, colognes, and oils on their skin do not realize that it is just like eating them, for they reach the bloodstream as though they had eaten them," cautions Dr. Sherry Rogers.

But with secondhand or "sidestream" exposure to perfumes, cosmetics, and other scented products, more and more people are being sickened by what they are inhaling from skunk mail and from others' use of personal-care products like scented detergents and fabric softeners, which continue to outgas from users' clothes. A Castro Valley, California, survey found that all of the following symptoms from perfume exposure were reported by more than half of the 427 people responding to the survey: headache, sneezing, inability to concentrate, spaciness, mood changes, sinus troubles, watery eyes, restlessness, dizziness, nausea, depression, short-term memory lapses, and sleepiness. Contact dermatitis? No. But plenty of indications of nerve-related problems and possible nerve-cell damage—whether temporary or permanent, no one knows. One person who suffered similar symptoms is a San Diego woman who became ill when a co-worker repeatedly wore a new perfume, Knowing, marketed by a billion-dollar cosmetics company. After she asked her co-worker not to wear it, the other woman retaliated by wearing more the next day and reapplying it. Ignoring requests by their supervisor, she continued wearing the perfume, and the affected woman had to leave her job. Unable to hold any job because of perfume and other exposures, she is now unemployed and on general assistance. Because of her sensitization, exposure to any similar fragrance can cause her such symptoms as headaches, choking, nausea, diarrhea, tunnel vision, burning and throbbing in her nose, depression, and muscle weakness. She feels that her life has been shattered. Like many people in industrialized countries who have been sensitized by exposures to certain chemicals in perfumes and other modern products, she now has EI/MCS.

Across the country, on the train from New York to Albany, Amy Solomon, communications director for State Senator Martin Connor, developed a "raging migraine headache" while reading a women's magazine with perfume-scented inserts. Her boss promptly introduced a bill to require smell-proof sealants. "The only hazard New Yorkers should have to face when leafing through a magazine or opening their mail is the threat of a nasty paper cut, not a migraine headache or, worse, a severe asthmatic attack," Connor said at his November 22, 1989, hearings on perfume inserts. Chemically sensitive Richard Zachary, wearing a mask as he testified in favor of the bill, said that everyone "should have the right to decide whether he or she wants to sample a chemical product. It's almost ludicrous to think of an aspirin sample reaching our blood stream without our knowing about it. Yet that is what happens with the molecules from fragrance samples."

Asthma

Another significant health effect related to perfume exposure is asthma, which can be life-threatening. A 1987 Swedish study of 680 patients with asthma or rhinitis found that perfumes and tobacco smoke caused irritation in 98 percent of the asthmatics and 67 percent of the rhinitis patients. In the U.S., a controlled study by two pulmonary physicians found that four asthmatic patients experienced substantial declines in lung capacity when exposed to a perfume frequently mentioned as causing asthma. Their survey of sixty patients discovered that fifty-seven found their asthma worsened by one or more odors, including insecticide, household cleaning agents, perfume and cologne, cigarette smoke, fresh paint smell, automobile exhaust or gas fumes, and cooking smells. Twenty-three patients had gone to emergency rooms for treatment, with nine being hospitalized. Several reported experiencing asthma attacks at home or at work and then finding out from others that someone nearby was wearing a heavy perfume. Yet "the odors that caused asthma were not necessarily unpleasant, and many noxious odors failed to produce asthma," the researchers wrote. Pure noxiousness, evidently, is not the test. Nevertheless, "you'd never want to stand next to an asthmatic if you're wearing a perfume," says Eleanor Newhouse, of the Los Angeles chapter of the Asthma & Allergy Foundation of America. At least that's what the nation's estimated ten million asthmatics might wish.

Yet denial, that ever-present psychological phenomenon, fogs the issue in the U.S. Both a spokesperson for the American Academy of Allergy and Immunology and Dr. Harold Nelson, of the National Jewish Center for Immunology and Respiratory Medicine in Denver, say that "no evidence exists that shows odors can cause ill effects in healthy people." Michael Petrina, spokesman for the Cosmetic, Toiletry, and Fragrance Association, says that "fragrances bother relatively few people and that their hardship is offset by the benefit to advertisers, magazines, and interested consumers."

Would New Yorker Deborah Martorano agree? In 1989 she spent eleven days in a hospital in critical condition with an asthma attack after a Bloomingdale's employee spritzed her with perfume without her permission. Though Martorano heard a voice behind her in the store, she was sprayed before she had a chance to respond. Winning $75,000 from her lawsuit against the store, Martorano nevertheless feels she is still not back to normal. "Getting sprayed turned my whole life upside down," she said. "It's wrong of Bloomingdale's to spray people." And "odors in general seem to be getting more and more aggressive," a reporter who covered Martorano's story felt moved to add. "I'm talking about cabbies who keep a bottle of high-smelling red stuff on the dash, publishers who infuse magazines with perfumed inserts, and those new wall gadgets you press to release a whiff of air freshener."

The Aroma Industry

Perfume. Scent. Fragrance. For most people, these words are pleasant, suggesting beauty, romance, allure, glamour, sex appeal. Since the ancient Egyptians, both men and women have used perfumes and cosmetics to enhance their lives. For some, however, these words are no longer attractive; they suggest pain instead. Perfume molecules—tiny, invisible bits of matter—are what are affecting some people's health. But why now? Why in the twentieth century?

One reason is that we now have more perfumes and cosmetics available to us, with new, celebrity perfumes introduced almost daily, it would seem. In the U.S., the aroma industry is flourishing. Despite the inflationary forces of the 1980s, the 1988 sales figures for fragrances were amazingly high, according to perfume researcher Paul Bedoukian. "Not too long ago, the fragrance market was less than a billion dollars a year. Now in excess of $4 billion, it has become a major business indeed." While a hundred years ago perfume was only dabbed on skin and seldom added to anything else, the fragrance industry now derives only 20 percent of its revenues from pure perfumes. Instead, a major trend of the 1980s was to increase perfume levels in many product categories, particularly powdered laundry detergents.

Another reason is that we have more advertising—and more powerful advertising—inducing us to buy these products. But possibly most important is that modern perfumes and cosmetics now tend to be made from petroleum and coal—not flowers and plants. Humans are inventing these modern products, and the human body has a hard time coping with them. Some of the ingredients in these products are "xenobiotics"—alien, foreign substances, not natural, familiar ones that our bodies are used to handling and detoxifying. Hence some of us are getting sick from them—and some of us just don't like the way they smell. Through our noses and our skins, these xenobiotics are constantly adding to our total chemical load, putting all of us at risk.

Fortunately for many of us, there has also been a recent increase in *un*scented products—66 out of 774 new health and beauty aids introduced in the first four months of 1993 contained no added fragrance. Many magazines, often the worst source for unwanted, smelly "skunk mail," have followed the same trend. *TV Guide* stopped running scented inserts after receiving complaints from over a thousand readers. The *New Yorker*, after receiving several hundred complaints about scent strips, started sending unscented copies to readers. And *Smithsonian* stopped using scented ads after receiving numerous letters from readers, including one from "a fairly upscale lady on Long Island [who] said, 'Your magazine came smelling like a bordello in May.'"

All of this is good news for us, and for a Long Island woman who suffered severe headaches, a stiff neck, fainting spells, and tingling sensations in her hands for seven years before discovering their cause. Having been tested and unsuccessfully treated by neurologists, psychiatrists, and neck and blood specialists, she heard about a pediatrician who had helped many patients by recommending avoidance of certain common products. "After spending thousands of dollars on doctors and tests," she figured, "what would it hurt to buy new soaps and deodorants?" She threw out all of her familiar personal-care products, washed all her linens and clothes several times, and stopped using her heavy musk perfume. Now much better, she has no more fainting spells, headaches, or stiff necks. Once, however, she tested herself with a dose of musk perfume and in an hour had a massive headache. For her and for many others, the effect of scented products on her health was apparently reversible—as long as she avoids exposures.

What, exactly, is in a particular perfume that could be causing unpleasant or even devastating health effects? "Exactly" is something very few know. So-called fragrance houses know the ingredients of their perfumes, but they do not have to reveal them on the label or to the FDA. One major cosmetic manufacturer, Avon, supplies consumers with a brochure listing approximately five hundred natural and synthetic ingredients in its products, but does not specify which ingredients are in which products. An ingredient list in a catalog for a mail-order firm called Beauty Boutique gives for most perfumes only "alcohol, water, and fragrance." The "fragrance" is either essential oils or aroma chemicals. According to the *Atlantic*, "the perfumer works with a palette of about 5,400 raw materials— 400 natural oils, extracted from flowers, roots, and grasses, and 5,000 aroma chemicals, which are either reconstitutions of natural scents or scents, such as hawthanol and hexalon, that do not occur in nature." The overwhelming trend is toward synthetic aroma chemicals, which can cost less than $10 a pound compared to more than $10,000 a pound for natural scents like tuberose or jasmine. It takes a lot of rose petals to make a true rose perfume. Actually, in 1988 about 95 percent of all ingredients in most fragrances were thought to be "synthetic compounds, chemically about as romantic as polyvinyl chloride."

The FDA

Again, you may wonder, what is our government doing about the problem? The 1938 Food, Drug, and Cosmetics Act, under which the FDA operates, has only one page (out of 156) on cosmetics. By law, the FDA can inspect cosmetics manufacturers, collect sample cosmetics for examination and investigation, and ask the Justice Department to remove adulterated cosmetics from the market. But it cannot require the manufacturers to test ingredients for safety. Nor can it require them to register their plants or cosmetics, file data on ingredients, or report cosmetics-related injuries. "Due to some adroit lobbying years ago by the cosmetics industry, the FDA has to beg for safety rather than demand it" is Ralph Nader's acerbic observation. The Cosmetics, Toiletry, and Fragrance Association, industry's own organization, has pledged to improve its self-regulation and voluntary testing.

In California in the 1980s, an accountant had to quit her job because of intense reactions to the perfume Opium and many other odors in her work environment. She first complained to the manufacturer, then to the FDA, and, receiving no satisfaction from either, finally to Representative Wyden. In 1989 Representative Wyden heard from then-FDA-Commissioner Frank Young that Opium's manufacturer had not reported her adverse reaction to the FDA under the FDA's "voluntary cosmetic product experience reporting program." So much for voluntary reporting: who knows how many other complaints perfume manufacturers have received?

Actually, some *have* been reported under the FDA's self-policing program for the cosmetics industry. In 1989, 133 of 850 cosmetics manufacturers registered with the FDA (out of an estimated four thousand to five thousand such manufacturers) disclosed 12,915 adverse consumer reactions to 1,513 products. That's an average of twelve complaints per product from a tiny fraction of the total number of cosmetics manufacturers. Yet John E. Bailey, in 1991 acting director of the FDA's Colors and Cosmetics Division, said "We are not aware, nor is there any obvious evidence that cosmetics pose significant risk to consumers. Yes, people are injured by products, but when you compare cosmetics to other products the numbers aren't cause for alarm." Heinz J. Eiermann, in 1989 director of the same division, wrote that "the number of people reacting to strong perfume odors is still very small and consumers not adversely affected by these fragrances should not be deprived of their enjoyment. You and I will have to and can avoid such exposures."

And you and I can write to the Office of Cosmetics and Colors, FDA, Washington, D.C. 20204, to complain about a particular perfume or cosmetic. In the years 1992 to 1993, that office received only sixty letters "documenting individuals having a sensitivity to fragrance products," according to a response to one woman who complained about a specific perfume. Actually, the phrase should have been "documenting fragrance products causing chemical injury," placing the blame where it belongs—on the product, not the sufferer. The response also said that "no clear scientific correlation between causative chemicals and specific adverse reactions has emerged that would allow the FDA to assess whether or not a legal basis exists for proposing regulation." Bureaucratese for "we're not going to do anything."

Keeping toxic chemicals out of scented products will take new laws. However, this may not be as difficult as it sounds; people tend to complain of the same scents over and over. While listing all perfume ingredients may be impossible (one perfume, Red, is said to contain more than six hundred ingredients), Congress could mandate a testing of the most suspect perfumes and cosmetics for toxicity. As Representative Wyden says, "It's incredible that the $18-billion cosmetics industry can urge millions of Americans to apply chemicals to their bodies daily and not be held responsible."

One Person's Skunk

Obviously, people react differently to different scents, and to different amounts of them, something that researchers are only now beginning to investigate. According to Charles Wysocki, of the Monell Chemical Sensing Center in Philadelphia, there are no universally good or bad smells. "What smells good to one nose may be unpleasant to another. There are some people who very much enjoy the smell of skunk, and I'm one of them." One person's lily-of-the-valley is another person's garbage dump.

For all of us, however, scent molecules travel the same paths. When you smell anything—perfume or not—you need to realize that molecules of that substance are in the air, floating away from it and landing in your nose and on your skin. When you apply perfumes or cosmetics to yourself, the molecules enter your body through both your nose and your skin. Those on your skin can move into your bloodstream. Those you inhale can move from your nostrils along the sensory nerve to the brain's olfactory bulb, with some going on to the brain's limbic system to be translated into memory or emotion. (Memory, of course, can be tricky: the scent that triggers pleasant memories in one person may bring back horrible memories in another). In 1988 a Johns Hopkins brain expert, Dr. Solomon Snyder, discovered a "carrier protein" that apparently ferries odor molecules from the nose to the brain. By following up this discovery, he and other researchers hope to find out, for instance, why some people "cannot smell jasmine while others are unable to detect hydrogen cyanide" and why people "can smell odors in such tiny amounts as one part per trillion in air."

Dr. Alan Hirsch, founder of the Chicago-based Smell & Taste Treatment and Research Foundation, had a woman patient whose ability to smell was "100,000 times greater than yours or mine. People who suffer from this have a very difficult time. They can be overpowered by odors from everything that surrounds them, like cleaning fluids in carpets and drapes or whatever." A more ominous note is sounded by Dr. Richard Doty, director of the smell and taste center at the University of Pennsylvania School of Medicine, who says that the nose "is capable of transporting harmful agents into the brain, including polio viruses and many larger molecules." Both Alzheimer's disease and Parkinson's disease, he suspects, might be caused, in some cases, by breathed-in environmental contaminants.

Secondhand Scents

Even more ominous for those who get sick from inhaling perfumes is the increasing threat of secondhand scents. At a 1991 meeting of the American Association for the Advancement of Science, fragrance scientists reported studies funded by the Fragrance Research Fund, an industry-supported organization, showing that whiffs of peppermint or lavender increased people's concentration and vigilance, which implies that these scents could be used to increase workers' productivity. "Pleasurable" scents were already being tested, it was reported, on "clerical workers in Japan, straphangers in the London subway, and patients having to endure brain scans." (Perfume-sensitive patients would thus have to endure more than the fearsomeness of the process.) This emerging new field, known as "aromacology," has had its start in Japan, "ahead" of us, as usual. One of Japan's large construction companies, Shimizu, has patented the first computerized odor dispenser, a machine designed to be attached to an office air conditioning system. In this country, a company called AromaSys has been hired to place scents in the Miami Marriott hotel, St. Croix Valley Memorial Hospital in Minnesota, and in other businesses. If such companies have their way, soon you will not be able to enter any public building without being subjected to someone's else's idea of what smells pleasant. And that includes fabric stores. In 1990 the government patent and trademark office registered its first trademark for a scent, a "high-impact, fresh floral fragrance reminiscent of plumeria blossoms," to be used on embroidery yarn and sewing thread. The company receiving the trademark already sells a kit for making a scented skunk. The Japanese, not to be outdone, are marketing lavender-scented stockings and pine-and-eucalyptus-scented alarm clocks.

Skepticism as to the wisdom of all this "progress" occasionally surfaces. Robert Baron, a Rensselaer Polytechnic Institute psychologist, found that commercial air "fresheners" in a conference room made discussion participants more likely to "compromise and make concessions." *Washington Post* writer William Booth observed that "Baron did not speculate if the subjects in the room with air 'fresheners' just wanted to hurry up and get out of the room, because some people say they find air freshener odors unappealing." But Baron is not the only one perceiving a political danger. Henry G. Walters, a former chairman of International Flavors & Fragrances, termed by the *Wall Street Journal* the world's largest flavors-and-scents company, acknowledged that "the dark side is mind control. This could be misused to conceivably make a population more compliant or more militant. There always will be people who overstep."

Psychologist Baron also said that he "personally found many [commercial air fresheners] to be quite hideous. On the other hand, this is a multi-billion-dollar industry. So some people must like them." Or the industry has hired an aggressive sales force. More and more public washrooms have air "fresheners" bolted to the wall—some timed to spew their nauseating contents into the air periodically. Many air "fresheners" contain the pesticide paradichlorobenzene, thus contributing to our total pesticide exposures. According to psychologist William Dember, another participant in the fragrance conference, no one has yet investigated the effect of unpleasant smells.

Only us guinea pigs, being tested without our consent. Some of us, however, have rebelled. In California, Tulare County officials shut down a factory making a sweet-smelling air "freshener" from flower petals, spices, scented wood chips, and methanol. The action was taken after neighbors complained of "horrible headaches" and nausea from the plant's emissions. Fined for violations of air pollution and environmental laws, the company, Aromax Inc., fought to stay open, but company executives lost the case partly because they came to the hearings exuding the strong odor of their product. "We always knew the people from Aromax," said Marcie Williams, head of a local environmental group. "You could smell them a mile away."

Less ominous than aromacology and its implications is aromatherapy, the use of "essential oils" to produce physiological and psychological responses, a practice currently being revived from ancient Chinese, East Indian, and Egyptian cultures. Essential oils are oils distilled from flowers, bark, roots, and other plant life. As such they are somewhat safer than commercial perfumes. In the U.S., a Minneapolis-based company, Aveda, started in 1978 by hair stylist Horst Rechelbacher, is the leading dispenser of essential oils. But even Rechelbacher warns that the aromatherapy movement "needs to be controlled. The FDA needs to step in. [Essential oils] are potent, volatile natural chemicals. In the wrong dosage and the wrong concentration, they can be toxic." One FDA official has pointed out that some natural perfume ingredients, such as civet, galbanum, patchouli oil, and asafetida, can cause reactions in chemically sensitive people, but the FDA has not taken steps to ban them or require warning labels. "More research is needed" is the standard defense.

In fact, the fragrance industry ignores nobody: women, men, even babies. Observes Dr. Fernando Aleu, president of the Fragrance Foundation, "[Babies] feel at ease in a familiar olfactory circumstance [such as near a mother's smell] and often fuss in an environment with strange odors. If a mother wears a fragrance, her infant might, or might not, like it, but it's a bond. If baby-sitters smelled like the mothers, the babies would feel more comfortable." (Is he implying that baby-sitters should spray themselves with the mother's perfume as soon as they come in the door?) Babies, of course, are the quintessential captive audience: until they can crawl, there is no way they can get away from a fragrance they don't like. This makes them especially vulnerable to such abominations as children's perfumes. A new Babar perfume, named after the popular children's-book elephant, is available in a special formula for babies, packaged in pink and blue bottles. Pity the poor child who gets that scent but doesn't like it!

Babies, of course, are not the only captive audience for fragrances. Some hospital emergency wards are using perfumes to "cover the smell of anesthetics and other wafting odors that frighten some people." Some airlines add a "pleasant" scent to cabin air "to help passengers relax." With scents, there are increasingly few "safe" environments.

For the chemically injured and all those affected by perfume exposures, the issue—rapidly becoming the secondhand smoke issue of the 1990s—is one of choice. In San Rafael, California, Richard Conrad, a biochemist, found that his neighbor's use of Tide and a perfume called Anaïs Anaïs was making him ill—so ill that he traded his $320,000 house in San Rafael for a house on five acres in an agricultural community. But "I have a right to choose how to make myself smell," asserts the neighbor. "Someone should have the choice whether to smell a particular item," counters Amy Solomon, New York State Senator Connor's assistant. Susan Molloy, of the San Francisco-area Environmental Health Network, has to take an oxygen tank to meetings in order to breathe safely in a perfumed atmosphere. "I know people have a right to choose their personal-care products," she says, "but the air is shared. I'm a gregarious person, not someone who will be driven out of society." To *New York Times* writer Katherine Bishop, the medical problems that chemically sensitive people experience from perfume encounters constitute "a form of toxic terrorism."

Fortunately for the chemically sensitive, a movement toward safer cosmetics has taken off in this country and elsewhere. The Body Shop, an English company founded in 1976 by Anita Roddick, pioneered the movement by marketing products derived "mainly from plants grown organically by Third World farmers and [which] are not tested on animals. They come in simple plastic containers, which can be returned to the stores for recycling and are not enclosed in boxes." Another pioneer is Californian Debra Lynn Dadd, whose books tell you not only which cosmetic products are safest, but also how to make your own. *Nontoxic & Natural: How to Avoid Dangerous Everyday Products and Buy or Make Safe Ones* and *Nontoxic, Natural, & Earthwise* are indispensable for people who want to improve their health by using safer products. Though still a small part of the market, less-toxic cosmetics are a growing trend. As cosmetics retailer Ed Forristall says, "People get sick of the hype, the claims that are unfounded, and the hefty prices that mainly pay for advertising."

Coping with Fragrance

If you are sensitive to perfumes, cosmetics, or other scented products, what recourse do you have? How can you be protected from what one office worker has termed "industrial-strength perfumes"?

- You can file a lawsuit. According to the *Indoor Pollution Law Report*, "lawsuits grounded in product liability, negligence, and workers' compensation claims due to chemical hypersensitivity [another name for EI/MCS] are no longer anomalies and are expected to continue to influence legislatures and local communities." In New York, Martorano's case against Bloomingdale's was primarily a negligence suit because the perfume demonstrator was temporarily distracted when spraying perfume in her face, says her lawyer.

- You can complain to your local post office. The U.S. Postal Service's new, industry-approved regulations stipulate that fragrance advertising samples must be "reasonably designed" to prevent people from being involuntarily exposed to the sample and that samples must adhere to Postal Service rules for their mailability. Skunk mail may indeed be on the way out—but the final test lies in the sniffing. The chemically sensitive are finding that the new regulations aren't good enough; perfume in scent strips escapes from its tiny capsules and contaminates magazines and catalogs before they can arrive at your door.

- You can refuse to pay scented bills. An Atlanta couple wrote that they had cut up their credit card from a store that sent them heavily perfumed bills and mailed the pieces back with a note stating that "we objected to the store stinking up our mailbox to advertise a perfume that it was promoting." The couple soon received a note from the store's credit manager assuring them that "it would be no problem to flag our account and send us regular bills that wouldn't stink up our mailbox." Worked like a charm, they said.

- You can patronize stores, restaurants, and hotels that cater to those bothered by perfumes. There aren't many yet, but their number may be growing. The Embassy Suites hotel in Alexandria, Virginia, will furnish air purifiers and scrub walls with baking soda for chemically sensitive patrons. "Clean has no smell," says the hotel's housekeeper. At Charlie Trotter's, an expensive

Chicago restaurant, hosts unobtrusively sniff customers and seat scented ones where they will not disturb wine connoisseurs, who don't want anything to interfere with *their* sniffing. (Another Chicago restaurant, Jimmy's Place, had to give up asking prospective customers, when they called for reservations, to refrain from wearing scented products—too many decided to eat elsewhere.) You can even find a church with perfume-free pews: the First Unitarian Church of San Francisco.

- You can become an activist. A grass-roots movement is already underway, primarily in Marin County, across the Golden Gate Bridge from San Francisco. There, a coalition of environmental groups has already succeeded in having fragrance-free areas set up at a few public meetings. The coalition has also succeeded in having some offices and meeting notices request that people not wear perfume or other scented products to those sites. "Our basic premise is that we who are disabled because of our chemical sensitivity need to have access, just like people in wheelchairs need to have access," said Julia A. Kendall, of Citizens for a Toxic-Free Marin.

- If you're curious about the toxicity of a specific product, you can ask the manufacturer for an MSDS, or material safety data sheet. Though such documents don't tell all, you may learn something.

- You can ask your doctor to help. Allergist Robert W. Boxer wrote a letter to the editor of a major metropolitan daily, which printed it: "People who wear strong perfume or other scented cosmetics often become insensitive to their odor and are unaware of how much they reek. This is especially inconsiderate when they attend events where expensive seating is assigned, particularly at theater, concert, opera, and sports events. Many people become ill from being exposed to these heavily scented cosmetics. The organizers and promoters of events with designated seating should request in their advertising, tickets, and programs that patrons avoid scented cosmetics." A valiant try, though we know that this will be a long time a-coming.

- You can, politely but persistently, ask friends to change smelly habits. In public, one can usually move away from scented strangers; at home and in the workplace, it's a different matter. Most chemically injured persons have had to wrestle with the difficult social problem of how to protect themselves from unwanted and dangerous exposures without offending or permanently alienating friends and relatives, especially those who believe "it's all in your head." How do you say, tactfully, "Your perfume is making me ill," or "I don't like the way you smell," or "What deodorant are you using?" We have all been brought up not to say such things, however delicately put. Yet to maintain their health, the chemically sensitive often have no choice but to break the taboo.

- For your health, you can and you *must* READ LABELS, READ LABELS, READ LABELS. (Perfume labels don't even give you a clue.) Even if a cosmetic product says "unscented," check the back of the bottle or tube; it may say "masking fragrance added." If the label reads like a chemistry textbook, don't buy it. Remember that no one knows the toxicity to humans of all those chemicals—either by themselves or reacting with each other (not all are toxic—but we don't know which are the safe ones). Instead buy cosmetics with fewer ingredients—ones that sound like plants or herbs. A centuries-old remedy, flaxseed oil, taken internally, will give you not only soft smooth skin but also essential nutrients. You'll save money and you may feel better.

- Finally, you can work to change your own attitude and values. Both men and women are now being targeted—nay, assaulted—by subtle, expensively produced, motivationally researched perfume and cosmetic ads. You aren't virile or attractive unless you spritz yourself with "Hocus Pocus" every morning, and you'll never be happy unless you use "Mask Everything" deodorant. But really, what is more important—health or a false sense of allure? Inner attractiveness and charm (based mainly on caring for others) or a skin-deep layer of goo? Acquiring a modicum of depth (based mainly on learning to be your own person) or being as superficial as almost everyone else? Do you want to let advertising continue to terrify you about growing old? Get off the commercial bandwagon, free yourself from our monstrous,

modern marketplace tyranny—you will find yourself feeling better not only physically, but emotionally.

* * *

To Find Out More

- *Nontoxic & Natural: How to Avoid Dangerous Everyday Products and Buy or Make Safe Ones*, by Debra Lynn Dadd, Los Angeles, Jeremy P. Tarcher, 1984.

- *Nontoxic, Natural, & Earthwise: How to Protect Yourself and
  Your Family from Harmful Products and Live in Harmony with
  the Earth*, by Debra Lynn Dadd, Los Angeles, Jeremy P. Tarcher,
  1990.

- *The Safe Shopper's Bible*, by David Steinman and Samuel S. Epstein, MD, New York, Macmillan, 1994, in press.

- *A Consumer's Dictionary of Cosmetic Ingredients: Complete Information about the Harmful and Desirable Ingredients Found
  in Men's and Women's Cosmetics*, third revised edition, by Ruth
  Winter, New York, Crown Publishers, 1989.

- *Natural Organic Hair and Skin Care*, by Aubre Hampton,
  Tampa, Florida, Organica Press, 1987.

- *Being Beautiful: Deciding for Yourself*, by Katherine Isaac,
  Washington, D.C., Center for the Study of Responsive Law,
  1986 (selected readings, including an article by Ruth Decker,
  "The Not-So-Pretty Risks of Cosmetics," from *Medical Self-
  Care*, Summer 1983).

- *The Beauty Myth: How Images of Beauty Are Used Against
  Women*, by Naomi Wolf, New York, William Morrow and Co.,
  1991.

- "Safely Gorgeous: You Don't Have to Poison Yourself to Look
  Good," by David Steinman and Samuel S. Epstein, MD, in *Environment & Health*, editor Joanne Bahura, July/August 1992
  (available from the Organization for the Advancement of Envi-

ronmental Health, P.O. Box 41057, Santa Barbara, California 93140).

A Few Mail-Order Stores and Catalogs (see Chapter 4 for more)

- InterNatural (pure products for personal care), P.O. Box 680, Shaker Street, South Sutton, New Hampshire 03273; 1-800-446-4903.

- SelfCare Catalog (taking control of your health), 349 Healdsburg Avenue, Healdsburg, California 95448; 1-800-345-3371.

- The Natural Choice, from Eco Design Co., 1365 Rufina Circle, Santa Fe, New Mexico 87501; 505-438-3448 or 1-800-621-2591.

- Greenhome, Inc., 3705 N. Spaulding, Chicago, Illinois 60618.

- Body Elements/Terressentials, 3320 North 3rd Street, Arlington, Virginia 22201-1712; 703-525-0585.

10

Who Is Most at Risk

- In the early 1980s, an Oregon couple, Ken and Jan Nolley, were worried about a frightening decline in the health of one of their two adopted sons, then four years old. Writing for the *Journal of Pesticide Reform*, they described him as nearly unmanageable in the daytime and often waking at night "drenched with sweat and screaming from nightmares." He began wetting the bed repeatedly every night. Increasingly aggressive and unhappy, he complained of stomachaches and joint aches. Fortunately, the Nolleys happened to read an article by Dr. Randolph and soon realized that their son's disintegration had begun when he started sleeping on a plastic mattress and pillow cover prescribed for dust allergy. Once these plastic covers were removed (without his knowledge), he began getting better. Later he told his parents that a lot of things in his world "smelled funny." Among them were polyester sheets, which he could always tell from cotton sheets by their smell. A subsequent accidental pesticide exposure brought on seizure-like episodes and loss of consciousness. The process of avoiding these harmful exposures has forever changed the Nolleys' lives.

- Daniel, a ten-year-old patient of Dr. Sherry Rogers, became "strangely wild" after Saturday morning cartoons, and his grades began deteriorating as he developed a nasty streak. When she tested him for phenol, a common chemical found in many modern products, he began scribbling and ripping up the paper he was working on. Questioning revealed that a new teacher was wiping the desks in his classroom with a common phenol-containing cleaner and that the family had a new television set, which was emitting phenol from heated wires. Daniel's family was lucky: his hyperactivity problem was solved by a note to his teacher and the installation of a fan in the television room.

• Kevin Ryan, an Illinois schoolboy, was eleven years old when he testified before a Senate environment subcommittee in 1990. Kevin was first exposed to pesticides as an infant playing in his sandbox during repeated sprayings by a lawn-care company on a neighbor's property. Reading from four pages of lined school paper, Kevin described how his current neighbors' lawn spraying brings on "numbing and tingling in my arms and legs, muscle and joint achiness, chest pressure, respiratory problems, nausea, severe stomach pain, diarrhea, brain symptoms, loss of memory, lack of concentration, irritability, depression, and fatigue. . . . What are these chemicals doing to the other kids if this is what is happening to me?" Before the family moved to a less-sprayed area, he, his brother, and his mother, who is also chemically sensitive as a result of unwanted pesticide exposure, had to uproot themselves every spring when the lawn-care trucks started rolling and move to an unsprayed area in the Colorado mountains. When a representative of a national lawn-care company testified after Kevin did, Kevin reacted so violently to the pesticide residues on the man's clothing that he had to be led from the room and treated with oxygen.

ALL THREE OF THESE BOYS have EI/MCS, in varying degrees. Indeed, all children today are very much at risk from the chemicalization of our environment. Parents of school-age kids like these three grew up during the post-World-War-II chemical revolution, taking plastics and other synthetic products for granted. Although these kids' grandparents knew a world without TV, detergents, fabric softeners, synthetic fabrics, and petroleum-based pesticides, the parents did not, and tend to use such products as if they had always existed, rarely questioning their safety.

But are children more at risk than others? In *Chemical Exposure: Low Levels and High Stakes*, Ashford and Miller state that children and infants in contaminated communities, as well as pregnant women and fetuses, may be affected first or most by exposure to environmental toxins. The authors of the OTA's 1990 neurotoxicity report agree, adding that while all of our nervous systems are particularly vulnerable to toxic substances, some populations bear special risk: "fetuses, children, the elderly, workers in occupations involving exposure to relatively high levels of toxic chemicals, and persons who abuse drugs." Let's take a closer look at some of these special-risk populations.

Fetuses

Like the canaries that used to alert coal miners to the presence of poisonous gases in the mine tunnels, fetuses have a message for us. Research biochemist Beverly Paigen says that "the most sensitive segment of the population is the developing fetus. Not only is this the period of most rapid growth, but during the first months of fetal life, the major organ systems develop. Any interference with critical biological processes during organ development, roughly the first three months, can lead to birth defects. . . . We now know that many chemicals can cross the placental barrier, and that the human fetus is capable of metabolizing these chemicals into harmful forms." Indeed, careful research has discovered the presence of industrial chemicals in the umbilical cords of newborn babies in America. And, unexpectedly, asbestos has been found in the lungs of stillborn fetuses. "This is a particularly significant finding, since the child never breathed atmospheric air," said Dr. Abida Haque in the *Annals of the New York Academy of Sciences*. "If fetuses are being exposed to asbestos, then they could also be exposed to any number of environmental toxics once believed not transferred through the placenta."

Statistics from at least three contaminated communities—Woburn, Massachusetts; an area in San Jose, California; and Love Canal, New York—point to possible connections, Paigen reports.

Each community experienced temporary increases in miscarriages and birth defects following exposure to chemicals in soil or water. Woburn was studied by the Harvard School of Public Health, San Jose by the California Department of Health Services; there was no follow-up study of Love Canal.

Approximately 250,000 children are born with birth defects each year in the U.S., with only 20 percent of the defects thought to be genetically caused. In 1982 Betty Mekdeci, of Orlando, Florida, formed the Association of Birth Defect Children, an information clearinghouse and support group for parents of children with birth defects. Soon after her son David was born, in the 1970s, with a shortened right arm and a deformed right hand, Mekdeci began suspecting the anti-nausea drug Bendectin, which her doctor had prescribed during her pregnancy. (Thought to have been prescribed for as many as thirty-three million women, Bendectin was removed from the market in 1983.) Her research has since led her to broaden her focus to other chemicals and to sue the pharmaceutical firm that manufactured the anti-nausea drug. During this period, Mekdeci fell ill with infections and neurological symptoms that she finally traced to pesticide spraying for fleas in her own home—an ironic confirmation of the information she was then gathering.

Unfortunately, not all birth defects show up immediately. One possible example of a delayed effect occurred in Taylorville, a small central Illinois town, where three children under twenty-two months were diagnosed with neuroblastoma, a rare cancer usually found in only nine of every million children. An abandoned coal factory is suspect; though coal tar and contaminated soil were removed from the site in 1988, "residents could have been exposed before and during the clean-up," according to the state EPA. And though the exact cause of neuroblastoma is unknown, Holly Howe, chief epidemiologist for the Illinois Department of Public Health, says that an environmental factor might be involved.

On Agent Orange, the dioxin-tainted herbicide used by the U.S. to defoliate Vietnam's trees, evidence of related birth defects continues to mount. Ever since 1962, the year that the U.S. Army began its defoliation program, Vietnamese doctors have noted an increased incidence in sprayed areas of birth defects such as cerebral spine defects, anencephaly, spina bifida, and hydrocephaly, as well as stillborn infants, immune deficiency diseases, and learning disabilities (these overworked doctors, however, have had neither the time nor the funds for large-scale documentation). A study of 1,964 pregnancies reported in the *American Journal of Public Health* in 1990 by the Boston University School of Public Health found that fathers who served the longest in Vietnam and who saw combat had the highest risk of having a baby with a birth defect. The researcher, Ann Aschengrau, concluded that Agent Orange must be viewed with suspicion.

None of this is good news for the children and families affected. What is cheering, however, is the now broadly increased awareness of fetal risk. Mekdeci's association started with only eighty families and now reaches thousands of parents and professionals in eight countries. Even mainstream physicians are also more aware of the dangers from the medications they have been prescribing. In 1990 medical columnist Allan Bruckheim, MD, wrote in response to a worried correspondent, "No type of medication is exempt [from possible damage to a fetus]. . . . Any preparation, liquid or in capsule form, injected or taken intravenously, eye drops, skin creams, or in fact by any route of administration, must be considered in the light of the possible risks to the unborn. Each medication should be carefully researched, using the publications of the U.S. Pharmacopoeial Convention, the *Physician's Desk Reference* [PDR], or package inserts provided with the medications. . . . All things [including caffeine and castor oil] must be suspect, and that will continue into the breast-feeding period as well." A study reported in the February 23, 1994, issue of *JAMA* found that mothers' exposure to secondhand smoke can be passed on to the developing fetus. Some infants of the passive inhalers had cotinine (a breakdown product of nicotine) levels "as if the mother had really smoked five to six cigarettes a day."

You can find the PDR, which lists possible side effects of virtually all currently used prescription drugs, in the reference room of your local library. (While you're there look at *Clinical Toxicology of Commercial Products*, which gives toxicology ratings of thousands of common products like soaps.) Whether you are pregnant, nursing, or neither, ask your doctor to write on the prescription he or she gives you an instruction to the pharmacist to give you the package insert. While these publications can be hard for the layperson to decipher, you will get some clues. Better still, while pregnant or nursing avoid all medications, prescription or otherwise; all alcohol and caffeine; and, yes, even cosmetics, at least synthetic ones. In fact, while pregnant or nursing, be very careful about everything you put on your body, in your body, and near your body. Children, unborn and born, cannot speak for themselves: adults must look out for them.

And adults, in this case, includes men. In 1985, in *The Poisoned Womb: Human Reproduction in a Polluted World*, John Elkington cites studies showing the presence of modern chemicals, such as PCBs, pesticides, and a flame-retardant used with foam-filled furniture, in semen, with an associated drop in sperm count and sperm density. Men who smoke or work with lead, paints, wood, textiles, pesticides, auto exhaust, rubber chemicals, anesthetics, and industrial solvents such as benzene, vinyl chloride, trichloroethylene, and butadiene or who work as janitors, electricians, and drivers are more likely than other men to be sterile or to father babies with low birth weight, birth defects, certain cancers, and other adverse effects. In 1993 the British scientific journal *Chemosphere* reported that dioxin has been found in the semen of Vietnam veterans. Scientists have even found residues from cigarette smoke in the seminal fluid of men who smoke. Says Dr. Alan R Gaby, "If we do not start cleaning up our environment for our children, we will not be able to have children for whom to clean up the environment."

Infants and Children

With an immature immune system and a liver not completely functional, a newborn baby is particularly vulnerable to chemical exposure. So perhaps the first question that we must ask is, should women breast-feed their newborn infants? In recent decades women have returned to breast feeding in droves, as the emotional and physical health benefits have become well known. Yet, according to Peter Montague, in *RACHEL's Hazardous Waste News*, "if breast milk from American women were bottled and sold commercially, it would be subject to ban by the FDA because it is contaminated with more than a hundred industrial chemicals, including pesticides. The

FDA has set limits on contamination of commercial milk by pesticides, and [according to a 1980 article in the *NEJM*] human milk routinely exceeds those limits by a wide margin." For new mothers, this is clearly a difficult risk/benefit decision.

But, as Dr. Rogers points out, such decisions can have lifelong ramifications. "Take a newborn infant, whose detoxification system is not fully mature," says Rogers. "What do you do with that kid? You put him in a plastic bassinet with plastic bumpers, you have him breathe benzene [and] toluene, you put him in polyester clothes with fire retardant. . . . And then they wonder why the kid is learning disabled, why he's foggy-headed, why he doesn't grow."

Infants can also be exposed to toxins in common baby products. A 1991 study by researchers at Loyola University Medical Center, in Maywood, Illinois, found that ten of the eighty chemicals in shampoos, powders, and other baby products were at least "moderately toxic" to animals. "Repeated exposure of an infant to so many chemicals in combination may not be very beneficial," says Dr. George Lambert, associate professor of pediatrics and an expert on environmental toxins. "A newborn baby more readily absorbs chemicals placed on its skin than does an adult." Avoid perfumes and additives, say the researchers; use only bland, simple products, and sparingly. A clean washcloth and warm water are often all that is needed.

Children of all ages are more susceptible to toxic chemicals than adults. This is so, says Paigen, because children take in more food, water, and air per pound of body weight—and thus more toxics—than adults; because their growing bodies and rapidly dividing cells are easily damaged by toxins; because some of their organ systems, especially their immune and reproductive systems, are immature; and because their lifestyle is more likely to bring them into contact with contaminants. Children are more likely than adults to roll around in the grass, play in mud and toxic waste sites, and put their dirty fingers in their mouths. In Love Canal, New York, children used to ride their bikes on a polluted dirt trail, raising clouds of dust which they breathed and brought home on their clothes. A seven-year-old Love Canal boy died three months after playing in an oily creek behind his house The autopsy found chemical damage to his kidney, lung, liver, and brain. Later the creek was found to be heavily contaminated with dioxin and other chemicals.

Cancer is often the greatest fear in contaminated communities, yet Paigen feels more concern about neurotoxins—chemicals, such as those in many pesticides, that affect the brain and the nervous system: "They cause symptoms such as severe headaches, dizziness, memory loss, clumsiness, depression, vision and hearing problems, loss of balance, and tingling or numbness in the hands and feet. In children, neurotoxins can cause learning problems at school, hyperactive behavior, and seizures. If exposure to neurotoxins continues long enough, permanent brain damage can result."

Providing one of the many pesticide exposures in our oversprayed world, parents often spray insect repellents on their children, not realizing that these "bug sprays . . . can cause toxic reactions in young children, such as slurred speech, staggering walk, agitation, tremors and seizures," said University of Michigan pharmacist Cary Johnson. Infants and toddlers can also pick up pesticides, especially older, persistent ones, in house dust, according to the EPA's 1990 Nonoccupational Pesticide Exposure Study (NOPES). And according to researchers at Rutgers University and Robert Wood Johnson Medical School, use of "flea bombs" can cause measurable toxicological responses in infants. Entering fumigated rooms too soon and spraying repeatedly can make the problem worse. Does this mean that you have to keep your house super-clean or learn to live with bugs and fleas? Not at all. It simply means that to protect your children you need to find alternatives to toxic pesticides (see Chapter 7).

According to the OTA's *Neurotoxicity*, the NAS estimates that 12 percent of the sixty-three million children under the age of eighteen in the U.S. suffer from one or more mental disorders, with exposure to toxic substances before or after birth one of several risk factors. Lead is one of those toxic substances—another neurotoxin that can affect children's ability to think and learn. The dangers of lead poisoning, especially to black and other minority children eating peeling paint in dilapidated housing in the inner cities, have been known since the 1930s, though little was done about it. In 1971 Congressman William F. Ryan said that lead poisoning "is totally manmade and a totally preventable disease. It exists only because we let it exist. Lead poisoning has sentenced thousands of young children to lives of misery, disease, and even death." Finally, in 1991, as it was becoming clear that lead was also affecting white children in affluent suburbs, Dr. William Roper, director of the CDC, announced that "lead poisoning is the No. 1 environmental problem facing America's children." In October 1991 the CDC lowered its lead exposure guidelines by 60 percent—from 25 micrograms of lead per deciliter of blood to 10 micrograms.

Once again children (and probably pregnant women) are most at risk: "Children absorb 50 percent of lead in their food, whereas adults absorb only 8 percent to 15 percent." How many children have high blood levels of lead? A surprising number, according to the National Center for Health Statistics (NCHS): "88 percent of American children younger than six have sufficient lead in their blood to retard their mental, physical, and emotional development."[36] And according to a 1992 EPA report, from three million to four million children—many black and Hispanic children living in urban areas—are affected by lead poisoning.

At a mid-1980s meeting of the International Conference of the Association for Children with Learning Disabilities, scientists presented findings indicating a possible link between learning disabilities and toxic substances, such as lead, PCBs, pesticides, and mercury. At the meeting, Dr. Herbert Needleman, of Pittsburgh's Children's Hospital, presented the results of his study of the effects of lead on school children: "the mean IQ score of children with high lead levels was four points below that of children with low lead levels . . . teachers tended to describe children with high lead levels as 'distractible, not persistent, not organized, and hyperactive,' traits commonly associated with learning disabilities." Not an encouraging report.

Mercury is another highly poisonous chemical element, present in soil, water, and food. It is used by dentists in "silver" fillings, and for years it was put in interior latex paint as a preservative and fungicide. It attacks the nervous system and the kidneys. It can lead to brain damage or loss of muscle control when ingested or inhaled in even minuscule amounts. It is also another particular hazard to children. The EPA has now banned mercury in interior latex paint, following the 1989 hospitalization of a four-year-old Detroit boy with near-fatal poisoning from exposure to mercury vapors from paint. Obviously, the child did not do the painting, but was a passive victim of something that did not affect the adult painter. If you intend to paint in the presence of children, the EPA suggests that you check paint can labels in order to avoid older paint containing mercury; ventilate your house well; schedule interior painting over an extended period of time; and not use exterior latex inside because it still contains mercury. Check Chapter 4 for a list of least-toxic paints.

You would also be wise to ask your dentist about alternatives to silver/mercury amalgams for your children's fillings (amalgams are about 50 percent mercury). Research teams at the University of Calgary School of Medicine and the Royal Dental College in Denmark discovered that mercury from amalgam fillings "could be found in the blood and tissues of pregnant [animal] mothers and their babies within a few days." And according to a 1991 University of Nebraska study, "trace amounts of mercury can be measured in the urine of patients up to a year after their teeth have been filled with mercury amalgam." Research such as this has ignited controversy within dental circles, because for over a hundred years dentists have put millions of silver/mercury amalgams in children's (and adults') mouths.

Smoking, of course, should never be done around children. The EPA's January 7, 1993, pronouncement about secondhand smoke noted that smoking poses special risks to the captive audience of children. Later that year, EPA head Carol Browner said that secondhand smoke causes 150,000 to 300,000 respiratory infections in infants that result in 7,500 to 15,000 hospitalizations a year. How much anguish and money would be saved if adults refrained from smoking around children!

Schools: a Chemical Soup

Are children any better off when they get in school? In 1989 the head of the EPA's TEAM study of indoor air pollution, Lance Wallace, said that in "public buildings such as offices, schools, and nursing homes, eight common chemicals were increased [over outdoor air levels] by factors of about a hundred."

Yes, schools. Our children are living and breathing nearly every day in buildings where pollution can be up to a hundred times greater than in the smoggy, smokestack air outside. What is causing this condition? In a 1985 survey of schools for the Toronto Board of Education, Bruce Small, a Canadian consulting engineer, found ninety-seven sources of health-threatening pollution. Among them were carbon dioxide, carpet glue, felt pens, cockroach and termite sprays, brush cleaner, floor polish, particleboard shelving, photocopy paper, and the fumes from art supplies and school buses. A similar study in the Wauconda, Illinois, schools in 1968 found the chief culprits to be aerosol sprays; janitorial and scholastic supplies; heating, ventilating, and cooking equipment; building materials and furnishings; cosmetics and toiletries; smoking; and school buses. Recall those pungent, unpleasant odors you encountered on the first day of school each year, after the janitors had spent the summer spiffing up the place? Ever heard of school phobia? Could there be a connection?

In 1990, in Wimberley, Texas, more than forty families joined in a product liability suit against nineteen defendants—including architects, air-conditioning contractors, and carpet suppliers—who were responsible for an unsafe elementary school. Several parents and children had rushed outside and vomited after touring the school just before it opened. Angie Button, who began coming home from the school with terrible headaches, nosebleeds, and ear and throat infections, has since become so chemically sensitive that a whiff of cigarette smoke, perfume, gasoline, or fabric softener makes her ill. Because Angie cannot tolerate the industrial cleaners used in her middle school, her parents have been teaching her at home.

School carpeting can make the chemically sensitive ill; in closed classrooms it can give students persistent chemical sensitivity problems. Karla and Kristin, daughters of a North Dakota Lutheran minister, both developed chemical sensitivity from exposures to new carpeting in two different high schools. Karla reacted so severely that she had to become a homebound student; Kristin had to be transferred to a safer high school. Both have had to take extensive precautions in order to be able to attend college. As their concerned father eloquently wrote, "There is one thing I have had to accept: The problem is real. It will not go away. Thousands of people are being adversely affected by hazardous chemicals commonly found indoors and out. Those affected need the church's ministry and need to know their suffering is real."

Despite strict laws requiring school districts to test their water for lead, government auditors report that many children continue to ingest "harmful amounts" of lead in school drinking water; state agencies and the EPA, say the auditors, simply fail to enforce existing lead laws. Perhaps in response, the EPA in 1991 lowered its standard for lead in drinking water from 50 to 15 parts per billion, with water utilities having twenty-one years to put this new standard into effect—by which time a new generation of schoolchildren will have grown up drinking lead with their water.

Diesel exhaust from school buses in Benton-Harbor/St. Joseph, Michigan, made eleven-year-old Matthew Pikorz sick, but it is not the only thing. When Dr. Randolph tested him after other doctors had failed to help him, he reacted to perfume, cigarette smoke, ethanol, formaldehyde, dry-cleaning solvents, auto exhaust, pesticides, hairspray, phenols, gasoline and its byproducts such as polyester, and many foods. Life has become very difficult for Matthew and his parents, who must now teach Matthew at home. His mother, herself a teacher, often feels helpless: "You can't see plasticizers. You can't see perfume or mold spores. You can see measles. You can see a runny nose. You can see these things, but you can't see outgassing and all the pesticides and you're breathing and eating them all the time. You have to play detective and you have to be informed."

Just as when they were infants, schoolchildren bear more risk not only because they are not informed, but because they have no control over their surroundings. For awareness and help, they must depend on adults, including their teachers, who *are* becoming more aware. In 1993 New York State United Teachers reported that internal air pollution afflicts buildings in about one in ten of New York State's public school systems. Students, teachers, and other employees in these buildings were suffering from respiratory illnesses, skin rashes, dizziness, and headaches. On average, Florida health officials receive five sick school complaints every day—not from children, of course, but from concerned adults. Former teacher

Irene Wilkenfeld, sensitized by formaldehyde, conducts safe-school workshops for parents and teachers. "Some students who appear to be sick OF school," she says, "are actually being made sick AT school because of a toxic school setting."

Pesticides are yet another hazard for school-age children. A 1990 study of pesticide use in Texas classrooms done by the consumer group Public Citizen echoed the findings of its 1988 study of pest control practices in Washington, D.C., which concluded that "children are unknowingly entering a veritable 'poison zone' of pesticide exposure in their classrooms." Fortunately, educators nationwide are becoming more aware of the dangers of routine spraying. Sierra Club National Defense Fund lawyer Victor M. Sher has suggested that school districts doing routine spraying could be subject to lawsuits: "If you stop and think about it, spraying kids in schools or in any state program is like grabbing them and giving them a very lethal drug. They can't say no." After Eastchester High School, in an affluent New York City suburb, was closed for three weeks in 1992 following a pesticide application that sickened students, teachers, and staff, the school employees' union filed a complaint with the State Department of Labor. In 1993 New York Attorney General Robert Abrams issued a report calling attention to the fact that children in New York schools are routinely exposed to high-risk pesticides without prior notification. Ironically, while many school nurses are not allowed to dispense aspirin to children without parental permission, toxic chemicals are usually allowed to be sprayed around schools without parental permission or even notification.

As word of possible legal and health dangers gets around, schools, school districts, and even states are opting for IPM, which uses pesticides only as a last resort and only as needed. Examples: Texas has mandated schools to have IPM in place by September 1995; the Eugene, Oregon, school system has adopted IPM; and Dade County (Florida) public schools have gone to IPM. The National Education Association (a teachers' union) and both state and national parent-teacher associations have passed resolutions backing reduced use of pesticides. One especially successful parent effort, in Glendale, Arizona, won two EPA demonstration grants, developed an education program called "Hug-a-Bug," and managed to convince one highly skeptical school administrator of the dangers from pesticides. "Hug-a-Bug" teaches children to develop their own—safer—pest management plans. How much better than making them helpless victims of poisonous fallout!

Still, even within individual schools, certain classrooms and activities can present particular problems. Fluorescent lighting, so prevalent in schools, has been found to affect students' behavior and health. In her 1980 book *At Highest Risk: Environmental Hazards to Young and Unborn Children*, Christopher Norwood cites the work of John Ott, pioneer in the relationship of light to health. His studies have found that students in classrooms lighted with full-spectrum light (which reproduces the balance of natural light) behaved better and had fewer cavities than students in classrooms lighted by cool-white fluorescent tubes. Striking photos of students' behavior with and without fluorescent lighting can be seen in Ott's book, *Light, Radiation, and You*.

Another activity worth special mention is arts and crafts, a component of nearly every elementary school's curriculum. Many chemicals used in arts and crafts are extremely toxic; yet many artists routinely pay little heed to warnings and, reports Michael McCann, director of the Center for Occupational Health in New York and author of *Artist Beware*, teachers often appear not to realize the toxicity of such materials as rubber cement, permanent felt-tip markers, pottery glazes, enamels, spray fixatives, and wheat wallpaper paste. When both the teacher and students fell ill with respiratory and other symptoms in an industrial arts classroom in Piscatawny Township, New Jersey, the teacher first complained, then sued, eventually winning a $60,000 settlement.

The Center for Safety in the Arts, in New York City, has this advice for choosing children's art materials: no dust or powders; no chemical solvents or solvent-containing products; no aerosol spray cans or air brushes; nothing that stains the skin or clothing; no acids, alkalis, bleaches, or other "corrosive" chemicals; no donated or found materials unless the ingredients are known; no old materials. Words to the wise . . . for their children.

Finally, children also appear especially vulnerable to a more recent twentieth-century threat, one often associated with schools. This time it is electromagnetic fields (emfs)—not chemicals as such, but the energetic emissions from chemicals. (Keep in mind that all matter is composed of chemicals. Electromagnetic fields are generated by the movement of electrons within, through, and near matter.) In the late 1970s, epidemiologist Nancy Wertheimer's independent research linked childhood leukemia to electric feeder lines from transformers near houses. The connection between emfs and illness, meticulously laid out by environmental health writer Paul Brodeur, first in the *New Yorker* and later in his book *Currents of Death*, continues to be confirmed by later studies, such as a 1992 Swedish study that showed a close relationship between emfs and cancer, especially childhood leukemia. Though such conclusions are tentative, Brodeur has written that while research is in progress "interim preventive measures should be undertaken to reduce magnetic-field exposure of children in hundreds of schools and day-care centers across the nation which have been built perilously close to high-voltage and high-current power lines. That can be accomplished by rerouting such lines, or burying them in a manner that will prevent hazardous magnetic-field emissions. Needless to say, such measures should be supported by the parents of schoolchildren, by members of parent-teacher associations, and by officials of school districts, of city and state health departments, and of the federal Environmental Protection Agency." Concerns like these have led activist Cathy Bergman, of the National Electro-Magnetic Radiation Alliance, to observe, "It is not unusual for parents to hear about the emf issue one afternoon, hire an attorney that evening, and have litigation filed in the morning."

Yet more and more schools are providing emf-generating computers for students, with little thought given to possible long-term health effects. We used to consider computers and other electronic marvels progress, but now some of us are not so sure. And in the words of Dr. Richard Jackson, chairman of the Academy of Pediatrics' environmental hazards committee, the U.S. hasn't been "keeping an eye on the canaries in our population, the children."

The Elderly

According to the OTA's neurotoxicity report, "the elderly are more susceptible to certain neurotoxic substances because decline in the structure and function of the nervous system with age limits its ability to respond to or compensate for toxic effects. In addition, decreased liver and kidney function increases susceptibility to toxic substances. Aging may also reveal adverse effects masked at a younger age."

Perhaps the most startling statistic, for both children and the elderly, however, comes not from the field of neurotoxicity but from the NCI: a "dramatic rise" in brain cancers has occurred during the last fifteen years in Americans over sixty-five, in children, and in adults aged thirty to thirty-four; the incidence of brain cancer in the elderly is doubling every nine years. The years 1973 to 1988 saw a 4.1 percent increase in the rate of all forms of cancer in children. At this point, researchers can only speculate as to causes.

Modern drugs can be especially dangerous for older adults, who take more of them than younger people. Although people over sixty-five make up only about 12 percent of the U.S. population, they take about 30 percent of the nation's prescription drugs and 40 percent of nonprescription drugs, according to the American Association of Retired Persons. HHS reports that people age sixty and older represent 17 percent of the U.S. population but "account for *nearly 40 percent of drug-related hospitalizations and more than half the deaths from drug reactions* [emphasis added]. Common adverse effects include depression, confusion, loss of memory, shaking and twitching, dizziness, and impaired thought processes."

Overprescribing and misprescribing are common in nursing homes and hospitals. A 1988 *JAMA* article suggested that "elderly patients in nursing homes may be getting risky and inappropriate medications intended to make them easier to control rather than to treat a genuine illness. . . . Although anti-psychotic drugs had been prescribed for one-third of the 850 patients studied, only thirty-six of those patients had been diagnosed as being psychotic. A study reported in the *Journal of the American Geriatrics Society* in 1990 found that "hospital records erred 60 percent of the time in listing important medications that patients older than age sixty-five were taking when admitted, raising a risk of serious treatment errors." A study of nursing home patients by Johns Hopkins researchers published in the *American Journal of Epidemiology* in 1991 identified medications such as sedatives and hypnotics with producing "strikingly higher risks" of falling than was true with patients not receiving such medications.

According to *Modern Maturity*, magazine of the American Association of Retired Persons, "thousands of older Americans are getting hooked on substances that are perfectly legal: the drugs prescribed by their doctors. . . . A federal report released in 1989 stated that two million older adults were addicted or at risk of addiction to sleeping pills or tranquilizers." There's even a new medical "specialty": at least thirty-one American doctors specialize in helping people withdraw from tranquilizers, such as Xanax.

Often patients, including the elderly, are not told of possible side effects or properly instructed in the use of medications. A 1991 University of California study estimated that "20 percent of Americans sixty years and older have suffered adverse reactions to prescribed drugs, primarily because their physicians did not tell them what side effects might occur and how they might be avoided." Pharmacist Forrest G. Hester says that according to the National Council on Patient Information and Education, "at least sixty thousand Americans lost their lives needlessly in 1986 alone as a result of not taking prescription medication properly." His advice: (1) Always ask your doctor and pharmacist questions, such as, What is this drug supposed to do? How and when do I take it and for how long? What should I eat or not eat, do or not do, while taking it? What are the side effects and what should I do if they occur? (2) Always get all your prescriptions at the same drug store so that your pharmacist can monitor them. (3) Take all your prescription drugs with you to your doctors so they can see what you are taking. (4) Follow label instructions exactly, report unexpected side effects to your doctor, and throw out all unused drugs. Sensible advice, and not just for the elderly.

Finally recognizing the special needs of the elderly, the FDA in 1990 proposed new physician labeling regulations for prescription drugs spelling out their effects on people over age sixty-five. "Patients [can] lose a third or more of their kidney function between the ages of thirty and ninety, so drugs may not clear the body as fast," said Dr. Louis W. Sullivan, then HHS secretary. "A dose of a muscle relaxant that might work fine in a young man or woman might so relax an older woman that she would fall and break a hip." However, you will look in vain for information about such effects on most labels or package inserts: "It's an imperfect world," commented John Hazard, of the FDA's Center for Drug Evaluation and Research, in 1993, when he was asked what had happened to the proposed regulations. Nevertheless, whatever your age, it is wise to ask your doctor to write on any prescription a request for the pharmacist to give you the package insert.

While overmedication of the elderly can occur both in and out of nursing homes and is fairly well recognized, a less-publicized hazard in nursing homes is the overuse of strong, sometimes toxic, cleaning products. In their zeal to have nursing homes bacteria- and odor-free, nursing-home administrators often unwittingly select products that are toxic, that make chemically sensitive patients sick, and that are unhealthy for both workers and patients. Formaldehyde, a suspected carcinogen, is in, among other things, bed sheets, disinfectants, air fresheners, mildew preventatives, soap dispensers, drugs, deodorants, toothpaste, casts, and bandages, according to the Formaldehyde Institute. An FDA panel has questioned the safety of antimicrobial "deodorant" soaps, declaring "not safe" or "not proved safe" those containing chloroxylenol (PCMX), cloflucarban, dibromsalan (DBS), fluorosalan, hexachlorophene, phenol, tetrachlorosalicylanilide (TCSA), tribromsalan (TBS), triclocarban, or triclosan. (These substances are present in many heavily advertised soaps.) The panel, according to environmental writer Debra Lynn Dadd, "could find no evidence that these potentially hazardous substances actually helped stop body odor any more effectively than did plain soap. It also warned that deodorant soaps should not be used on infants under six months of age."

If such products are bad for infants, they are surely bad for the elderly . . . and for you.

Women

Though the neurotoxicity report did not cite women as being most at risk, there is some reason to believe that women are more endangered by environmental pollutants than men. According to NCI figures, the lung cancer rate is sharply up in nonsmoking women. A study by NAS researcher Devra Lee Davis found that the death rate from lung cancer among nonsmoking women is higher than the total lung cancer death rate in women thirty years ago. The reasons, she speculated, could be exposure to secondhand smoke and to radon, asbestos, and possibly air pollution. Female smokers may run about twice the risk of lung cancer that male smokers do for a given number of cigarettes smoked during their lives, according to a study by epidemiologist Harvey Risch, of the Yale University School of Medicine. Epidemiologist Samuel Epstein has pointed out that "virtually the entire U.S. population consumes, without any warning, labelling, or information, unknown and unpredictable amounts of hormonal residues in meat products over their lifetimes. . . . Left unanswered is whether such chronic and uncontrolled estrogen dosages are involved in increasing cancer rates (now striking one in three Americans), particularly the alarming 50 percent increase in the incidence of breast cancer since 1965 [emphasis added]." Radiologist S. Boyd Eaton and others researching primitive tribes in Africa and Australia suggest that American women may be one hundred times more vulnerable to breast cancer than their Stone Age ancestors, because of markedly different modern lifestyles.

While researchers caution against any rash assumptions as to cause, environmental physicians find that most of their patients are women, both those who work in the home and those who work out of the home. Few statistics are available, but one such physician, Dr. Gerald Ross, has documented that 78 percent of his chemically injured patients are women, with the most common age of onset being the twenties. One clue: a Vancouver consulting firm reported at the conference Indoor Air '90 in Toronto that because of exposure to household cleaners, housewives have a 55 percent higher risk of cancer than women who work outside the home. Many household cleaning products are known to contain toxic chemicals.

Questions arise: Are women perhaps more apt to seek medical help than men? In 1986 the proportion of women teachers in elementary through high school was 68.8 percent: could this be a factor? (Dr. Randolph, who diagnosed and treated more than nine thousand chemically sensitive patients in over forty-five years of practice, considers teaching a hazardous occupation.) Are more women than men working in tightly closed, energy-efficient but inadequately ventilated buildings that recirculate perfumes, copier fumes, and the fumes from inks, carpets, cosmetics, detergents, synthetic fabrics, pressed wood, pesticides, and so on? One theory, from the director of the National Institute of Environmental Health Sciences of the NIH is that "women are more susceptible to toxins due to the physiological changes brought on by menstruation and menopause. Many of these toxins replace natural estrogen in cells, sometimes stimulating the production of various hormones or blocking such hormones. The toxins are absorbed into fatty tissue—such as the breast, where they can influence cellular function over decades." But no one knows for sure.

Help!

By now you may be thinking that this is too much. It's too grim. You want to stop reading. Actually, you're right; it is grim. But before you stop reading, consider Lawson's Laws:

Lawson's First Law: *You can never know too much about this stuff.* There is a lot to know, and more is turning up every day. It's hard to keep up—but what alternative do you have, if you want to stay healthy?

Lawson's Second Law: *You have to be your own personal environmental protection agency.* This is sad, but true. With the environment (read "health"), our leaders are asleep at the switch. The EPA is playing tiddledywinks with corporate America. You have to learn how to protect yourself. Just remember that we're all different: what helps one does not always help another.

Lawson's Third Law: *You have to be your own private detective agency.* Look for clues everywhere, especially in labels on products. Be sure to read the label on the back as well as the front of the bottle or can. The front may say "unscented" and the back "masking fragrance added." If a label says "turpentine" or "petroleum distillates" or "keep out of reach of children," find something that doesn't. It will probably do the job just as well.

Now read on. Your children (and maybe your parents) are counting on you.

* * * *

To Find Out More

- *Poisoning Our Children: Surviving in a Toxic World*, by Nancy Sokol Green, Chicago, The Noble Press, 1991.

- *The Poisoned Womb: Human Reproduction in a Polluted World*, by John Elkington, Penguin Books, 1985.

- *At Highest Risk: Environmental Hazards to Young and Unborn Children*, by Christopher Norwood, New York, McGraw-Hill, 1980.

- *Taking Care of Your Baby and Young Child: Birth to Age Five*, American Academy of Pediatrics, New York, Bantam, 1991.

- *Is This Your Child?*, by Doris Rapp, MD, New York, William Morrow, 1991.

- *The Impossible Child: In school, at home*, by Doris Rapp, MD, 1986; available (plus audio and video tapes) from Practical Allergy Research Foundation, P.O. Box 60, Buffalo, New York 14223-0060.

- *Artist Beware*, by Michael McCann, New York, Lyons and Burford, 1992.

- *The Artist's Complete Health and Safety Guide: Everything you need to know about art materials to make your workplace safe and comply with United States and Canadian right-to-know laws*, by Monona Rossol, New York, Allworth Press, 1990.

- *Making Art Safely: Alternative Methods and Materials in Drawing, Painting, Printmaking, Graphic Design, and Photography*, by Merle Spandorfer, Deborah Curtiss, and Jack Snyder, MD, New York, Van Nostrand Reinhold, 1992.

- *Air Pollution in the Schools and Its Effects on Our Children*, by Kathleen A. Blume, 1968; available from the Randolph Clinic (Terrell Haws, DO), 121 South Wilke, Suite 111, Arlington Heights, Illinois 60005.

- *Neurotoxicity: Identifying and Controlling Poisons of the Nervous System*, U.S. Congress, Office of Technology Assessment, OTA-BA-436, 1990 (write Superintendent of Documents, U.S.

Government Printing Office, Washington, D.C. 20402-9325; $15, GPO stock number 052-003-01184-1).

- *Neurotoxicity Guidebook: Neurotoxicology for the lay person and the scientist*, by Raymond Singer, New York, Van Nostrand Reinhold, 1990 (also *Neurotoxicity Screening Survey: Self-administered symptom questionnaire*, available from Raymond Singer, 50 Monte Alto Road, Santa Fe, New Mexico 97505).

- *How to Raise a Healthy Child . . . in spite of your doctor*, by Robert S. Mendelsohn, MD, New York, Ballantine, 1984.

- *Healthy Homes, Healthy Kids*, by Joyce Schoemaker and Charity Vitale, Washington, D.C., Island Press, 1991.

- *The Toxic Time Bomb: Can the Mercury in Your Dental Fillings Poison You?*, by Sam Ziff, New York, Aurora Press, 1984.

- *Currents of Death*, by Paul Brodeur, New York, Simon & Schuster, 1989.

- *Cross Currents*, by Robert O. Becker, Los Angeles, Jeremy P. Tarcher, 1990.

- *Power Over People*, by Louise Young, New York, Oxford University Press, 1973, updated 1992.

- *Worst Pills Best Pills II: The Older Adult's Guide to Avoiding Drug-Induced Death or Illness*, by Sidney M. Wolfe, MD, and Rose-Ellen Hope, RPh, 1993; available from Public Citizen Health Research Group, 2000 P Street NW, Suite 700, Washington, D.C. 20036.

Other Sources of Information

- Association of Birth Defect Children Inc., 3526 Emerywood Lane, Orlando, Florida 32812.

- National Lead Information Center (sponsored by the National Safety Council), 1019 Nineteenth Street NW, Suite 401, Washington, D.C. 20036-5105: Clearinghouse 1-800-424-LEAD and 24-hour Hotline 1-800-LEAD-FYI, both in English and Spanish.

- To test for lead paint, try your local hardware store or two home kits rated as effective by Consumers Union: LeadCheck Swabs, by HybriVet Systems (1-800-262-LEAD) and Frandon Lead Alert Kit, by Frandon Enterprises (1-800-359-9000). Before removing lead paint, consult sources such as David Steinman's book *Diet for a Poisoned Planet* (Harmony Books, 1990).

- New York Coalition for Alternatives to Pesticides (NYCAP), 33 Central Avenue, Albany, New York 12210; 518-426-8246 (NEA and PTA position statements; packet of articles; sample indoor IPM contracts).

- Office of Public Information, New York State Department of Law, 120 Broadway, New York, New York 10271 (reports by New York Attorney General Robert Abrams, "Pesticides in Schools: Reducing the Risks" and "The Secret Hazards of Pesticides").

- U.S. Environmental Protection Agency, Public Information Center, Washington, D.C. 20460; 202-382-2080 or 202-260-7751 (ask for EPA booklets "Lead Poisoning and Your Children," "Environmental Hazards in Your School" and "Pest Control in Schools: Adopting Integrated Pest Management"; the latter includes sample school IPM policy and model set of contract performance specifications).

- Residents for Alternative Pest Policy, 1408 Rosemonte Drive, Phoenix, Arizona 85024 (for information on Arizona law and Hug-a-Bug curriculum).

- Foundation for Toxic-Free Dentistry, P.O. Box 608010, Orlando, Florida 32860-8010.

- Dental Amalgam Mercury Syndrome Inc. (DAMS), P.O. Box 9065, Downers Grove, Illinois 60515.

- Center for Safety in the Arts, 5 Beekman Street, Suite 1030, New York, New York 10038.

- Arts, Crafts, and Theater Safety (ACTS), 181 Thompson Street, #23, New York, New York 10012.

- Chem Safe Consulting, Inc., P.O. Box 332, Mapleton, Maine 04757 (ask for its publication "Parents Guide to Curricular-Based Chemicals in Schools").

- National Electro-Magnetic Radiation (EMR) Alliance, 410 West 53rd Street, Suite 402, New York, New York 10019; 212-554-4073.

- *EMF Resource Directory*, available from Micro-Wave News, P.O. Box 1799 Grand Central Station, New York, New York 10163; 212-517-2800.

- "How Environmentally Safe Are Our Schools?," a two-hour workshop designed by former teacher Irene Ruth Wilkenfeld, 52145 Farmington Square Road, Granger, Indiana 46530; 219-271-8990.

11

Recourse

I F   Y O U   A R E   A   P E R S O N who is severely chemically sensitive, you are a person with serious problems in living. If you have a job, you probably will not be able to keep it; you may have to move; you may lose friends and family; you probably will have less energy; for a while you will need more money; you may not be able to go to stores and other public buildings; you may even become completely homebound. In short, you will have to give up a great deal—or experience the continued deterioration of your health as you go on living as you have been.

As you give up these things, you will probably begin feeling better. In time, you may feel fairly well. You may even be almost "cured," though you will probably have to be careful about chemical exposures the rest of your life. When Dr. Randolph was asked in 1987 if there is a cure for EI/MCS, he said "No, there cannot be a cure because new chemical hazards are multiplying faster than we can deal with them."

But what do you do while trying to recover? Your needs can be overwhelming. You need help—mainly money and safe housing. You don't look disabled, but you are. What recourse do you have? For the short term, you will have to rely on family, friends, and savings. For the long term, there are now a few bright spots in a once dismal picture.

Social Security Disability

Many disabled people look to social security disability benefits as their first hope. For people with EI/MCS, however, obtaining such benefits has not been easy. Often it has required legal action. In 1979 the U.S. District Court for Hawaii ruled the illness disabling and ordered the U.S. Department of Health, Education, and Welfare (now Health and Human Services) to provide social security disability benefits to Marna Slocum. (She now maintains a toxin-free rental apartment in Hawaii for recovering EI/MCS patients who are able to travel. Renters are asked to use washable luggage that they must wash in an outdoor machine before entering the apartment, to rid it of possible contamination from the plane trip.)

In 1988 the Social Security Administration (SSA) added a section on multiple chemical sensitivities to its disability manual, thus giving official recognition to the illness and opening the way for more of the chemically injured to obtain social security benefits. According to Earon Davis, a lawyer and long-time advocate for chemical victims, this means that "it makes it an error for SSA to say that the illness does not exist and/or that it is psychosomatic. If violated, the Appeals Council or any competent administrative judge would review it. Therefore, it should be easier to contest attempts to have the claimant evaluated by a psychiatrist."

With many claimants it was only too easy for SSA officials to assume that the illness is psychiatric. "The stresses of being a chemical victim, as well as neuropsychiatric effects of many substances, often contribute to the appearance of psychiatric disturbance," Davis wrote in his newsletter *Ecological Illness Law Report*, in which for several years he thoroughly covered legal actions relating to EI/MCS in the U.S. and Canada. Actually, some chemical victims, though they and their physicians knew better, had to accept a psychiatric diagnosis in order to obtain benefits. This may change as officials become more aware of the work of researchers like Linda Davidoff, clinical psychologist at Johns Hopkins University, who has demonstrated the flaws in studies purporting to show EI/MCS as psychological in origin. "At present," she says, "there are no credible data supporting any of these observations."

Before 1988, acceptance by the SSA was spotty at best. Many

EI/MCS claimants were turned down repeatedly by the system and finally gave up after long, time-consuming efforts. Some found themselves too ill to prepare the extensive paperwork, obtain the essential supporting documents, and attend the necessary consultations with their own lawyers and the opposing physicians—or too ill to attend hearings in unsafe locations. Some who made it to the final stage, a hearing before an administrative law judge, found themselves confronted with hostile professional "experts" and a basic lack of understanding of this complex, little-known condition. Even since the SSA's 1988 landmark action, some petitioners have had to resort to the courts. In 1990, in a Minnesota case, the U.S. Court of Appeals overruled the SSA and upheld MCS as a disabling condition.

Some petitioners' problem lay in the difficulty of convincing officials that they were fairly healthy at home but sick in workplaces, whether offices, stores, factories, or conveyances. A Denver secretary, Janet Carlson (not her real name), had suffered for ten years from severe, incapacitating headaches. When she quit her job, stayed home, and rid her house of petrochemically based products, her health improved, though she was still unable to tolerate printer's ink, correction fluids, typewriter ribbons, and typewriter cleaning solutions. Unable to work either at home or in an office, she applied for social security disability benefits. Her claim twice denied, she proceeded to the next step, a hearing with an administrative law judge. There, at a hearing in 1988, just before the SSA's acceptance of EI/MCS, she found herself and her environmental physician the object of a vicious verbal attack by a traditional allergist hired by the court (not an appropriate expert in toxicity cases). When she and her physician tried to explain the illness to the judge, he stopped them: "I don't want to get involved in the medical controversy surrounding this illness," he said. (How could he avoid it?) Months later came his decision: claim denied. Carlson's lawyer submitted the claim to a U.S. District Court, at which stage no new evidence can be admitted. After this court denied the claim, Carlson's lawyer—and Carlson—gave up.

Some workers who developed EI/MCS had had the foresight to sign up for their employer's private disability insurance. Proving the existence of this usually invisible illness is no easier with private insurance than with governmental insurance, but a few sufferers have been successful in obtaining at least temporary benefits.

With either form of insurance, the social costs of our society's reliance on toxic chemicals are mounting. Unknowingly, we foot the bill for increased disability payments with our taxes and find ourselves saddled with increased premiums for our private insurance plans. How much better if companies could be persuaded to substitute safe—or less toxic—ingredients for the toxic ones in their products and workplaces.

Workers' Compensation

Workers with job-induced injuries and illnesses often turn to workers' compensation for redress. For those with chemically induced illness, that road is not easy either. Commenting on New York State's workers' compensation system, environmental physician James M. Miller said that "if you cut off a finger or break a leg on the job, or are overcome and must be carried out from a toxic dose of some chemical, the workers' compensation system will probably perform as intended with a minimum of delay and red tape. If you become sick or disabled from the daily incremental injuries of a chronic chemical exposure and develop an acquired multiple chemical sensitivity, you can expect an entirely different course of events. The system that was designed to handle occupational injuries and occupational illnesses seems to be thrown for a complete loss when confronted with an individual with multiple chemical sensitivities."

Workers' compensation was originally set up as an insurance program designed to protect companies from lawsuits, by means of a fair and expeditious compensation of workers for job-induced injuries and illnesses. State-run workers' compensation programs represent a compromise between labor and business—one reached before today's flood of toxic and untested chemicals. On-the-job injuries and their causes are fairly obvious, but workers with job-induced illnesses are often left high and dry. Their private insurance companies are only too eager to decide that the illness is job-related, which leaves them without their usual coverage; and the workers' compensation insurance companies do what they always do: resist the claims as much as possible and hire physicians as "independent examiners." For the chemically sensitive patient, the "independent examination" can be torture. "It is bad enough that a physician, merely by being ignorant of the illness, can destroy a valid claim; but in addition the examiner's office environment often makes the patient sick," says Dr. Miller. "It is quite obvious when one enters the office—to find smoking in the waiting room or among the staff, the floor carpeted, the furniture plastic, and the staff and doctor wearing perfume—that the establishment is not one that is capable of helping the patient. The resulting illness may last for days and yet remain invisible to the medical examiner and to the administrative law judge [who hears the case]."

In Dr. Miller's eyes, the system functions badly for the chemically injured patient because of "physician ignorance and intellectual dishonesty. The insurance carrier knows quite well which physicians are ignorant of the problems of chemical sensitivity and which physicians are willing to prostitute their medical degrees for the generous payments offered. Some of my patients have encountered physicians who saw their role as that of an advocate for the insurance company and an adversary of the patient, rather than that of an expert who might help to reveal truth."

In individual states the system does not appear to be working any better. In Illinois, where studies suggest that thousands of Illinois workers become ill or die from workplace-caused diseases each year, only a minuscule number turn to the workers' compensation system for financial relief. Less than 2 percent of the 54,088 claims filed before the [state's workers' compensation review board] in 1987 were for occupational diseases. Most of those were for such ailments as dermatititis and hearing loss, few for "the nation's leading occupational disease killer: cancers caused by exposure to airborne toxic substances on the job." One reason is that, in Illinois, disease claims must be filed within three years of the worker's last exposure and within three years of the onset of the disease. Cancer, like EI/MCS, often develops slowly, the result of repeated low-level exposures to toxic chemicals. Other reasons are that (1) an estimated 80 percent of the chemicals used in commerce have never been tested for toxicity, (2) many workers do not know the toxicity of the chemicals they are working with that have been tested for toxicity, and (3) their doctors are tuned into the disease, not the cause. Also, contested workers' compensation claims can hold up doctors' payments for years, while workers' private insurance companies will pay up more promptly, thus providing an incentive for the treating doctor to overlook a possible environmental cause for the illness.

One Illinois worker has fought for ten years for compensation for her workplace-induced disabling illness. Nine months of employment in a Chicago picture-framing shop, beginning in 1984, changed this victim's life forever. Previously healthy, when she started using lacquer paints and spray adhesives in the poorly ventilated shop she soon began experiencing sporadic, severe head and eye pain; lack of coordination and muscle strength; intermittent numbness in her face, arms, and legs; incoherence and memory loss; severe mood swings; and menstrual, digestive, respiratory, and sleep problems. On a Sunday night in February 1985, the day two newspaper articles about workplace injury and lack of toxicity data on chemicals appeared, the shop owner called her and fired her— for "low productivity." Deprived of her income and unable to hold other jobs because of her continuing health problems, she applied for and received unemployment benefits and, later, nearly bedridden, social security disability benefits. In February 1985 she filed with the Illinois Industrial Commission for workers' compensation, an expensive, frustrating, time-consuming action that required lengthy visits to the new State of Illinois building in Chicago's Loop. "Each time I walked into that building for a hearing," she said, "I immediately had a 'floating' sensation, and as the day went on I got more and more disoriented. Severely intoxicated by the chemical environment, I was unable to give coherent, cohesive testimony." Nevertheless, she eventually won both temporary total disability (TTD) and permanent total disability (PTD) from the workers' compensation judge. Though relieved when the employer involved decided not to appeal, in 1993 she found herself once more going to court to try to get workers' comp to cover her extensive medical bills. Because of the PTD, her social security benefits have been dramatically cut, leaving her permanently below the poverty line.

During the proceedings, she discovered that she had been working with fifty-six different chemicals, including benzene (a known human carcinogen), and such neurotoxic chemicals as toluene, xylene, butadiene, methylene chloride, and styrene. Uninformed as to their toxicity, she and other workers poured solvents like these onto rags to wipe picture frames. When she complained to the owner about the poor ventilation, he made promises but did nothing. A company-hired doctor recommended that she wear a respirator, but she could still smell and taste the chemicals through the mask. Not believed by the doctor (his tests proved negative), she was fired three weeks after MSDSs for the solvents arrived on the scene. Though permanently disabled, she now feels better physically, especially when she uses oxygen to assist her breathing and to prevent seizures. She takes no medication.

In Colorado things are much the same—"simply another case of the system penalizing the victim," according to Benjamin Kramer, a Boulder attorney. Sometimes the problems of his EI/MCS clients become too large and complex for him, particularly when employers stonewall his requests for information about workplace chemicals. Attorneys like Kramer, "too often saddled with sketchy diagnoses by doctors who don't fully understand the disease, and stalled by combative employers, spend almost three times as long investigating environmental illness cases [as investigating more conventional cases]." And even if they stick with their clients, the results are often discouraging: "Most workers' comp cases have a win ratio of 60 to 70 percent, but with MCS it's way below 50 percent," Kramer says. "How do you prove it was something a person was exposed to at work, that they aren't otherwise exposed to outside work?" The system needs serious reform, he believes. "As long as the employer or the insurer decides who the doctor will be to perform the diagnosis, well, how in hell are you going to fight that?"

In Washington State, chemically injured workers find that workers' compensation doctors give short examinations and do not perform any kind of tests. Yet "we can prove that patients have chemical sensitivity," said Dr. Gordon Baker, the Seattle allergist who has treated many such patients, "with the immune tests, with the neuropsychological tests, with the PET [positron emission tomography] scans, with the SPECT [single photon emission computed tomography] scans, and QUEEGs [quantitative electroencephalograms], [and] the antibodies to formaldehyde" and other chemicals.

Although a medical consultant at the Washington Department of Labor and Industries, which has denied most EI/MCS claims, has testified that there is no physiological or organic base for chemical sensitivity, there is a growing body of published evidence demonstrating the usefulness of such tests in diagnosing chemical injury. A research team headed by Los Angeles physician Gunnar Heuser, MD, PhD, found that objective immune-system, neurological, SPECT, and pulmonary-function tests on 135 patients proved to be valid diagnostic markers for EI/MCS. (SPECT and PET scans measure disruptions in cerebral blood flow.) Careful quantitative evaluation of electroencephalograms (QUEEGs) has shown certain components to be valid indicators of brain injury and functional impairment in chemically sensitive patients after exposure to perfumes in a controlled setting. A study of thirty-three people exposed to formaldehyde, pesticides, and VOCs found that 94 percent had abnormal SPECT scans, 91 percent had abnormal perception thresholds, 33 percent had abnormal nerve conductance velocities, and 29 percent had abnormal magnetic resonance imaging. Many of these patients were chemically sensitive. A study of 289 computer workers exposed to such chemicals as trimellitic anhydride, phthalic anhydride, and isocyanates found significant immune activation or suppression compared with control subjects. These researchers, led by Aristo Vojdani, PhD, consider the computer workers chemically injured. While many doctors seem unaware of how many tests are available to show physiological changes in the chemically sensitive, "laboratory abnormalities have now been demonstrated in so many parameters in chemically sensitive patients that the physician's difficulty is to select the best tests: those that are most sensitive, specific, and best correlated with clinical status and prognosis," says Grace Ziem, MD, DrPH, co-chair of the Multiple Chemical Sensitivity Task Force of the American Public Health Association.

In other states a few EI/MCS claimants have succeeded in obtaining workers' compensation benefits, though with difficulty and sometimes through court action. In 1986 the Oregon Court of Appeals ordered workers' compensation benefits paid to furniture store employees on the basis of MCS; and in 1987 the California Court of Appeals awarded benefits to an employee who was found to have developed MCS from long-term exposure to PCBs. Also in 1987, total disability benefits were awarded under South Carolina's workers' compensation laws to a woman whose physician wrote that "the constant exposure over nineteen years to the petrochemicals in her workplace dysregulated [her] immune system resulting in an allergic or hypersensitivity cascade [sic] to her total environment, including all foods, chemicals, and her own microbiological flora." (Chemical injury often manifests itself as an immune-system dysfunction.) A Florida appeals court in 1987 upheld a worker's compensation award based on an immune-system injury caused by a coolant used in his workplace. Though the worker showed no signs of illness elsewhere, the injury was considered a permanent disability.

Despite workers' difficulties in obtaining benefits, workers' compensation is big business in the U.S. In 1987, for example, companies paid $38 billion for workers' compensation insurance, and the insurance companies paid $27.4 billion for treatment of workers and for time-off or damage payments. The National Council on Compensation Insurance estimated that in 1993 total workers' compensation claims will reach $70 billion. Though not all job-related injuries or illnesses are preventable or caused by chemical exposures, surely this enormous and skyrocketing cost—which is of course passed on to consumers in increased prices for goods and services—can be reduced by companies learning to avoid toxic chemicals in the production process.

Legal Action

Some people with EI/MCS have bypassed social security and workers' compensation and gone directly to lawsuits, with varying degrees of success. In the 1980s an employee of Browning-Ferris Industries was awarded $275,000 after developing central blind spots in both eyes. For eight years he had worked with toxic chemicals such as benzene and toluene—all under the maximum allowable levels, but together causing disabling damage. In 1990 an Iowa district court jury awarded $1.5 million to five women permanently disabled by exposure to the pesticide Dursban (chlorpyrifos). After exposure in the county office building where they worked, these women were diagnosed with peripheral neuropathy, central nervous system effects, and immune dysfunction.

Often cases are settled out of court, or decisions are reversed. The *Wall Street Journal* reported in 1990 that "Boeing [aircraft] had settled out of court a case brought by an employee alleging that his leukemia was caused by exposure to ELF [extremely low frequency] fields." In an extraordinary first admission by a company that electromagnetic fields had harmed an employee, Boeing agreed to pay Robert Strom and his family more than $500,000 in cash and an additional annuity. The successful suit alleged in part that Boeing, "while knowing that the very high levels of electromagnetic fields might be harming lab workers, arranged for repeated physical examinations without revealing that the purpose of the exams was to study possible health damage." In Missouri, a jury awarded $49 million to community residents claiming numerous adverse health conditions resulting from toxic waste from a nearby chemical plant. The judge set aside the verdict, an action affirmed by the appeals court. The case was then settled out of court for an undisclosed amount.

Chemical injury suits address a huge variety of exposures. A 1991 suit on behalf of twenty-one thousand residential, commercial, and industrial painters asked for more than $2.1 billion from paint manufacturers as compensation for health damage from lead in the paints. In 1990 the American Psychological Association (APA) filed a friend-of-the-court brief in a case involving a family's claim of brain damage from an improper application of the pesticide aldrin in their home. The suit alleged that this brain damage "led to psychological problems, including permanent impairment of their cognitive abilities." A lower court had ruled that previous testimony by a licensed psychologist was not medically valid; the APA's brief argued that psychologists are "leaders in the scientific investigation of industrial and pharmacological agents' effects on the human nervous system and neuropsychological functioning." In 1991 seven airline flight attendants, alleging that they had contracted cancer, heart disease, and respiratory illnesses from exposure to passengers' cigarette smoke, sued several tobacco companies for $5 billion in punitive damages on behalf of sixty thousand airline employees. All said that they did not smoke and had become sick before Congress outlawed smoking on flights in the forty-eight contiguous states in 1989. One plaintiff, Marilyn Mittan, said, "I couldn't breathe through my nose. I had to sleep sitting up." She claimed that after she returned to her job following a six-month leave to recuperate, she was fired because of her condition.

Together with eight others, a former Westinghouse employee, whose 3,450 parts per billion of PCBs in the blood was "the highest ever recorded in a human," sued the company in 1991. (Animal studies link PCBs to cancer, liver damage, and birth defects.) Despite decades-old internal memos about possible PCB toxicity, a Westinghouse plant manager was reported to have "washed his hands and face in what he told workers was liquid PCBs to convince them not to worry." For Westinghouse and other companies, the suit raises the question of whether they should warn workers and risk exposing themselves to "financially crippling liability suits," or instead "keep mum until all the evidence is in." The PCB-loaded employee would no doubt have an answer to that question. Another answer would be for companies to find safe (or safer) substitutes for toxic chemicals like PCBs.

How many lawsuits involving EI/MCS have been filed? No one knows for sure. According to attorney Earon Davis and writer/advocate Mary Lamielle, there is no centralized data base for arriving at a figure. Nevertheless, they estimate hundreds, or even thousands: "In fact, it is likely that a majority of personal injury and product liability cases related to indoor air quality actually involve MCS. . . . Often, health symptoms more traditionally verifiable than MCS have been the focal point of these cases." In the *Indoor Pollution Law Report*, they cite as typical a landmark sick-building case, a formaldehyde case, carpeting cases (including a suit by EPA employees who developed EI/MCS from the EPA renovation), a school-roofing case, and the case of a family poisoned by pesticides in their own home.

"The legal stakes are high indeed," say Davis and Lamielle, "[and] the potential devastation of MCS raises questions about new and different measures of damages. . . . People with environmental disabilities may be capable of traveling, of going to restaurants, movies, and public buildings. Their nemesis is not the absence of handrails in a bathroom, but the presence of pesticides, disinfectants, or perfumes in modern buildings. The legal system is accustomed to addressing compensation for fixed disabilities. However, it has not dealt with the tremendous isolation and frustration caused by the variable loss of functioning caused by environmental disabilities." The Chemical Manufacturers Association agrees about the high stakes: in 1990 it sent to its 182 members a warning of the "potentially enormous cost" that might follow legal and medical legitimization of EI/MCS. The CMA may be right: in 1992 a Mississippi jury awarded $3.2 million to two landowners who feared developing cancer from eating catfish from a river contaminated by dioxin from a wood-pulp company. In 1993 New York State's highest court ruled that owners of property near high-voltage power lines can be awarded damages when "cancerphobia" lowers their property value, even without proof of a health risk. "We got an award for fear," said the Mississippi plaintiffs' lawyer. For chemically sensitive people, however, it's not a matter of fear, it's a matter of knowing what has made and is continuing to make them sick.

Lawsuits involving chemical injuries are on the increase, according to South Florida attorney Bryan Henry, who in 1989 had forty such cases. Speaking to a group of heating, refrigerating, and air-conditioning engineers about sick building syndrome, Henry attributed the increase to the fact that 90 percent of Florida's buildings are "sealed up for energy efficiency. . . . Victims of severe ecological illness suffer increased intolerance to a host of chemicals, like pesticides, formaldehyde, natural gas fumes, perfumes, and cigarette smoke." Two types of legal actions are possible, Henry has found: "breach of contract and negligence. If someone leases a building, they are providing an implied warranty that the building is safe for people to work in or habitate. If it can be shown that the building is related to a medical problem or personal injury, then that building is longer habitable. Therefore, the implied warranty of habitability has been breached." Negligence, he says, is a matter of the standards of care taken to assure habitability

Across the country, workers are paying the price for tightly constructed buildings holding in hundreds of noxious chemicals—and wanting to be reimbursed for the cost to their health. In Du Page County, Illinois, 125 workers made ill by the county's new $53-million courthouse are suing the building's engineer and architect and several other companies involved; the county is suing two of the companies. In Martin County, Florida, an $11-million courthouse remains abandoned because of poor indoor air quality, with a resulting "triangle of lawsuits" among workers, builders, and the county. Forty-three workers and their spouses, claiming they were poisoned by pesticides used at three New York State office buildings, have sued four corporations for $82 million. In what is thought to be one of the first awards of this kind, the state of Wisconsin in 1992 awarded more than $2,300 in workers' compensation benefits to two state employees for time off because of illness from SBS.

Winning chemical-related lawsuits is not easy, however. Take a typical case: former workers at a rubber-making plant in Texas allege that the butadiene in the plant causes cancer. A corporate epidemiologist says that one can't extrapolate from mouse studies to humans. The plaintiffs' lawyers argue that emissions from the plants years ago sowed the seeds of diseases that are only now showing up. Experts disagree; judges are not trained in science; scientists are reluctant to testify; and neither scientists nor doctors are trained in adversary proceedings. A 1989 workshop for doctors and lawyers on improving procedures for scientific evidence in toxic torts (lawsuits involving allegations of health or property damage from toxic or allegedly toxic substances) noted "an avalanche of multimillion-dollar verdicts in toxic tort cases." Workshop participants found that the courts have no systematic way to evaluate the validity of evidence presented by expert witnesses. Judges, for instance, may be "reluctant to bar testimony from 'outliers' whose views contradict those of the majority of scientists for fear they may be silencing a new Galileo."

Regarding a "junk science" case decided by the U.S. Supreme Court in 1993, Harvard University paleontologist Stephen Jay Gould said, "Almost every generally accepted view was once deemed eccentric or heretical." Gould was one signer of a friend-of-the-court brief arguing that judges and juries should not base their decisions solely on testimony about the conventional wisdom. The

Court, in a complex ruling, nevertheless charged judges to become "gatekeepers" to weed out witnesses clearly outside orthodox science. Though judges can appoint their own scientific experts, few do. How do judges unsophisticated in medicine or science know whom to appoint? In a medical issue as controversial as EI/MCS, appointing experts—and other, similar steps—is fraught with the possibility of loading the dice one way or the other. The chemically injured can easily be unlucky in court—and often are.

Another factor that is not helping EI/MCS plaintiffs is the secrecy surrounding some legal settlements. In 1989 residents of a town east of Rochester, New York, wondered why neighbors were moving out and no one was moving in. "We're in the dark," said one resident of a group of houses across the road from a Xerox plant. Finally they learned the truth. Alleging health problems, two families on the block had sued the company because of its groundwater and air contamination. Sources familiar with the case confirmed that Xerox had paid the families about $4.75 million and relocated them; under terms of the settlement, however, a New York judge sealed all records of the lawsuits and prohibited those involved from discussing them. Violation of the judge's order could have resulted in prosecution for contempt of court. The company settled after learning that medical specialists were ready to testify that the plant's air and water discharges were a likely cause of neurological problems experienced by seven members of the two families and a probable factor in a rare form of cancer found in one teenage girl. Hence the "covenant of silence."

Secrecy in this and other cases is seriously hampering the development of scientific knowledge about the health effects of toxic chemicals, according to Je Anne Burg, of the ATSDR, the federal agency charged with collecting and assessing such data. And Arthur H. Bryant, director of the Trial Lawyers for Public Justice, a public-interest group that helps plaintiffs in environmental cases, says that "by making sure that nobody knows about injuries that are caused [by the environment and] by controlling access to the data on which scientific opinions are based," manufacturers can influence the state of scientific knowledge. Secrecy—one more hurdle in the ongoing fight for environmental justice.

Housing and Urban Development

Safe housing is a primary need for people severely ill with EI/MCS. Some chemically sensitive people have lived temporarily in their cars, which proved less toxic—if also less comfortable—than their apartments. One young woman, unable to tolerate her parents' home, discovered she could not tolerate living in a shelter for the homeless in Lawrence, Kansas, because of the cleaning products, smoking, and perfumes she encountered there, or in housing for people with disabilities, because of the pesticides and carpeting there. Thus she became doubly—or triply—homeless.

For help, some people with EI/MCS have turned to HUD, which administers two laws that recognize multiple chemical sensitivities as a disability entitling people with this condition to *reasonable accommodation*: Section 504 of the Rehabilitation Act of 1973 and Title VIII of the Fair Housing Amendments Act of 1988. As written, however, these two acts only recognize. While they hold promise, they deliver only after great effort by the needy. According to a 1990 letter from HUD to Senator Frank R. Lautenberg (D-NJ), "because of the unique nature of MCS and the limitless variety of chemical sensitivities possible, *HUD has not written a policy that sets forth specific required reasonable accommodation for this disability* [emphasis added]." Instead, HUD handles appeals on a "case-by-case" basis, which, though daunting, may not be altogether bad. In a 1991 letter, HUD said that it can do nothing about new housing: only Congress can establish design and construction requirements for new housing to benefit the chemically sensitive. (With the Fair Housing Act, Congress did make provision for new housing to be accessible for handicapped people in wheelchairs.) Providers of existing housing, however, are required by the Fair Housing Act to provide reasonable accommodations for people with EI/MCS or to allow people "to make, at their own expense, reasonable modifications to the existing premises, if the proposed modifications are necessary to afford them the full enjoyment of the housing premises." Successful cases under the Fair Housing Act include one that asked that an apartment's hallways be off limits for smoking and one that asked for laundry doors to be kept closed. Another accommodation achieved the use of integrated pest management and

less-toxic cleaning products and restricted the janitor's use of tobacco and other toxic materials in a workroom below the complainants' apartment. In 1993, in a case that HUD was unable to
resolve, the U.S. Department of Justice sued and won similar concessions for a Hawaii resident, the first time such a case had been
won in a federal court.

Section 504 of the Rehabilitation Act of 1973, which applies to
any program or activity receiving financial assistance from HUD,
requires recipients "to operate their programs in a manner which
does not discriminate against individuals with handicaps, including
persons with MCS." Under Section 504, housing modifications to
accommodate the handicapped must be paid for by the recipient of
the financial assistance, not the handicapped person.

By now it should be fairly obvious that HUD is quite correct in
speaking of the "limitless varieties of chemical sensitivities possible." It should also be obvious that society as a whole is nowhere
near ready to deal with the implications of these sensitivities for
public health or public policy. Yet small victories are possible.
Using the Oakland, California, post office should be a little safer for
the chemically sensitive, following a complaint filed in 1989 by the
Berkeley-based Disability Rights Education and Defense Fund
(DREDF) on behalf of Joya Salzman, an Oakland woman. Post
office employees had refused to provide her service by coming outside so that she could avoid perfume exposure. The complaint alleged discrimination on the basis of handicap in violation of Section
504, which requires reasonable accommodation, and of a postal
regulation allowing for special arrangements for handicapped customers.

That same year, DREDF also helped Marcia Fisher, a chemically
sensitive member of Kaiser Permanente, the country's largest health
maintenance organization, obtain access to health care in Kaiser's
newly carpeted facilities in Oakland. When Kaiser failed to respond
to her requests for help in obtaining care without exposure to the
carpeting, DREDF suggested that she warn the organization that
they were in violation of Section 504, which entitles her to reasonable accommodation of her disability. This time Kaiser responded:
"Ambulatory services directors will assist you in gaining access to
your medical care provider with as little delay as possible in areas

where you will be exposed to carpeting. Please be assured that we sincerely wish to make whatever reasonable accommodations are possible to make you as comfortable in our setting as we can.' "

Popular Epidemiology and Other Individual Efforts

Across the country, the chemically injured have tried a variety of individual actions to achieve some measure of environmental justice. Some with EI/MCS have handled the problem of accommodation of their disabilities by approaching state human rights agencies. In 1987 a Pennsylvania realty company refused to renew Sally Atkinson's lease after she complained about pesticides that the company used in and and around her apartment complex. A former nurse, Atkinson realized in 1984 that she was sensitive to many modern chemicals; when she moved into the complex in 1986 she was assured that her avoidance needs would be met. Her attorney appealed the company's refusal to the Pennsylvania Human Relations Commission, and for three years she lived with her bags packed, expecting eviction. But in 1990 the Commission, in a precedent-setting decision, ordered the complex manager to "cease and desist from discriminating on the basis of handicap" and to accommodate her needs by doing such things as removing her dishwasher and sealing the piping to prevent odors from seeping into the apartment; installing a fan in the laundry room to exhaust the odors of chlorine bleach, fabric softener, and soaps; permitting her to remove her carpeting; and using the least toxic methods for controlling pests and weeds. Predictably, the company's management, calling the ruling "scary," claimed it would keep them from providing their tenants attractive, sanitary, comfortable housing. However, one of the commissioners said that "one must strain to even attempt to understand why [the realtor] never attempted to design a pest management strategy that at least attempted to implement some of Atkinson's suggested alternatives." While the Commission was considering Atkinson's complaint, someone sprayed an industrial pesticide in the halls of her building and on her door, knocked on the door, and ran. Atkinson stepped out in the hall, collapsed, and broke her wrist. "If I knew who it was [who did it], I would have that person up for attempted murder," said Raymond Cartwright, the Commission's director of housing.

In 1991 three women filed charges with the Illinois Department of Human Rights against the Village of Hinsdale, an affluent Chicago suburb. They believe that, on the basis of laws guaranteeing handicapped people equal access to public property, the village's pesticide spraying of parks and other public grounds discriminates against them. Two of the women and the son of the other woman suffer severe headaches, nausea, and flu-like symptoms when exposed to pesticides and other potent chemicals. "We're like the warning lights on the dashboard of a car," said Marilyn Hamilton, one of the women. "I wouldn't have gotten involved if I didn't think this was a greater issue involving more people than myself." By March 1993 the village had spent $46,000 to fight the agency's preliminary finding in favor of the complainants. Meanwhile, the three have joined with other suburban women to fight the overuse and misuse of pesticides. "Most of them are mothers. Some have kids that got sick from being exposed to toxic chemicals, and the others are concerned that their children will get sick," according to Mary Ross, head of the Chicago-area Sierra Club's pesticide-education committee.

In southern California, bus driver Randy Humber developed disabling chemical sensitivities from the routine pesticide spraying of the buses, the toxic solvents used to clean them, and the outgassing of their plastic upholstery. Angered and no longer able to work, in 1989 Humber began circulating a petition for safe working conditions, which eventually was signed by almost five hundred drivers. "Pesticides and other chemicals," said the petition, "are causing more and more people to become sensitive and severely impaired. There are many other nontoxic alternatives for use. In the long run it would save [the bus company] money because work productivity would increase and absenteeism would decrease substantially. Many drivers, passengers, or others don't realize that these chemicals, especially the pesticides, are the cause of their health problems. THEY ARE!"

In 1989, largely as a result of efforts by EI/MCS activist Susan Molloy, who persuaded people with other disabilities to join her, a hospital in California's Marin County opened a new wing designed to be mostly free of toxic building materials and furnishings and then proceeded to "bake out" the wing to try to rid it of any remaining toxins. "Safe materials don't cost any more than the kind that pollute, and they make everyone more comfortable," said Molloy. "We can avoid the . . . perfume counter and we can avoid restaurants and office buildings if we have to, but we can't avoid hospitals if we get sick." Obviously, if you are chemically sensitive and need to be hospitalized, Marin County is the place to be.

Near the Hanford Nuclear Reservation in Washington State, a farm family became concerned about what seemed to them excessive numbers of heart attacks among relatively young local farmers leading healthy outdoor lives. Suspecting radiation in the land these farmers plowed and cultivated, Lenita Andewjeski created a "death map" of the area downwind of the Hanford plant. Her map led reporters and others to press for information under the Freedom of Information Act, thus uncovering what some federal officials now acknowledge was a major Cold War cover-up by the producers of plutonium for America's nuclear weapons. Washington scientists are now studying local residents for evidence of other conditions— cancer and thyroid problems—possibly related to the radioactive emissions, mainly iodine 131. Similarly, a group of concerned parents of autistic children did their own research and discovered that they had all lived near a Leominster, Massachusetts, plastic sunglasses factory. The factory's pollution had been obvious; one father recalled knowing from the factory's smoke just which color of sunglasses was being made that day. On the Mexican border, in Nogales, Arizona, an organization of poor and Hispanic residents called "Living Is for Everyone" (LIFE) has drawn up a map illustrating an incidence of cancer five times higher than the ACS's "normal" rate, an incidence the group attributes to the air and water pollution from U.S.-owned electronics and plastics firms just across the border. "Something is very wrong," says Dr. Bill Kraus, executive director of the American Lupus Society, investigating the excessive number of lupus cases in Nogales. Enterprising efforts such as these have been called "popular epidemiology" by Brown University sociology professor Phil Brown, who says that "the lay public is doing what should be done by corporations, experts, and officials."

In the Puget Sound area of Washington State, residents of Whatcom County organized to defeat an initiative on their 1990 ballots. Naming their group "Neighbors Opposing Power Encroachment" (NOPE), by a two-to-one margin they said "no" to a proposed high-voltage power line whose possible health effects they feared. Never before had a power line issue been put to a popular vote, according to NOPE and power company officials. Apparently the company had not spent enough money to defeat the initiative. During the same election month, November 1990, agricultural, pesticide, and timber industries spent $16.5 million to successfully defeat "Big Green," the California initiative that, if passed, would have banned cancer-causing pesticides, curbed offshore oil drilling in state waters, reduced carbon dioxide emissions, and halted the felling of ancient forests. A spokesman for the Sierra Club, which supported the broad initiative, mourned that "we succeeded in uniting the polluting community."

But as one effort fails, another springs up. In 1989 the Los Angeles Labor/Community Strategy Center set up its WATCHDOG committee to appeal to "nontraditional environmental constituencies," such as the 71 percent of Los Angeles-area blacks who live in the region's most polluted districts. Eric Mann, a former auto worker who co-authored *L.A.'s Lethal Air* with WATCHDOG, blames Big Green's defeat on the environmental movement's failure "to address the realities of class and race."

Corporate Crime

Despite such setbacks in the 1990 elections, there's a "tremendous increase, statistically, in the number of environmental crimes now being investigated," said Carol Dinkins, a Houston attorney formerly with the U.S. Department of Justice. "The whole environmental law area is quite active now and there are many more lawyers who practice in this field than there were twenty years ago. Now the regulated community knows better what's expected and there's more of an opportunity for prosecutors to make a criminal case and say somebody knew what the law was and violated it." The year 1989 saw a 70 percent increase in corporate criminal indictments, with a corresponding increase in the amounts of fines levied, according to the Justice Department, which, together with the FBI and the federal EPA, has expanded its role in investigating environmental crimes. Since 1982, for instance, the EPA's office of criminal investigations has convicted 587 defendants, 20 percent of them corporate managers who end up serving fifteen to twenty-one months in prison, if not given probation. Judges in several states have sentenced some corporate criminals to support environmental advocacy groups by contributing or joining and attending meetings, according to the *Wall Street Journal*. In a Clinton administration crackdown, EPA head Carol Browner announced in July 1993 that twenty-four civil cases seeking millions of dollars in penalties had just been filed against hazardous waste violators across the country.

One La Jolla, California, company, Science Applications International, has felt the increased heat. In 1991, after a three-year investigation by the EPA, this federal contractor pleaded guilty to falsifying results of its testing of toxic waste dumps and was fined more than $1.3 million (to be paid out of its $1.16 billion revenues). "This company handled analysis of soil and water samples from all over the country," said Brooks Griffin, EPA divisional inspector general, who also said that he had "no way to evaluate health effects from the problems."

In Canada, the full health effects of 180 buried drums of chlorinated industrial solvents near Toronto are probably not known either, but in 1990 a business executive was jailed for six months and his company fined $76,000 for polluting drinking water with the chemicals trichloroethane and trichloroethylene in those drums. Following an investigation undertaken after residents of the area complained of contamination of their wells, he became the first person jailed in Canada for an environmental offense.

States and cities are also taking up the fight, with California once again a leader. California's Proposition 65, the voter-approved 1986 measure which said that businesses must warn consumers of products that could cause cancer or birth defects, has had a national impact. Because manufacturers wouldn't want to be found selling such products to the rest of the country, several products, such as Gillette's liquid paper, Dow's K2R spot remover, and Kiwi's shoe waterproofing spray, have been reformulated for safety. In the banner year of 1989, the California Attorney General's Commission on

Disability recognized environmental illness as a disabling condition creating "new challenges that have yet to be addressed." The official listing of those challenges—new building codes, safe temporary housing, safe access to medical facilities and public services, clarification of existing laws, and educational workshops for state workers—was a major step forward. California also enacted a law—the Corporate Criminal Liability Act of 1989—making it a crime for a corporation or corporate manager to "knowingly fail to notify regulatory authorities of any concealed danger to consumers or workers." Employers must give workers written notice of the danger and could be jailed for failing to disclose life-threatening dangers. David Lapp, associate editor of the Washington, D.C.-based *Corporate Crime Reporter*, hopes that the rest of the nation will follow California, for "the social and economic costs of corporate crime are mounting yearly, as seen by taxpayer losses wrought by the savings-and-loan crooks, the thousands of injuries, illnesses, and deaths of consumers and workers due to corporate neglect and crime, and the ever-increasing damage to the environment."

Realtors are one group that has taken notice of the corporate criminality law. An article by Peter S. Young, president of a California air cleaning company, in the November/December 1991 issue of *Real Estate Today*, magazine of the National Association of Realtors, warns property managers and building owners to take immediate steps to see whether their buildings are causing health problems to occupants—and not only because of the possibility for Californian realtors of fines and imprisonment. "Businesses occupying buildings that have fallen victim to indoor air pollution suffer many economic losses, mostly from workers' compensation, employee absenteeism, overtime pay to employees filling in for absent co-workers, production slowdowns, and damage to particle-sensitive equipment, such as computers," said Young.

"Ecocops" now patrol Illinois highways, following passage in 1981 of that state's Environmental Protection Act. The HAZMIN (Hazardous Materials Investigation) unit of the Illinois State Police, traveling in vehicles equipped with computers, reference books, and laboratories, is authorized to look for illegal hazardous waste dumping. By 1991, the state had generated thousands of dollars in fines and sent six people to jail. According to Lieutenant Gary Long,

HAZMIN coordinator, the unit targets "company presidents and people calling the shots." Iowa is also cracking down on polluters. A detective from the state's Division of Criminal Investigation and an environmental specialist from its attorney general's office began in 1989 to "cruise the state in an ethanol-fueled sedan, on the lookout for criminals who violate water pollution and hazardous waste dumping laws." So far, they feel, they have "seen things to suggest that environmental crime in Iowa is much worse than anyone suspects."

Portland, Oregon, hired Lee Barrett to enforce its law prohibiting restaurants and retail food vendors from using containers made of polystyrene foam, the petroleum-based product that can damage the earth's ozone layer. Nicknamed "Styro-Cop" by Portland residents, he walks his beat, in his first four months inspecting 140 establishments and finding six violations. Passionate about his job, he says that "to use plastic to drink eight ounces of coffee for two minutes and then throw it away where it will take up space forever is absurd." Maybe some day he and Portland's legislators will also realize that the coffee—and the coffee drinker—are likely to have absorbed styrene, known to cause damage to the central nervous system, from that container.

The Americans with Disabilities Act

Perhaps the governmental action offering the most hope to the chemically injured is the far-reaching Americans with Disabilities Act of 1990 (ADA). At least six chemically sensitive people were among the 3,300 people invited to the ADA signing ceremony at the White House, and the final regulations for implementation of the act do mention the illness (the Act itself does not define disability). However, despite strenuous efforts by two environmental leaders— Mary Lamielle, president of the National Center for Environmental Health Strategies (NCHS) and Susan Molloy, of the San Francisco-based Environmental Health Network—the Department of Justice, which, together with the Equal Employment Opportunity Commission (EEOC), is charged with enforcing ADA, declined to state categorically that these types of allergies or sensitivities are disabilities. Instead, with EI/MCS it will resort to a case-by-case analysis. The government's Architectural and Transportation Barriers Compliance Board sidestepped the issue pending further studies, though it took note of suggestions sent in by EI/MCS sufferers—windows that open; better heating, cooling, and ventilating systems; less-toxic building materials and furnishings. (Ironically, Lamielle, one of the six chemically sensitive people invited to the signing, could not attend because of her disabilities; her husband went in her place.)

Basically, the intent of the ADA is to extend to the disabled the civil rights protections already available on the basis of race, sex, national origin, and religion. It attempts to guarantee equal opportunity for the disabled in employment, public accommodations, transportation, state and local government services, and telecommunications.

What do ADA and its regulations say that might help people with EI/MCS? Concerned mainly with employment and accessibility, the regulations define an individual with a disability as a person who has a physical or mental impairment that substantially limits one or more major life activities, such as caring for oneself, performing manual tasks, walking, seeing, hearing, speaking, breathing, learning, and working. While ADA and its regulations are overwhelmingly concerned with employment, accommodations, and transportation for the mobility-impaired, vision-impaired, and hearing-impaired, they do recognize the necessity of breathing, a life activity fraught with varying degrees of danger to the chemically sensitive and others whose reactions to chemicals take the form of breathing difficulties. (In 1993, using the ADA, sufferers from asthma and lupus sued to try to force McDonald's and two other fast food chains to ban smoking.) Under ADA, employers must reasonably accommodate the disabilities of qualified applicants or employees, unless doing so would cause "undue hardship." Despite the ADA's broad scope, "there still appear to be some gaps in coverage, such as full protection for people with environmental illness," according to the National Council on Disability in its report "ADA Watch, Year One," which advocates legislation to help those "severely adversely affected by secondary smoke or other pollutants in public places."

Many of the chemically injured well know that at present their employers do not accommodate their special needs, that they cannot fully enjoy much in our present society, and that government services are often unavailable to them. When, or whether, or how much ADA will help them remains to be seen. "Sometimes respiratory or neurological functioning is so severely affected that an individual [with EI/MCS] will satisfy the requirements to be considered disabled under the regulation," says the Justice Department. "In other cases, individuals may be sensitive to environmental elements or to smoke but their sensitivity will not rise to the level needed to constitute a disability. For example, their major life activity of breathing may be somewhat, but not substantially, impaired. In such circumstances, the individuals are not disabled and are not entitled to the protections of the statute despite their sensitivity to environmental agents."

This, then, is the case-by-case approach. Actually, according to San Francisco Independent Living Resource Center official Herb Levine, the Justice Department and the EEOC will probably have to handle *any* disability by the same approach. Disabilities other than EI/MCS may not always make a person "substantially impaired." The first suit against a private employer under the ADA—filed by the EEOC on behalf of a man fired after his employer learned he had cancer—had spectacular results: a settlement of $572,000, of which the plaintiff is allowed under the ADA to keep no more than $300,000. One ADA regulation defines a person with a disability as one who "is regarded as having such an impairment." Thus, since government agencies such as the SSA, HUD, and the EPA regard EI/MCS as a disability, it is, says Levine dryly, "safe to say that it is regarded as a disability."

ADA and its regulations make no provision for new safe buildings for people with EI/MCS; that will take a mandate from Congress. However, in existing buildings ADA requires, according to Levine, that "places take a look around and see what the barriers are to folks using the place and that they remove everything that is readily achievable, which means that it is easy to do and doesn't cost much." For the chemically sensitive, this could mean things like removing air "fresheners" in bathrooms, removing or changing fluorescent lighting, or relocating perfume counters away from doors in order to provide safe access to the store. Or, if the store was completely inaccessible, it still might be able to provide goods and services at the door, at the sidewalk, at the curb, or by home delivery. For the provider, there would have to be significant difficulty or expense, in legal terms called an "undue burden," to win exemption from ADA mandates. There would probably *not* be undue burden in, for example, no-smoke/no-scent policies, elimination of "carbonless" carbon paper, provision of air filtering systems, clear notification and posting of areas to be tarred or painted, use of non-toxic cleaning products, rearrangement of workspace, or allowing employees to work at home. In fact, a national survey of ten thousand employers who have made employee accommodations found that most of them cost little or nothing and were viewed as a "sound business investment."

With ADA, as with all government entitlement programs, the chemically injured encounter two major problems in proving their case. One problem is that their disabilities tend to be invisible, non-measurable, and intermittent. At any given time they may look healthy—and even feel healthy, until exposed to toxics. They may be able to function at home, but not in most workplaces. With few exceptions, a person in a wheelchair cannot walk without help or without the wheelchair; persons with EI/MCS can usually walk, see, hear, and talk "normally"—until overcome by VOCs emanating from paints, perfumes, pesticides, fabric softeners, copy machines, furniture, or furnishings. The other problem is exactly that: because public places are filled with hundreds of VOCs, it is difficult, if not impossible, to identify the chemical culprit or culprits that are making a person sick. And without a known culprit, benefits are hard to obtain.

Nevertheless, under the ADA possibilities are opening up. The more that people with EI/MCS claim their rights under ADA, the more those who administer it will become familiar with their needs. Victories will be won, and precedents will be set. The future looks more hopeful.

EPA: the History

Almost from our birth, in this democracy, we are told that the government is us, or that it represents us, or that it is protecting us.

"Write the President," "write your representative," "write the EPA," we are exhorted. But how much good does contacting, say, the EPA, do? How much is it protecting us?

One answer lies in the history of the EPA, which did not exist before 1970. The late 1960s produced great ferment in American society. Students and many others were protesting American involvement in Vietnam. People everywhere were concerned about the catastrophically increasing pollution of land, air, and water—and about the twentieth-century population explosion. Across the U.S., college students flocked to classes on the environment or on ecology, a newly popular word. On the first Earth Day, April 22, 1970, professors and other experts held "teach-ins," seminars devoted solely to the deteriorating condition of the earth. Garrett De Bell has summed up the era this way: "In 1969 the U.S. woke up to the fact that the richest country in the world is in the middle of an environmental crisis. We said goodbye to pelicans, realized that the ubiquitous automobile was the cause of smog and of the Santa Barbara oil slick, and meditated on the fact that our burgeoning multiplicity of air conditioners, clothes dryers, and other aids to gracious living meant another ugly power plant. Mother's milk, we were told, wasn't fit to drink. . . . We learned the meaning of scientific doubletalk. We learned that when scientists said, 'We have no evidence that DDT is harmful to humans' they meant that the study was still in progress, and we were the experimental animals. In fact, many experiments were being conducted on us . . . simultaneously—smog, tranquilizers, calcium cyclamate, monosodium glutamate, hair spray, deodorants, lead, strontium-90, noise—to name only a few. Statisticians had a peculiar worry: they wouldn't be able to tell exactly how much of the increases in cancer, emphysema, mental illness, deafness, and other diseases to attribute to any particular environmental insult." Words to ponder in the 1990s: are the statisticians still worrying? Some of us know more now: does everyone?

What did emerge from the 1960s ferment was new regulatory and enforcement agencies. In 1970 Congress created EPA, OSHA, and NIOSH. In 1972 it set up CPSC, and in 1976 it passed TSCA, the first comprehensive legislation on toxins. The government and the alphabet were now ready to do battle with polluters and pollutants. The EPA, staffed by government careerists but also by idealistic, concerned scientists attracted to the new agency, was at first the center of "frenetic, exhilarating, and often confused activity," recalls EPA senior scientist Bill Hirzy. For many it was exciting; finally, something was going to be done about pollution. But early enthusiasm soon gave way to disillusionment, as pure science began losing out to politics, the familiar Washington game. "Somewhere along the line," Hirzy says, "a decision was made to limit the caliber and number of scientists employed by the Agency. Rule writing was emphasized over scientific investigation." Lawyers began furthering the interests of industrial and governmental (policy-making) clients. Under President Reagan "EPA epidemiologists were fired en masse. . . . Enforcement activities were diminished and piecemealed," says Hirzy. "Even lawyers were told, 'If you can't serve this Administration in conscience, get out!'" During the Reagan years, when a chemically sensitive citizen called the EPA for information, he was first put on hold and then asked, "What company are you with?" (That is beginning to seem like a standard response from government agencies.) Reagan's environmental policies were so bad that his daughter, Patti Davis, on hearing that her father would not be welcome at Earth Week 1990 activities in Hollywood, is reported to have said, "I agree with that. His environmental policies were not only unsound but mean-spirited."

The Bush administration was no better at protecting the environment, and possibly worse, for President George Bush appointed Vice President Dan Quayle to head a newly created entity, the Council on Competitiveness, set up to subvert Congress's intended curbs on industry. Fortunately, one of President Bill Clinton's first acts in office, in 1993, was to disband this ill-conceived and possibly illegal council. More than that action will be needed, however: "For the past decade," wrote Peter Montague in 1992, "the effect of White House policy has been to drive out good people and replace them with functionaries. Today EPA has few talented, committed employees left, and fewer still who are competent managers. Today many employees simply look upon the agency as a place to do time while awaiting an opportunity for a lucrative trip through the revolving door." A sad state of affairs for a once hope-filled agency.

EPA: the Good and the Bad

Can anything good be said for the EPA? Yes, one can praise the honesty and courage of those within the organization who have put their careers on the line to expose corruption and coverups, both in Washington and in the agency's ten regional offices. During the Reagan years, for instance, EPA employees in Chicago determined that the Dow Chemical Company was dumping dangerous dioxins into a Michigan river. When EPA headquarters wanted this information deleted from their report, which they considered accurate and professional, Valdus Adamkus, Region V director, categorically refused. His refusal and subsequent testimony before Congress put his career on the line. Both Adamkus and Milton Clark, the scientist assigned to investigate the Dow plant in Midland, Michigan, had begun their careers in the EPA as idealistic environmentalists. Both watched Reagan's appointee to head the EPA, Anne Gorsuch, "undermine what they felt was the agency's purpose. Corporate profits, they said, started to take precedence over health and environmental concerns." Nevertheless, courageous employees Valdus Adamkus and Milton Clark, and others like Steve Shapiro, Bobbie Lively-Diebold, and Bill Hirzy, go on trying to hold the line against intransigence, spinelessness, and indifference.

Why, apart from the Reagan/Bush depredations, is the EPA the way it is? Some would say that the problem really starts at the top. The President of the United States, whoever he [or someday she] may be, usually gives first priority to national security, foreign affairs, the economy, and the budget. Other needs, like housing, education, welfare, transportation, and the environment come second. What he wants from his top-priority appointees is performance; what he wants from his second-level appointees is peace and quiet. Don't rock the boat.

In this light, the consequences for EPA are perhaps predictable. William Sanjour, a veteran whistle-blower who has worked for the EPA as both employee and contractor, sums them up this way: "people who like to get things done, people who need to see concrete results for their efforts, don't last long at EPA. Hundreds of people in EPA have spent tens of millions of dollars and have advanced their careers by being very busy drawing up work plans, attending meetings, making proposals, writing reports, giving briefings, conducting studies, and accomplishing nothing." When something does get accomplished, it is because organizations like the Environmental Defense Fund and the Natural Resources Defense Council have sued to make EPA employees "do what the law already requires them to do and for which they are already being paid. Taxpayers' money is used to defend EPA against such suits to protect their right not to do what the taxpayers are paying them to do."

According to Sanjour, whose special area of expertise is toxic waste, those influencing hazardous waste policies are, in decreasing order of importance, (1) the waste management industry, (2) state governments, (3) powerful waste-producing industries, (4) important congressmen, (5) national environmental groups, and (6) the media. Consequently, EPA more often than not *opposes* Congress passing really tough environmental laws. Individuals and grass-roots groups have no power unless they go through their elected representatives, starting at the state level. Though most EPA employees, like everyone else, have their own hidden agenda—advancing their careers within and after EPA—the individual concerned citizen or member of a grass-roots organization does have "the power to affect the pocketbooks and careers of people who in turn can affect the pocketbooks and careers of EPA [employees]."

The EPA is a follower, not a leader. What can be done about it? Sanjour has some suggestions, mostly for Congress: enact laws with "hammer provisions" (deadlines with penalties falling on the people the EPA regulates); promote enlightened self-interest (e.g., giving lawyers access to information that can lead to a windfall for them); make the EPA the enforcer of regulations, not their author (often the EPA writes regulations to thwart Congress's intentions); expand companies' liability; encourage states to set up "bad boy" laws that keep them from doing business with violators; block the revolving door that allows EPA employees to move into higher-paying jobs in the industries they have been regulating; pass a conflict-of-interest law that forbids agencies to both regulate *and* promote products or services; wield the carrot and the stick (reward employees for succeeding or whistleblowing, not for failing); and eliminate consent agreements, which allow companies to pay fines without admitting guilt.

Should agencies like the EPA be abolished? No; society would be chaos without them. Nevertheless, it is folly to trust them. It helps to realize that the people in them are only people: "Behind the awesome visage of the magnificent Wizard of Oz, there is a fragile little man pulling the levers." The right approach, Sanjour says, is to create a balance, one with the minimum use of institutions, relying instead "on the maximum use of the people who have the most at stake." His most fascinating example of this occurred in the 1970s in Albuquerque, New Mexico, where as part of the settlement of a lawsuit regarding strong odors from a local sewage plant, a "sniffing committee" dominated by local residents was set up to monitor future sewage odors. Enforcement of the law was in their hands, not those of bureaucrats. In the Land of Oz, Dorothy *can* prevail.

A Bill of Rights for the Chemically Injured

Though the possibilities for recourse are improving, reality can be disappointing. Victories can be hard-won and insubstantial. Disappointed by government inaction, EI/MCS sufferers occasionally turn to churches or charities for sanctuary (literally—one unemployed person with EI/MCS slept for a while on church pews) or succor. Some have gotten financial or other help, an indication that such recourse is worth a try.

If you are chemically sensitive and need to lift your spirits until the millennium arrives, consider Susan Molloy's bill of rights for the chemically injured:

- **THE RIGHT** to medical care by enlightened medical practitioners.

- **THE RIGHT** to hospitalization in facilities free of pesticides, scented personnel, toxic furnishings, and toxic cleaning products.

- **THE RIGHT** to adequate insurance reimbursement for medical expenses.

- **THE RIGHT** to safe temporary housing, such as nontoxic halfway houses or recreational vehicles, for those fleeing paint, tobacco smoke, pesticides, or other contaminants in their permanent housing.

- **THE RIGHT** to safe permanent housing, free of such unhealthful contaminants as formaldehyde emissions; fluorescent light emissions; natural gas combustion products; pesticide and tobacco smoke residues; perfume and toxic cleaning product residues; outgassing carpeting; detergent and fabric softener fumes; chlorine vapors from swimming pools; gasoline vapors from garages; and neighbors' barbecue smoke.

- **THE RIGHT** to reasonable accommodation in an adequately ventilated workplace provided with any necessary protective devices or measures, including flexible hours, permission to relocate during renovation, and permission to work at home whenever possible, and with adequate education of co-workers and supervisors so that negative attitudes do not compound the problem.

- **THE RIGHT** to safe access to public buildings and services.

- **THE RIGHT** to a proportional amount of taxpayers' money to be spent on research into the causes, treatment, and prevention of this disability.

- **THE RIGHT** to equal treatment from government entitlement programs such as social security, workers' compensation, rehabilitation, and the Americans with Disabilities Act.

But until society catches up with your needs, you might try the nuisance factor. To EI activist Helen Moore the nuisance factor requires that each of us approach the appropriate top government and business officials with demands for protection of our individual rights. When Moore first wrote the North Carolina authorities for protection from roadside herbicide spraying, she received a public relations brush-off that she termed "a blatant disregard for [her] health and an insult to [her] intelligence." Later, when one official said, "Imagine if we got a hundred such letters," she replied, "Yes, you'd have to stop spraying, wouldn't you?"

Using carefully reasoned arguments to refute any nonsense, and with the help of her attorney, she persisted and is now able to travel the North Carolina highways safely. Her advice: (1) insist on going to the top person in the department in question, (2) keep documentation of letters and phone calls, (3) be persistent and insistent, (4) remember that while you can do little about what others do on their own property, you have the right to protect yourself from what others do that harms you. "Be a nuisance," says Moore. "You have nothing to lose, and what we all stand to gain is invaluable."

* * * *

To Find Out More

- Equal Employment Opportunity Commission, 1801 L Street NW, Washington, D.C. 20507; 202-663-4900 (voice); 1-800-3302 (TDD).

- Office on the Americans with Disabilities Act, Civil Rights Division, U.S. Department of Justice, P.O. Box 66118, Washington, D.C. 20035-6118; 202-514-0301 (voice); 202-514-0381 (TDD); 202-514-0383 (TDD).

- Housing and Civil Enforcement Section, Civil Rights Division, U.S. Department of Justice, P.O. Box 65998, Washington, D.C. 20035; 202-514-8038.

- Office of Fair Housing and Equal Opportunity, Room 5116, Department of Housing and Urban Development, 451 Seventh Street SW, Washington, D.C. 20410-2000; 202-708-2878 (its booklet "Fair Housing: It's Your Right" tells how to file a complaint with HUD).

- The President's Committee on Employment of People with Disabilities, Suite 636, 1111 Twentieth Street NW, Washington, D.C. 20036; 202-653-5044.

- Disability Rights Education and Defense Fund (DREDF), 2212 Sixth Street, Berkeley, California 94710; 510-644-2555; 510-644-2629 (TDD); 1-800-466-4232 (also 1633 Q Street NW, Suite 220, Washington, D.C. 20009; 202-986-0375).

- National Council on Disability, 800 Independence Avenue SW, Suite 814, Washington, D.C. 20591; 202-267-3846 (its booklets

"ADA Watch, Year One" and "Health Insurance and Health-Related Services" mention EI/MCS).

- *Indoor Air Pollution Law Report,* published by Leader Publications, 111 Eighth Avenue, New York, New York 10011; 212-463-5709.

- *The Health Detective's Handbook: A Guide to the Investigation of Environmental Health Hazards by Nonprofessionals,* M.S. Legator, B.L. Harper, and M.J. Scott, editors, Baltimore, Johns Hopkins University Press, 1985.

- *L.A.'s Lethal Air: New Strategies for Policy, Organizing, and Action,* by Eric Mann with the WATCHDOG Organizing Committee, 1991; available from the Labor/Community Strategy Center, 818-781-4800.

- *Hazardous Substances in Buildings: Liability, Litigation, and Abatement,* by C. Jaye Berger, New York, John Wiley, 1992.

- *New Immunologic Markers for Diagnosis of Toxic Chemical Exposure,* by Aristo Vojdani, 1991; available from Immunoscience Lab Inc., 1801 La Cienega Boulevard, Suite 302, Los Angeles, California 90035; 310-287-1884.

- Copies of William Sanjour's talk "Why EPA Is Like It Is" may be obtained by sending $3 to Citizens Clearinghouse for Hazardous Wastes, P.O. Box 6806, Falls Church, VA 22040; or for his article "Why EPA Is Like It Is and What Can Be Done About It" send $15 to the Environmental Research Foundation, P.O. Box 5036, Annapolis, Maryland 21403-7036; 410-263-1584.

For Legal Help

- Association of Trial Lawyers of America, 1050 Thirty-first Street NW, Washington, D.C. 20007; 1-800-424-2727 or, in the Washington, D.C., area, 202-965-3500.

- Earon S. Davis, JD, MPH, available through NCEHS, 1100 Rural Avenue, Voorhees, New Jersey 08043; 609-429-5358.

12

The Best Health-Care System in the World: Shooting Arrows at the Storm

EVEN IN THE CLINTON ERA of widely acknowledged dissatisfaction with the U.S. health-care system, we still hear that our health-care system is the best in the world. Government officials say so, physicians say so, medical writers say so. Certainly when it comes to medical technology, the U.S. leads the field. Patients come across the border from Canada and from much farther to be diagnosed by our sophisticated, high-tech machines and treated by those who understand the data these machines provide. Patients also come from around the world for complex, delicate, life-saving surgery. Miracles are wrought daily in operating rooms and emergency rooms. And when it comes to bacterial infections, thousands of antibiotics and other life-saving drugs have been developed and marketed in this century by American drug companies. In 1991 alone, the FDA had several hundred new-drug applications to review. Since World War II, pharmaceutical and medical supply companies have become a highly profitable growth industry.

The results of this outpouring of money, research, education, and manufacturing in an effort to keep Americans alive and healthy are not to be minimized. If you have broken a leg or need prostate surgery, you are going to be very grateful for your surgeon's knowledge and competence. If you have an acute infection that is closing your airway, you are going to be very grateful for steroids, IVs, and antibiotics. Modern technological medicine as practiced in the U.S.

has much to recommend it. For the management of traumas and infections, it is quite possibly unsurpassed anywhere.

But the twentieth century has also seen the rise of chronic, or degenerative, diseases, many of them life-threatening: heart disease, cancer, stroke, mental illness, high blood pressure, diabetes, arthritis, obesity, and addiction. "Although we no longer face the high rates of infant and childhood mortality from infection our forebears did, we are experiencing a new range of diseases resulting from fundamental changes in our environment, lifestyles, and nutritional habits during this century," says Dr. Joseph Beasley. Modern medicine, he says, because of its "classical science paradigm and methods of specific etiology [is] shooting arrows at the storm."

Thus, instead of hearing about infectious diseases like smallpox, diphtheria, and tuberculosis, we now hear about immune-system dysfunction and deficiency, chronic fatigue syndrome (CFS), asthma, chronic headaches, arthritis, panic disorder, fibromyalgia, multiple sclerosis, lupus erythematosus and other autoimmune diseases, and EI/MCS. These noninfectious diseases are not always life-threatening, but they can be profoundly uncomfortable and life-altering. Sufferers want and need medical help, but modern physicians, mostly untrained in nutrition, geriatrics, exercise, prevention, immune-system disorders, and environmental and occupational influences on health, have a hard time coping with these chronic, debilitating illnesses. Batteries of tests often turn up nothing. Instead of seeking basic causes in a patient's occupation or environment or food, doctors may end up treating the symptoms with a palliative, which masks the symptom without addressing the disorder itself. When symptom management does not work, the physician, feeling baffled and frustrated and assuming the illness is all in the patient's head, refers the exasperating (and exasperated!) sufferer to a psychiatrist, who follows the treatment he or she has been trained to provide, leaving the patient ultimately no better off. Or the doctor may simply say, as one chemically sensitive patient, a nurse, reported, "Medical science has failed you."

Since World War II, no branch of medicine has been more overlooked, more misunderstood, or more maligned than environmental medicine. Physicians looking for an environmental role in disease diagnose and treat patients who have baffled other physicians. Their ranks include over five hundred physician members of the American Academy of Environmental Medicine (more than half of whom are board certified in various specialties and a fifth of whom are also certified by the American Board of Environmental Medicine), and over eighteen hundred members of the American Academy of Otolaryngic Allergy, a society with representatives in the AMA House of Delegates. Many have turned to environmental medicine because they find themselves frustrated or even bored with conventional medicine.

Yet only in the past six or seven years has the diagnosis of EI/MCS—or chemical injury—begun to be accepted by mainstream doctors. Sometimes labeled "controversial" in the popular press and bitterly opposed by many traditional allergists, EI/MCS first began to achieve widespread recognition with the publication in 1987 of *Workers with Multiple Chemical Sensitivities*, a collection of papers both pro and con edited by Dr. Mark R. Cullen, of the Yale University School of Medicine (see Chapter 3). In 1988 the Institute of Medicine (IOM), policy arm of the NAS, said in its landmark *Role of the Primary Care Physician in Occupational and Environmental Medicine*: "There is increasing concern that our highly sophisticated health care system is not well prepared to address problems in an important sector of medicine, those related to occupational and environmental factors. This concern arises in the face of the public's growing recognition and apprehension of adverse health effects associated with exposure to hazardous substances in the home, the workplace, and the general environment." The IOM has followed up this report with two more: *Meeting Physicians' Needs for Medical Information on Occupations and Environments* (1990) and *Environmental Medicine in the Medical School Curriculum* (1993). Interested physicians may obtain these reports from the IOM, 2101 Constitution Avenue NE, Washington, D.C. 20418. Finally public concern about—and experiences with—toxic chemicals are being noticed by mainstream medicine.

Yet attacks on environmental physicians—mainly for being "unscientific"—continue, as though mainstream medicine were blameless. But evidence of the latter's failings continue to mount.

Inappropriate Medical Care

Contrary to often-expressed hyperbole, the U.S. may *not* have the best health-care system in the world. A Johns Hopkins study published in *JAMA* in 1991 evaluated health care in ten developed countries around the world on the basis of three measures: emphasis on primary care, favorable scores on health indicators such as infant mortality, and public satisfaction. The study found that Canada, Sweden, and the Netherlands ranked near the top on all three measures. The U.S. ranked worst or close-to-worst on them all—more indication that we, as a society, are not taking care of our citizens, especially some of our most vulnerable members.

Individual statistics help fill out the picture of a system in trouble. You may find some shocking, but, again, would you rather not know?

- In 1974 pharmacologist Milton Silverman, PhD, and Philip R. Lee, MD, former chancellor of the University of California in San Francisco, estimated in their book *Pills, Profits, and Politics* that on the basis of a six-year study of nine hospitals, there were more than 130,000 deaths per year from hospital-acquired adverse drug reactions. There is little reason to think things have changed much since then.

- In 1978, according to Lawrence C. Horowitz, MD, author of *Taking Charge of Your Medical Fate*, "roughly a third of the hundred most common drug uses in the country were for purposes not then approved by the FDA [and] because the U S. has no systematic program for monitoring prescription drug use, serious side effects, even eventually fatal ones, may go undetected for some time." Citing the prevalence of unnecessary surgery and unnecessary laboratory tests, Dr. Horowitz advises that patients question their doctors closely on every aspect of medical care.

In 1993, finally noting the medical profession's lack of information about what is becoming known as medical "outcomes," the State University of New York at Buffalo, funded by the FDA and the pharmaceutical industry, established a surveillance network to monitor drug side effects from 1,100 clinical pharmacists and 522 acute-care hospitals. But don't expect too much from the FDA: it has little history of vigilance in this area.

- In its 1978 report "Assessing the Efficacy and Safety of Medical Technologies," the OTA warned that "many technologies which have been used extensively have later been shown to be of limited usefulness. . . . It has been estimated that *only 10 to 20 percent of all procedures currently used in medical practice have been shown to be efficacious by controlled trial* [emphasis added]." Indeed, of the twenty-six full-scale assessments done by the Office of Health Technology Assessment in 1982, results from randomized clinical trials were available for only two.

- A 1991 study done for the nation's largest health insurer, Blue Cross and Blue Shield, concluded that "11 percent of the medical procedures doctors perform on patients are unnecessary, with the rate of inappropriate care as high as 27 percent for tonsillectomies and nearly 22 percent for the removal of the uterus." Unnecessary procedures not only put the patient at risk, they add millions to health-care costs, which is undoubtedly why Blue Cross/Blue Shield was looking at them.

- In 1991 the Public Citizen Health Research Group's *Health Letter* estimated on the basis of three studies that "between 150,000 and 300,000 Americans are injured or killed each year by doctor negligence. . . . The disciplinary actions that state medical boards take (3,123 in 1990) are trifling compared to the amount of injury done through poor medical practices." A random sampling of New York State hospital records done by Harvard University researchers found that 3.7 percent of patients suffered "adverse events," with about a quarter attributed to negligence. To fill what it sees as an informational gap, PCHRG has for three years published difficult-to-get data about doctors, dentists, chiropractors, podiatrists, and other doctors whose records make them questionable; in 1993 the report was entitled *10,289 Questionable Doctors.*

- A Brown University study suggested that "most doctors will tell little white lies—and some will even tell whoppers—if they think it will benefit their patients or themselves." One-third of the doctors polled said they would mislead the family of a very sick patient if they knew their treatment error had contributed to the patient's death.

• A study reported in *JAMA* in 1990 found that mortality rates for Medicare patients declined when hospital stays were shortened after cost-cutting measures were introduced. Another 1990 *JAMA* article reported that errors of prescription writing averaged 2½ a day in a large teaching hospital in New York State, and one in five of the mistakes could have have caused severe medical problems or death.

Drug Therapy

With such statistics, what is one to make of drug therapy—the kingpin of modern medical practice? Are the obvious flaws just a matter of the wrong words or wrong amounts on a prescription form? Or are there broader, more far-reaching concerns? The NAS's landmark 1984 study of toxicity testing was not reassuring; it found that 61 percent of drugs and excipients (fillers such as cornstarch) did not have even minimal toxicity information available. Because of this deficiency, Public Citizen Health Research Group's *Health Letter* regularly publishes reports of adverse health effects from prescription and nonprescription drugs. In recent years, drugs cited have included those used for arthritis, high blood pressure, depression, pain relief, ulcers, colds, allergies, nausea, and sedation.

One major concern raised by such reports has to do with insufficient or even dangerous testing of drugs. In 1991 Enkaid, a drug used to treat mild irregular heartbeats, was withdrawn from the market after studies by the NIH linked it with "startling" death rates; in 1993 doctors testing an experimental heart drug, vesnarinone, found that several patients died when given high doses of the drug. A study in the *Annals of Internal Medicine* in 1990 reported eleven cases of severe liver damage, including three deaths, in patients taking a widely used drug, labetalol, for high blood pressure. Yet the FDA estimates that "no more than one out of ten drug-induced adverse reactions that actually occur are reported to the FDA." This lack of reporting works the other way too: a 1992 study in *JAMA* found time lags of up to a decade in informing doctors of new effective therapies, such as the use of magnesium to reduce the death rate from heart failure. Finally recognizing a need to know more about the outcomes of what they are doing, cardiovascular specialists in 1993 joined in a new network aimed at improving the care of heart disease and keeping costs down.

Vaccines are another example of insufficient testing. In the early 1980s, Barbara Fisher's son, Christian, 2½, developed mysterious symptoms after receiving routine vaccinations. No doctor could help, but after the suburban Washington, D.C., mother saw a TV program that linked the whooping cough vaccine to cases of brain damage and death, she did her own research. After her son developed multiple learning disabilities, she and others organized Dissatisfied Parents Together (DPT) to work for safer and more effective vaccines . . . and the right to refuse some. "We just want to be able to say no," she said. In 1986 Congress set up a system to compensate parents for vaccine-related injuries or deaths.

In a classic case of insufficient testing, in January 1994 a jury awarded $42.3 million to eleven women whose mothers took the synthetic hormone diethylstilbestrol (DES) during pregnancy; the women were the first to claim that the drug caused reproductive problems not related to cancer. DES was prescribed for approximately five million women between 1947 and 1971 in an effort to prevent miscarriages. This case points up a major problem with drug testing: premarket testing cannot possibly predict long-term results. No one in or out of the drug industry knows what most modern drugs will do to us ten, twenty, or thirty years down the road.

Insufficient reporting to the FDA sometimes accompanies insufficient testing. In 1991 the British government banned Halcion, a popular and widely prescribed sleeping pill. Why is such a product on the market in the U.S.? According to PCHRG, the manufacturer of the drug omitted details of some patients' side effects, which may include amnesia, anxiety, depression, hallucinations, and bizarre and aggressive behavior, from a summary given the FDA during the drug approval process. In 1991 a murder charge against a Utah woman, Ilo Grundberg, for killing her mother was dismissed because of psychiatrists' testimony that she was intoxicated by the drug. Grundberg has since sued the manufacturer for $21 million, charging that the company failed to warn the FDA about Halcion's severe adverse effects. The company, attacking and now suing Dr. Ian Oswald, a Scottish psychiatrist who said that "the whole thing has been one long fraud," contends that "the drug's side effects are rare, and its benefits far outweigh the dangers." Again, benefits to whom? Dangers to whom?

Health Letter also has reported that a German drug company and several U.S. drug companies have pleaded guilty to withholding reports of life-threatening or fatal adverse reactions from the FDA. The drugs in question have since been removed from the market, "but only after hundreds of needless American deaths and injuries had occurred. These deaths and injuries were preventable because . . . it is very likely that the FDA would never have approved either of these drugs had they found out before approval, rather than after, how deadly the drugs really were." It is cases like these that prompted attorney George Burditt, a specialist in FDA law, to say that the public is mistaken if it thinks the agency's approval can guarantee safety. Also, though companies may test drugs on a few hundred to a few thousand patients before FDA approval, after approval "you may find a problem in one out of a hundred thousand people that you'll never find in your initial test." Caveat emptor indeed.

Another drug-related concern is "disease-shifting" and other unexpected results from drug therapy. Three drugs commonly used to treat schizophrenia—haloperidol, chlorpromazine, and thiothixene—produce symptoms similar to those of Parkinson's disease, according to researchers at the University of Colorado School of Medicine. Stanford University studies have discovered that X-rays and drug treatments that wipe out Hodgkin's disease (cancer of the lymphatic system) in women can cause breast cancer five to fifteen years later. Many of the asthma drugs now in use, such as cromolyn and theophylline, cause a variety of unpleasant symptoms, including tremors, nausea, vomiting, headaches, and drowsiness. In 1989, on the basis of reports submitted by doctors to the American Academy of Allergy and Immunology from 1980 to 1989, *JAMA* cited fourteen deaths following allergy shots and four deaths following skin testing for allergies (again, the FDA suspects a good deal of underreporting).

A concern of massive proportions is that of synergism, or additive effects, and interactions, not only of one drug with another, but also of drugs with any of the thousands of other chemicals we encounter in daily life. An extraordinary example of additive effects was reported by the *Wall Street Journal* in 1991. Thomas Latimer, a vigorous, successful petroleum engineer, developed dizziness, nausea, a runny nose, and a pounding headache after mowing his lawn in Dallas, Texas, in the summer of 1985. His symptoms persisted, and he developed testicular cancer that fall: "six years and twenty doctors later . . . Latimer, thirty-six, accept[ed] the diagnosis of doctors: that he was poisoned by an organophosphate pesticide used to treat his yard." But there was a complicating factor, according to his doctors: he was taking the prescribed daily dose of a popular ulcer drug, Tagamet. "A toxicologist, three neurologists, and two neuro-ophthalmologists who examined him all concluded independently that the [drug] suppressed the normal role of his liver in metabolizing the poison and expelling it." One expert, Alfredo A. Sadun, of the University of Southern California, who has treated victims of aerial organophosphate spraying, said that taking drugs like this one "can make a person a hundred to a thousand times more sensitive to organophosphate poisoning."

If prescription drugs often prove hazardous, what about nonprescription drugs? Take analgesics, known to millions of sufferers as painkillers. In one year alone, 1990, Americans bought almost $2.7 billion worth of analgesics, amounting to a fourth of the nonprescription drugs sold. Most of these were some form of aspirin, probably the single most popular drug in the world, though its mechanism of action is still not fully understood. In 1984 the NIH linked long-term use of over-the-counter combination drugs containing aspirin with a rise in kidney disease, including kidney cancer. A twenty-year study by Swiss investigators reported in the *NEJM* found that "women who used phenacetin [a frequent component of such drugs] regularly had a higher incidence of kidney failure, high blood pressure, and death from heart disease and cancer than women who did not use analgesics." Phenacetin is now off the market in the U.S.—too late to help those who took such combination drugs for years. Actually, there are many reasons to beware of aspirin and other painkillers. In 1992 the GAO reported health hazards from the abuse of aspirin (bleeding ulcers and hearing loss), acetaminophen (fatal liver damage when combined with alcohol, and kidney damage when taken over a long period of time), and ibuprofen (kidney damage when taken in large doses or over a long period of time).

Looking at the total picture, in 1990 U.S. consumers spent $11.2 billion on an estimated 125,000 to 300,000 different over-the-counter drugs. Under FDA guidelines, these readily available and yet potent drugs are regulated even more loosely than those requiring a doctor's prescription. To make matters worse, since 1972 the FDA has approved over-the-counter sales of forty-nine prescription drugs, according to the Nonprescription Drug Manufacturers Association. More drugs, including powerful painkillers and ulcer and allergy drugs with "potentially serious side effects and dangerous interactions with other drugs," are expected to make the same transition to over-the-counter status.

Concerned about potential abuse of over-the-counter drugs, from painkillers to diet pills, a growing number of pharmacists and other health advocates want the FDA to set up a third category, one for drugs in transition from prescription to nonprescription, to be available not on the shelves of supermarkets, convenience stores, and gas stations but only from a licensed pharmacist. With this category in effect, pharmacists would keep such drugs behind the counter, counsel patients about side effects, and keep records of adverse reactions. Patients could still obtain the drugs they want, but would be informed and monitored, not left to their own devices until such time as the drugs' safety and effectiveness are better known.

Because of the flaws in our current system of drug testing and evaluation, environmental physicians tend not to prescribe or recommend drugs unless absolutely necessary. As "third-line" physicians, they usually see only patients with chronic symptoms that traditional doctors and popular drugs have not helped. In fact, many of their patients have had their symptoms worsened by modern drugs, most of which are petroleum-based and can contain cornstarch, soy, milk, or other common food allergens. Hence most of the chemically injured try to reduce their chemical and allergen load by taking as few drugs as possible.

Still, drugs are tempting when you are suffering: it's so easy to just pop a pill with a glass of water. Hazards are relative and trade-offs must sometimes be made; fortunately, less-toxic solutions are available for some common conditions. Acetaminophen and ibuprofen, for example, were found by researchers at the Indiana University School of Medicine to be more effective in treating arthritis of the knee than expensive, heavily promoted, prescription anti-inflammatory drugs that can lead to severe stomach bleeding. (A 1993 study reported in the *Annals of Internal Medicine* found that the oils in evening primrose and borage seeds, available in health food stores, were a well-tolerated and effective treatment for rheumatoid arthritis.) One arthritis expert called the study, published in the *NEJM*, a landmark that might change medical practice. Another arthritis expert commented on the study: "If you can get away with something that the patient tolerates better and that has less hazard, by all means do it." For years doctors have prescribed anti-inflammatory drugs for the estimated 80 percent of people over sixty-five with osteoarthritis of the knee because they thought the condition to be the result of inflammation. They are now concluding that osteoarthritis is caused by a "poorly understood process that makes the cartilage that cushions the knee joint wear out." Thus do medical knowledge and medical fashions change.

Implants and Other Devices

Modern medicine has brought us the wonders of implants, some truly miraculous to the patients who receive them. According to the National Center for Health Statistics, an estimated eleven million Americans (4.6 percent of the population) had at least one medical device implant in 1988. Yet, measuring the use of only artificial joints, fixation devices, artificial heart valves, intraocular lenses, and pacemakers, the group found that 20 to 50 percent of all implanted medical devices resulted in one or more problems. Ten percent had to be replaced.

In 1974 the Dalkon Shield, billed as "the birth control device you didn't have to remember to use," became the birth control device you'd better not use, for it was removed from the market after being blamed for painful infections, spontaneous abortions, hysterectomies, and at least eighteen deaths among its three million users. After several women won multimillion-dollar suits against the manufacturer, the company went bankrupt.

Hearts that malfunction are worrisome things, but sometimes the devices that doctors use to treat the malfunction can be even more worrisome. In 1979 the FDA approved a heart valve known to have a history of fracturing. After several recalls of the valve, the manufacturer in 1986 withdrew it from the market and by 1990 reported a total of 389 fractures and 248 deaths (a Dutch study estimated 667 deaths). Though the company notified surgeons of possible risks, neither the company nor the FDA notified patients (or their family doctors) that a possibly defective device had been planted in their hearts. Said the *New York Times*, "many patients remain in total ignorance of the situation." In 1990, PCHRG sued the manufacturer on behalf of approximately eighty thousand people who had had defective valves implanted in their chests. In 1992 a federal judge approved a settlement of up to $215 million in damages. In a similar case, in 1993, involving at least one death, a manufacturer of heart catheters agreed to pay $61 million to settle a case involving 391 criminal counts.

Who in our government regulates such devices? The FDA, under authority granted it by the Safe Medical Devices Act of 1990, which reformed the 1976 medical device law. The FDA did not begin to implement the 1976 law until 1984, and when it did, it found, by using documents obtained through the Freedom of Information Act, "serious, unreported device problems in the files of thirty-five different companies" that manufacture medical devices. These "problems" included "at least 7 deaths, 109 serious injuries, 265 malfunctions, 77 malfunctions/serious injuries (not specified), and one design defect." Under the new law, the FDA cannot only recall devices, it can, in conjunction with the recall, ask the manufacturer to notify patients that the device they are using may injure them. If the manufacturer can't find them, the FDA has to make a public announcement about the risks. When it comes to enforcement, however, the FDA continues dragging its heels, says PCHRG, neither fining nor prosecuting manufacturers for failing to report serious problems with their medical devices.

PCHRG not only keeps track of such matters, it also takes a active role. In 1991 the public-advocacy organization announced that it had won its lawsuit to force the FDA to release thousands of pages of information regarding silicone gel breast implants, including scientific studies that may show serious adverse health effects. Calling the decision a major victory, PCHRG director Sidney Wolfe said, "We've been attempting since 1972 to get the courts to say that data on safety and effectiveness of drugs should be public." The FDA had argued that release of such documents would reveal trade secrets. About this, the federal judge in the case said that the FDA "would have this court believe that it is the most impotent agency in Washington, and that the only way it can protect the public's health and welfare is by begging manufacturers of possibly lethal devices to submit information voluntarily."

It was this decision, of course, that led to a series of dramatic disclosures about breast implants. When previously secret information about the implants became public in 1991 (medical literature had contained reports of adverse effects since 1979), some women raved about their implants, some women raged about their health problems from implants, and plastic surgeons said that the devices should remain on the market (plastic and reconstructive surgery is a $330-million-a-year business). In 1992 Mariann Hopkins, a California woman who received silicone implants after a double mastectomy, successfully sued the manufacturer of her implants for $7.3 million. She claimed that the silicone gel that leaked had damaged her immune system, causing joint pain, fatigue, muscle spasms, and connective-tissue disease. When she asked her rheumatologist if her illness might be related to her implants, he told her that people always need something to blame and "I might as well accept my illness." When she asked her lawyer, Don Bolton (whom she hired after she happened to hear him on TV talking about implant-related disabilities), why she hadn't heard about other women with this problem, he said that it was because "there have been suits filed against [the manufacturer] and they have settled out of court, and then all the documents are kept under lock and key." Believing that this was "criminal," Hopkins stuck to her guns and refused out-of-court settlements. The manufacturer, she said, "places absolutely no value on my life or the life of any other woman, as far as I can see." To give the other side its due, the chief executive officer of a major manufacturer of silicone implants said in a 1992 interview: "My overriding responsibility and that of [the manufacturer] in this whole matter [are] to the women who use [our] mammary breast implants."

By March 1993 more than 3,500 women, many of them claiming immune-system problems, had sued Dow Chemical, a Midland, Michigan, a leading maker of silicone implants. Also in 1993, U.S. attorneys representing women in nine other countries filed a class-action suit in Michigan. In 1992 a Texas woman won $25 million in damages; she claimed that the resultant illnesses had forced her to have a mastectomy. On September 9, 1993, lawyers for both defendants and plaintiffs announced a proposed $4.75 billion fund to compensate women with breast implant problems. In February 1994 three of the largest defendants—Baxter International, Dow Corning, and Bristol Meyers-Squibb—agreed to pay up to $3.7 billion to settle current and future claims over a period of thirty years. In March 1994 a jury awarded $27.9 million to three women whose breast implants had leaked.

In the meantime, an FDA advisory panel recommended in 1992 that silicone breast implants be allowed to stay on the market, but with severe restrictions. Women may still obtain them for cosmetic reasons, but only by participating in clinical studies. How did they get on the market in the first place? As the FDA was not given regulatory authority over medical devices until 1976, the implants, which had then been in use for at least a decade, were "grandfathered" onto the market without adequate investigation. The agency canceled its planned 1978 investigation of silicone breast implants after being assured by plastic surgeons that they were safe. In the thirty years or so that breast implants have been available, an estimated five hundred thousand to two million women have received them, with about 80 percent implanted for cosmetic reasons.

By October 1993 an estimated thirty thousand women had undergone "explantation," the removal of silicone implants. If you or someone you know has breast implants and is faced with this difficult decision, you may obtain more information by asking the

Public Citizen Health Research Group, 2000 P Street NW, Washington, D.C. 20036, for a copy of the March 1992 issue of their *Health Letter*, which contains questions and answers about silicone gel implants, or by calling the FDA at 1-800-532-4440 (for general information about breast implants) or at 1-800-638-6725 (to report a problem with implants). Also, MedicAlert (1-800-344-3226) operates a registry for people with any implanted device; for a small yearly fee you can be notified of recalls or problems with your implant. Silicone is not inert: researchers have found that the human body produces antibodies against it. For information about silicone-generated antibodies, your doctor may contact Immunoscience Lab, 1801 La Cienega Boulevard, Suite 302, Los Angeles, California 90035; 1-800-950-4648.

Drug Research and Marketing: the Bias Within

In managing acute bacterial infections and other conditions, twentieth-century medicine has come to rely heavily on antibiotics and other drugs. Who researches illnesses, drugs, and medical procedures and devices? Drug companies, of course, spend millions to study proposed new products by means of both animal (toxicological) studies and human (clinical) studies that are finally submitted to the FDA for drug approval. Their interest in these studies is obvious. Not so obvious is the government's interest, except presumably for the protection of public health. In 1990 our government spent more than $7 billion for NIH research, 62 percent of which went to colleges and universities (the NIH consists of thirteen tax-supported institutes that conduct and support biomedical research into the causes, prevention, and cure of diseases). Eventually, much of this research gets published in prestigious, peer-reviewed journals like *JAMA* and the *NEJM*.

Yet even scientists are not immune to common human weaknesses. The peer-review system can suppress innovation when personal egos get in the way. In a 1990 issue of *JAMA*, David F. Horrobin, DPhil, BM, cautions, "editors must be conscious that, despite public protestations to the contrary, many scientist-reviewers are against innovation unless it is *their* innovation." Further sources of research bias are two possible factors: data can be and have been cooked (this subverts the peer-review process, for the peers do not see the original data); and conflict of interest (scientists can have financial interests in the products involved) can bias results. A few flagrant examples of both kinds of distortion led a Congressional committee to conclude in 1990 that "the public may be misled and endangered by scientific misconduct and conflicts of interest."

As modern medicine lurches toward the twenty-first century, still larger issues loom—issues that discourage medical science from looking for nontraditional solutions for health problems. Scientists and doctors want grants to do research, but where can they get them? Some scientists believe that there are few totally "neutral" sources of funding. Drug companies, government administrations, and even advocacy groups and universities can have their own agendas and biases, in addition to the researchers' personal biases. With drug company research leaning heavily toward patentable products and with mainstream medicine drug-oriented, little money is available for research on prevention, natural remedies, and nutrition. It's hard to patent aloe vera or broccoli or vitamin C. Avoidance of toxic chemicals is not an exciting topic. Environmental physicians rarely get grants and seldom get their research published in the major peer-reviewed journals.

Another systemic problem is that we live in an age of specialists. Dr. Beasley again: "Tunnel vision is destroying American medicine. In order to obtain grants, one must know more and more about less and less. The narrower your research interest, the better chance you have of obtaining money. Super-specialization keeps taking us further away from fundamental factors like nutrition, the environment, and the way we live. Someone has to start dealing with the big picture." Those who already do are the environmental clinicians, who deal with chemically injured patients rather than statistics.

The emphasis on cure rather than prevention is a third factor stalling truly productive research. Epidemiologist Devra Lee Davis, who is among those documenting the worldwise increase in cancer, deplores the NCI's emphasis on cure instead of prevention. "The prevention of cancer on a big scale is going to require that we change our habits, change our lifestyles, clean up the environment, change the consumer products that contain hazardous materials," she says. "It's going to mean a whole new approach to everyday living." Yet her approach faces tough going. "When you treat cancer, profits are made through drugs or surgery," she points out. "But when cancer is prevented, nobody makes any money. There is almost no constituency for cancer prevention." Davis is well aware of scientific resistance to a new idea: "At first, people say it's ridiculous. Then they say, 'Well, it might be true, but it's not important.' Then they say, 'Well, actually, I discovered this myself.'"

Indeed, medical history records many such flip-flops. As recently as 1991, for example, a cancer patient interested in exploring unconventional treatments reported that "when I mentioned diet to my oncologist, he thought it was so silly that I didn't even bother bringing up visualization, acupuncture, or meditation, all of which I ended up doing on my own." Yet in 1992 a front-page headline screamed "New focus on diet in war on cancer," over a story reporting a major shift by the American Cancer Society. Such shifts inspire little confidence in modern medical therapies.

Once a drug is researched, developed, and approved by the FDA, it is marketed, and therein lie several traps for the unwary practitioner and patient. Although you, the patient, are the consumer, drug companies have for years hawked their wares only to doctors, by means of often flawed advertisements in professional journals, visits by salespeople loaded with freebies and colorful brochures, and—more sinister and seductive—free trips and vacations often disguised as "continuing medical education."

Further jeopardizing medical objectivity are such recent drug-company practices as "video news releases," TV spots put together by public relations firms for drug companies and slipped into newscasts as if they were impartial news reports. Sometimes edited to appear as if the anchorperson were interviewing a patient or a health expert (often one paid by the promoters), they induce viewers to believe that they are hearing real information. According to Eugene Secunda, professor of marketing at Baruch College, such videos "are meant to deceive in the sense that they do not represent themselves as a promotional message. When the television audience does not recognize that there is a promotional objective to be achieved, that is inherent deception." Newspaper and magazine ads are usually labeled as such; these videos are not. Until TV news directors "just say no" to these slick, inexpensive, convenient, but deceptive commercials, consumers be wary! Another technique used by drug companies is the funneling of money to health organizations. One drug company, the maker of Xanax, the only drug approved for the treatment of panic disorders, contributes regularly to the Anxiety Disorders Association of America, whose president has appeared on a video news release for the company.

Such practices led in 1990 to Congressional hearings, which revealed that the drug industry spends more than $5 billion a year on promotion (over half as much as the $8 billion spent on research and development, a figure which often includes marketing research) in the U.S. alone—undoubtedly a factor in spiraling health costs that create problems especially for the elderly, who often must choose between food and medication. In 1993 President Clinton charged that the pharmaceutical industry is spending $1 billion more each year on advertising and lobbying than it does on development of new and better drugs.

Doctors' testimony at the 1990 hearings shed light on drug company practices, evidence of which you can see when you visit many doctors' offices: golf balls with a company or drug logo, rulers, pens, pencils, note pads, mugs, glasses, cups, hats, caps, shirts, magnets, towels, tie tacks, clipboards, a large variety of anatomic models, games, puzzles, socks, visors, packages of candy, gum, popcorn, tennis balls. Some perks are hidden: tickets to shows, dinners, weekend getaways, golf fees, even cash. Though most testifying doctors agreed that relationships between the majority of physicians and drug-company representatives were ethical, others questioned this assumption. What about the drug company, asked one witness, that offered frequent-flyer points for each prescription? Dr. John Nelson, a Salt Lake City obstetrician, told of his two partners taking their wives on free trips, one to the Caribbean and one to a California golf resort, both paid for by a drug company. "Both doctors," he testified, "who previously had refused to prescribe the drug firm's new product, came back converted after attending company-sponsored lectures." The lure was hard to resist. Attempting a still higher level of sophistication, a large drug company, according to one of its former executives, introduced its new prescription tranquilizer by inviting doctors to a night at the opera in New York, one in which singers perform[ed] scenes from opera's greatest neurotic episodes and then to programs in which each of these medical conditions was carefully described and the new drug recommended as the cure. For this scam the doctors could claim continuing medical education credits (state certification boards require doctors to participate in continuing medical education programs). A Seattle internist testified at the hearing that drug companies now subsidize virtually all continuing medical education for doctors.

Doctors may think they are being ethical in their prescribing practices, but studies indicate that they are often unaware of the influence of drug company sales pitches. Like the rest of us, doctors can fall for advertising. One study by Harvard Medical School researchers determined that most doctors surveyed believed that drug advertisements exerted "minimal" influence over their decisions. But the doctors held beliefs about certain drugs that were not scientifically correct and could have been learned only from advertising. A University of Minnesota survey on drug marketing to doctors found that one-fourth changed their prescribing practices at least once in the preceding year based on talks with salespeople.

Where should doctors get their information on drugs? Not from salespeople, with their obvious conflict of interest. Several teaching hospitals have started informational sessions offering doctors unbiased information. Such programs have proved effective in cutting costs, though drug company reprisals are a possible hazard. One doctor testified that drug companies had threatened two teaching hospitals with the loss of research support because the hospitals' pharmacists had not recommended the companies' drugs.

Two groups have been closely following the drug-marketing scandal—Public Citizen and Consumers Union, publisher of *Consumer Reports*. Public Citizen's Dr. Sidney Wolfe testified at the Senate hearings about doctor-bribing which violates federal or state laws having criminal and civil penalties. As examples, he cited five specific cases: (1) frequent-flier bonus miles for frequent prescribing, (2) bribes of $1,200 in cash for prescribing expensive antibiotics and answering a few questions about patients receiving the drug—a "clinical study," (3) kickbacks for purchasing vaccines, (4) $100 for using a toxic drug for an unapproved indication, and (5) free $35,000 office computer systems (which would allow drug companies to tap into doctors' computers for information about what they are prescribing).

In response, the AMA, the Board of Regents of the American College of Physicians, and the Pharmaceutical Manufacturers Association (PMA) have adopted ethical guidelines for their relationships. The AMA's voluntary guidelines allow for small gifts that serve "a genuine function," recommend against "gifts with strings attached," and allow for industry-funded "reasonable" honoraria and "reasonable" travel while attending symposia or conferences. Violating physicians run the risk of ending up in a data bank, but one that is not open to consumers. The PMA's code calls for "complete candor . . . objectivity and good taste . . . and scrupulous regard for truth" on the part of drug companies.

Will these voluntary guidelines help correct current drug-promotion practices? No one knows. Will the government step in to stop them? Past experience is not encouraging: the FDA has not prosecuted a drug company for advertising and promotional violations for twenty years, according to Dr. Wolfe. Will drug prices go down? David Jones, a drug industry defector, thinks not: "The price of prescription drugs is determined by what the market will bear. Pain and suffering and desperation will support a high price indeed."

Meanwhile, an estimated 8 percent of the nation's office-based doctors are directly cashing in on the profits to be made from drugs. By buying (from drug repackagers) and selling (to their patients), these doctors are augmenting their already high incomes. Thus, says Representative Ron Wyden (D-OR), "there is a growing number of fast-buck artists who are telling doctors they can make $50,000 without any more difficulty than reaching for a prescription pad." In 1991 the pay of doctors in private practice averaged $191,800 (only $170,000 "average annual income," argues the AMA), according to Ron Pollack, of the advocacy group Families USA, with anesthesiologists averaging $221,000, radiologists averaging $229,000, and hospital chief executives averaging $235,000. (Data for 1992 from the Medical Group Management Association gave cardiovascular surgeons the top salaries, an average of $575,000.) In 1992 the AMA political action committee gave $2.94 million to candidates, second only to the National Association of Realtors. In the first half of 1993, health insurers gave $2.3 million to key Congressional members considering health reform.

For years, drug companies have been profiting from America's health problems. According to *Consumer Reports*, "the pharmaceutical industry has long been the nation's most profitable. The top ten U.S. drug companies averaged 16 percent profit on sales in 1990, more than triple that of the average Fortune 500 company. . . . Between 1980 and 1990, while general inflation was 58 percent, overall health-care costs rose 117 percent—and the cost of drugs rose 152 percent. Every unnecessary prescription, and every unnecessary choice of an expensive, brand-name drug over a cheaper alternative, contributes to these excessive costs."

Many drugs, of course, are now sold like detergents—on the mass media, at a cost of $70 million in 1970 and with the disapproval of most doctors. *Consumer Reports* quotes drug company-defector Jones about the common practice of sending doctors on media tours to launch new drugs: "We'd get a doctor who looks the part, send him to charm school to learn about sound bites, how to handle hostile questions, how to manipulate the media. Then we'd book him as a medical expert on the talk-show circuit." Usually the doctor's financial ties to the company were not disclosed. Another new marketing technique is toll-free hotlines set up by drug companies to promote their wares to unwary consumers. "Your patients call toll-free to hear a totally controlled, prerecorded, interactive event that inspires compliance," blatantly bleats an ad promoting this service. Reprints of *Consumer Reports'* two articles, "Pushing Drugs to Doctors" and "Miracle Drugs or Media Drugs?" (from the February and March 1992 issues) are available in bulk; write CU Reprints, 101 Truman Avenue, Yonkers, New York 10703. You might also ask whether reprints of CU's October 1993 articles "Do We Pay Too Much for Prescriptions?" and "How to Buy Drugs for Less" are available.

Environmental Medicine

The fight over health-care-financing dominates the present scene, yet a fundamental question remains: is our current medical system providing optimal care for Americans? Dr. Adriane Fugh-Berman says that the medical establishment "likes to pretend that a true *health care* system that emphasizes prevention and the most benign therapies is not possible. . . . The dirty secret in medicine . . . is that much of our practice today is based not on science but on the Hippocratic belief in clinical judgment and experience." Even in the age of science, the practice of medicine remains more the healer's art than the researcher's science. In 1991, for example, Washington State family practitioners were asked how they would treat a woman's uncomplicated urinary tract infection. Eighty-two physicians suggested 137 separate treatment regimens, ranging in cost from nothing to $250.

All of this is not to say that the great majority of U.S. doctors are not caring, dedicated, and hardworking. They are; and millions of patients are grateful for life-saving drugs and surgery, prescribed or performed by such doctors, who have spent hard, long, numbing years in medical school and hospital residencies. Such doctors may well deplore the abuses just enumerated. The problem, it would seem, lies in the system rather than the individual doctor, in what is and is not taught in medical school, and in the attitudes fostered by a dominant system resistant to new ideas.

Predictably, most physicians practice what they were taught, and medical schools are notoriously reluctant to accept new ideas. Dr. Randolph was dismissed from the faculty of Northwestern University Medical School in the early 1950s; his new ideas were allegedly "a pernicious influence on medical students." Later, turf battles within medical schools and between medical specialties obscured the issues and prevented chemical susceptibility (his term) from receiving the recognition it needed from traditional medicine. Medical schools have tended to focus on cure rather than cause, on treatment (by drugs) rather than prevention, on preparing doctors for private practice rather than public health and epidemiology, and on specific prescriptions for specific diseases, rather than holistic approaches to multiple symptoms. Since medical science has largely ignored EI/MCS or denied its existence, the major environmental organizations tend not to perceive the relationship between the environment and human health. Only recently have the major media noticed the illness.

Unfortunately, this vacuum has created a splendid opportunity for critics of environmental medicine, who use it to resort to several outworn attacks:

"The therapies are still unproven." By now you know that traditional medicine uses many "unproven therapies." And indeed, with many diseases what's "proven" and "unproven" is hard to tell apart. A 1991 study of cancer care regimens found that "terminally ill cancer patients treated at a clinic that emphasizes unproven treatments fare no better—and no worse—than people who get chemotherapy and other standard care." Dr. Kerr White, retired deputy director for health sciences at the Rockefeller Foundation reports that, taken as a whole, "only about 15 percent of all contemporary clinical interventions are supported by objective scientific evidence that they do more good than harm."

Realities such as these may be one reason that sufferers are turning to alternative medicine in large numbers. In its November 5, 1991, cover story, *Time* magazine reported that alternative medicine is a $27-billion-a-year business in the U.S. and that 30 percent of those surveyed reported having used some form of unconventional (by Western standards) therapy: acupuncture, biofeedback, shiatsu, chiropractic, homeopathy, and the like. A Harvard Medical School study found that in 1990 Americans spent $13.7 billion on alternative therapies, mostly out of their own pockets. In the face of this rising defection, an alarmed NIH in 1992 set up a new Office for the Study of Unconventional Medical Practices, now called the Office of Alternative Medicine.

Environmental physicians consider what they do as not "alternative," but arising out of centuries-old traditions. Many chemically injured patients, however, do prefer environmental medicine precisely because they see it as an alternative—one which is almost entirely noninvasive, nonsurgical, and nonpainful, and definitely nontoxic. The latter is especially true of the chief therapy, avoidance, the "treatment" most often prescribed by environmental physicians. The therapy can include vitamins, minerals, enzymes, amino acids, and other dietary supplements. Preferring to recommend avoidance and natural substances, environmental physicians tend not to prescribe drugs, which only mask symptoms "as if a headache were a Darvon deficiency," says Dr. Sherry Rogers. Also, they are especially aware of the dangerous side effects of most petroleum-based prescription drugs.

Environmental physicians do rely on extensive experience and testing to determine the appropriate course of therapy, and as a result their chief contribution is often their ability to diagnose specific causes for a patient's multiple symptoms. By testing for foods and chemicals, with the patient unaware of what he or she is receiving intradermally or sublingually (a "single-blind" test), the doctor can discover what patients are reacting to and should avoid. Sometimes the doctor will discover "neutralizing" doses that turn off the patient's reactions. A hyperactive child, for instance, can be first "revved up" and later calmed down by appropriate dilutions of a suspected food or chemical. A child's handwriting can go from legible to illegible and back again as test dilutions are changed. Regarding this "provocation-neutralization" controversy, Dr. James L. Bryant, president of the American Academy of Otolaryngic Allergy, has commented that there is "a medical turf battle in allergy today that is based mainly on economic considerations but has resulted in attempts to discredit testing techniques."

"It's too expensive." This is a curious complaint, one seemingly motivated by a genuine concern for the patient's pocketbook. Yet a sufferer often comes to an environmental physician after having fruitlessly spent thousands of dollars going from specialist to specialist, submitting to inappropriate test after test, helping to pay for modern medicine's high technology. It is true that for chemically sensitive patients, cleaning up their environment may prove costly at first, but these costs diminish with time and are often gladly shouldered as the patient finally begins to feel better. Also, these costs may be far less than those of surgical treatment or a lifetime of disability.

"It's all a dangerous waste of time." Here critics seem motivated by concern for the patient's health, arguing that patients are wasting valuable time by not seeking help from mainstream doctors. Actually, of course, it is often the other way around. People with symptoms like fatigue, headaches, nausea, dizziness, depression, and anxiety can spend years and large sums of money on psychiatrists without lasting relief of those symptoms, while testing by environmental physicians could have put them on the right track much sooner. In the experience of Earon Davis, a lawyer with long experience in the field of chemical injury, "psychiatric approaches have not worked with confirmed cases of MCS, except to assist them in the tremendously stressful process of coping with this illness and with physicians and insurers who insist that the illness is 'all in their heads.' "

Like psychiatrists, environmental physicians *do* spend more time with patients than most other doctors—more time asking questions, listening to answers, formulating individual solutions. One reason many patients prefer environmental physicians, when they finally get to them, is precisely this greater attention to details and to what the patient has to say. Patients are treated as individuals, not as members of a diagnostic group. Instead of "Here's a list of foods that cause headaches," the doctor asks many questions to elicit clues and then tests the patient to discover the *particular* foods to which the patient may be allergic. If a patient turns out to be chemically sensitive, doctor and patient become a pair of detectives in a joint search for clues and for remedies (the latter search mainly a hunt for alternative products, work, or lifestyles). In environmental medicine, the only quick fix is the occasional fortuitous discovery that a particular food or environmental toxin is what has been making the patient sick. In mainstream medicine, quick fixes like drugs can sometimes lead to future, and worse, fixes.

"There's only anecdotal evidence." This scornful attack, often applied to environmental medicine, reflects mainstream medicine's assumption that if something isn't proved by a randomized, double-blind, controlled scientific study, it doesn't exist. But how many anecdotes are needed before EI/MCS is fully accepted? And how many of mainstream medicine's practices have been "proved"? How many double-blind, controlled studies of the effectiveness of, say, psychiatry have been made? Some psychiatrists instead seem to prefer to concentrate on producing flawed studies of chemically injured patients. Actually, "anecdotal" means "clinical," and clinical observation is medicine's historic way of making discoveries. Careful observation is the basis of science; replication of the results of observation comes later—much later with environmental medicine, because of the lack of research funding. Yet thousands of people can testify to the existence of EI/MCS and the benefits they have obtained from environmental specialists. Their "anecdotes" are discounted by scientists who, while sympathetic, believe that the existence of the condition and the validity of its chief treatment (avoidance) have yet to be proved by scientific tests. Skeptics often become believers when the illness strikes them or their relatives or patients.

Are "scientific" tests really possible with EI/MCS? With more than seventy thousand chemicals, mostly petroleum-based, added to the marketplace since World War II—a thousand more every year—toxicity largely unknown, how is it possible to test for their combined effect on human beings, even if it were ethically permissible to do so? It's not like testing a new drug versus a placebo. For one thing, the drug is presumed to be beneficial, not toxic, to people's health (though drugs often prove to be quite toxic). Most modern industrial chemicals are not intended to be beneficial to anyone's health (except for the manufacturer's economic health) and may be toxic. Furthermore, how can any test reproduce in a controlled way the exposures to the hundreds of chemicals found in homes, workplaces, or public buildings? And how many people— chemically sensitive or not—would consent to sit in a room filled with vapors of formaldehyde, toluene, xylene, dioxins, PCBs, methylene chloride, or all of the above? Studies of the synergistic (additive) effects of such chemicals have yet to be done, though there is speculation that such effects can be far greater than the effects of each chemical acting alone.

Actually, a few studies of people with chemical sensitivity *have* been done. In 1988 a controlled study with thirty-six subjects indicated that while chemically sensitive people may not have heightened awareness of odors, MCS is "associated with depression, increased respiration rate, and decreased nasal airway patency." A study of workers exposed to mixtures of organic solvents found "a highly significant relationship" with a history of nausea, headaches, and subjective distress and a decrease in ability to learn and remember. Researchers at the East Carolina School of Medicine found nose and throat abnormalities in ten patients with MCS. Other researchers are developing a theory as to a possible mechanism of action in the olfactory-limbic system. Marco Kaltofen, former laboratory director for the National Toxics Campaign (NTC), has found that chemical sensitization shows a distinct dose-response relationship—in other words, as the concentration of a chemical in the air increases, more and more people develop symptoms—and that a chemical doesn't have to have an odor to cause symptoms. Carbon monoxide is a good example.

The issue of ethics in research is complicated. Controlled studies by traditional researchers have been stopped when it became evident that the drug being tested was so beneficial that it was not ethical to deny it to some subjects just for the purpose of collecting evidence. Conversely, unless subjects voluntarily give their fully informed consent it does not seem ethical purposely to expose humans to significant amounts of chemicals (or mixtures of chemicals) of known or unknown toxicity, nor does it seem ethical to presume, without overwhelming evidence, that symptoms have psychological rather than physiological causes. Actually, of course, we are all *involuntary* guinea pigs in this vast, ongoing twentieth-century clinical trial.

In the U.S. the number of *voluntary* clinical trials conducted by mainstream medicine is increasing, despite possible risk to patients. When five out of fifteen participants in an NIH pilot study of a promising hepatitis drug died, investigators stopped the experiment immediately, and experts on biomedical research questioned whether participants had been fully enough informed about possible risks. Dr. Wolfe, of Public Citizen, charged that the drug's manufacturer had covered up data on its liver toxicity. In 1992, worried by the increasing incidence of breast cancer, basically healthy women jumped at the chance to participate in a five-year study of the use of a highly risky drug, tamoxifen, to prevent the disease. Thus clinical trials—of drugs or of industrial chemicals, by traditional or by nontraditional researchers, controlled or not controlled—appear questionable as to both feasibility and safety.

Whether to continue using this common method of evaluating new treatments is a difficult question. In the past, most common treatments were not scrutinized by clinical trials. As a result, physicians have been fooled into adopting some therapies that later turned out to be useless or even harmful, such as the use of radiation

to treat acne or shrink tonsils. The year 1994 brought us the unfolding story of doctors using unsuspecting people as guinea pigs
after World War II, in the early days of nuclear medicine.

Actually, the closest that scientists can come to a controlled
study of chemical reactivity is the environmental unit pioneered by
Dr. Randolph and recommended by participants at a 1991 workshop on EI/MCS conducted by the NRC at the request of the EPA.
An environmental unit is a carefully monitored hospital-like environment kept as free of modern synthetic chemicals and other
pollutants as possible. If subjects' symptoms subside in this environment only to recur on the introduction of carefully monitored, small
amounts of such chemicals, one at a time or even in combination,
then a cause-and-effect relationship becomes apparent. According
to Nicholas Ashford, speaking at a 1989 American Public Health
Association workshop on EI/MCS, the test could even be double-
blind, though it is hard to imagine how it could approximate the
chemical soup we all live in or how, if the chemicals were inhaled,
subjects would not be likely to recognize what they were smelling.
Nevertheless, most people—patients and nonpatients—agree that
more research is needed. Epidemiological studies are another approach, though, like environmental units, they are expensive, time-
consuming, and cannot prove individual causation. Must
recognition of EI/MCS and help for sufferers await such studies?

"Nobody knows how the disease works." Critics say that nothing
can be done about EI/MCS until we know more about what's going
on inside the body. Yet medical progress has often been made before exact bodily mechanisms are known. In the 1850s John Snow
ended the cholera epidemic in London by removing the handle of
the Broad Street water pump, thirty years before the bacterium
causing cholera was discovered. "Fortunately, he did not need to
contend with a 'Cholera Institute' that demanded the pump keep
working until it was proven that water from the pump was causing
the cholera," says former Surgeon General C. Everett Koop. Fibromyalgia is the name given to aches and pains that cannot be
"pinned down by lab tests or physical exams," according to Dr.
Robert Bennett of the Oregon Health Sciences University. "An important lesson in the . . . 'fibromyalgia saga,'" he says, is "granting

patients credibility when symptoms and signs do not conform to contemporary medical prejudices."

The incidence of clinical depression has increased in developed countries since the 1940s, and this illness is now affecting nine million Americans annually, according to the American Psychiatric Association. "I'm pretty convinced that something rather profound happened in our society from about 1950 to 1980 and that it had its greatest impact on young people," said Dr. Gerald Klerman of the New York Hospital-Cornell Medical Center. "It could be some virus or some toxin in our food or water, or it could be these social forces that are changing the family, or urbanization, or the changing role of women, or stress." Whatever the cause, a common drug for one form of depression—manic depression—is lithium, which appears to correct a chemical imbalance in the brain, though its precise mechanism of action is unknown. Dr. Harold Klawans, a neurologist at Rush-Presbyterian-St. Luke's Medical Center in Chicago, pictures the doctor as a detective, "the skilled observer who meticulously gathers evidence and uses judgement, insight, and intuition in tracking and apprehending the source of an affliction or behavioral problem." Even today, he says, "with all the fancy equipment and diagnostic techniques, between 25 and 35 percent of all neurological diseases must still be established clinically, by observation." Finally, Nicholas Ashford wrote in the *NEJM* that "in the light of mounting evidence that suggestions of toxicity are for the most part ultimately confirmed by painstaking scientific inquiry, perhaps it is time to reexamine whether scientific standards of proof of causality—and waiting for the bodies to fall—ought not give way to more preventive public health policies that are satisfied by more realistic conventions and that lead to action sooner."

"EI/MCS is all in the mind." In 1991 the *Mayo Clinic Proceedings* said that "subjective tinnitus . . . is noise that can only be heard by the patient—but this doesn't mean it's 'all in your mind.' Although the exact cause of subjective tinnitus is unknown, it presumably results from electrophysiologic derangements in the auditory system." Similarly, EI/MCS often can be "heard" only by the patient, and, similarly, this does not mean "it's all in your mind," though this statement is heard all too often by the chemically injured. Yet, in one sense, a lot of EI/MCS *is* in the mind. Chemically induced headaches and other neurological symptoms such as convulsions, short-term memory loss, disorientation, and dizziness certainly originate or are located there. The OTA's book on neurotoxicity details the adverse health effects of industrial chemicals, pesticides, therapeutic drugs, "substance" drugs, foods, food additives, cosmetic ingredients, and naturally occurring substances like lead and mercury. The book has a drawing of the brain on its cover.

A Modest Dose of Self-Care

As a society, we have conquered many of the ailments that plagued human beings during recorded history. Diseases such as measles, scarlet fever, tuberculosis, and smallpox are almost a thing of the past (though tuberculosis seems to be making a comeback). Since Pasteur and Fleming, medicine has concentrated on infectious diseases and relied on medications, such as antibiotics, to cure them. "Miracles" have occurred, and great strides have been made. But we are now encountering adverse effects from the overuse of antibiotics with both humans and animals, effects such as the rampant development of resistant bacterial strains in hospitals and the overgrowth of *Candida albicans* in the human gut. And paradoxically, the strong, toxic disinfectants and air "fresheners" used in hospitals, nursing homes, and public washrooms in a misguided and overdone attempt to be "clean" are making some people sick. They are part of society's synthetic chemical overload that has become part of every person's body load.

Given the confusing state of modern medicine, with its multiple strengths and weaknesses, what is the layperson to do? Dr. Beasley has concluded that despite modern medicine's superb achievements, "our best hope for a healthy life is not medical care, but self-care." While nothing in this chapter is to be construed as medical advice, a few suggestions are possible.

- Avoid both over-the-counter and prescription drugs as much as possible. Many can do more harm than good, and some, like Darvon, the prescription drug that killed National Football

League player John Matuszak, can prove fatal. When buying any drug, read the package insert and pay attention to the fine print.

- When looking for a doctor, try to find one well-versed in both conventional and alternative medicine—or at least one open to new ideas. Look for one who listens carefully and respectfully and who is willing to work with you to better your health. Remember that in some ways you know your body better than your doctor does; you've been living with it longer. Realize that you cannot leave your health solely to your doctor; ultimately you must take responsibility for it yourself.

- Accept that if you are looking for medical alternatives, you're in good company. Harvard Medical School instructor David M. Eisenberg says that unlike the stereotype of the wacky patient seeking magic remedies, most people interested in alternatives are "bright, well-educated, critical thinkers." Join these thinkers in looking for doctors who do not take themselves too seriously. Dr. Richard J. Sagall, editing *Pediatrics for Parents* with tongue in cheek, lists his "medical school secrets" with the admonition to the reader not to divulge them to anyone. Here's one: "Half of what you will learn in medical school is wrong. The difficulty is we don't know which half it is." Doctors, he says, are "working with a constantly shifting body of knowledge that contains many contradictions and uncertainties." A refreshing attitude indeed. When looking for relief for a symptom, consider the profound differences between drugs and nutrients, the latter from food or from supplements such as vitamins, minerals, enzymes, and amino acids. According to Dr. Beasley, drugs are foreign to the body, which tries to eliminate them as fast as possible; never satisfy a deficiency of the body; interfere with the metabolism of the body; have immediate and specific therapeutic activity; can be dangerous when taken in combination; often do not work, particularly with susceptible people, such as the elderly; alleviate symptoms and, except for antibiotics, do not affect underlying causes; are toxicants in any dose and have sometimes serious side effects (they kill hundreds of people a day).

In contrast, nutrients are essential to the body, which either uses them quickly or stores them; can make up for deficiencies in the body; support the metabolism of the body; have broad, gradual therapeutic effects; work best in combination; always "work" and are particularly important to susceptible people; work only by dealing with underlying causes; are natural to the body and heal rather than sicken or kill.

Similarly, old-fashioned remedies like herbs and plant-based substances can alleviate symptoms without adverse health effects (though some, like deadly nightshade, comfrey, and sassafras root, can be toxic). In fact, thirty-seven of the hundred most commonly prescribed medicines in America contain active compounds derived from flowering plants or fungi, according to the Nature Conservancy. If Dr. Norman Farnsworth, director of the pharmacognosy program (pharmacognosy is a descriptive pharmacology dealing with crude drugs and medicinal plants) at the Medical Center of the University of Illinois at Chicago, were stranded on an island, he would want to have the following plants for coping with common aches and pains: eucalyptus, as a bronchodilator; willow (a source of aspirin) for headache, rheumatism, or arthritis; senna and cascara, for constipation; barberry, for diarrhea and infections; peppermint, for indigestion; chamomile, for insomnia; wintergreen, for joint stiffness or muscle aches; aloe, for burns and minor abrasions; ginseng, for anxiety. If you are chemically sensitive, you might be better off going with—or at least starting with—the simple, plant-based remedy: with plain eucalyptus oil rather than mixtures containing spirits of turpentine; with aloe vera rather than mercurochrome; with peppermint tea rather than promethazine.

Finally, the wise words of inventor Thomas A. Edison (1847-1931):

> The doctor of the future will give
> no medicine but will interest his
> patient in the care of the human frame,
> in diet, and in the cause and prevention of disease.

* * * *

To Find Out More

- *Pills, Profits, and Politics,* by Milton Silverman, PhD, and Philip R. Lee, MD, Berkeley, California, University of California Press, 1974.

- *Confessions of a Medical Heretic,* by Robert S. Mendelsohn, MD, Chicago, Contemporary Books, 1979.

- *The Politics of Cancer,* by Samuel S. Epstein, MD, Garden City, New York, Doubleday, 1981.

- *The Cancer Industry,* by Ralph W. Moss, New York, Equinox Press, 1993.

- *Taking Charge of Your Medical Fate,* by Lawrence C. Horowitz, MD, New York, Random House, 1988.

- *Role of the Primary Care Physician in Occupational and Environmental Medicine,* by the Institute of Medicine, Washington, D.C., National Academy Press, 1988.

- *Multiple Chemical Sensitivities: Addendum to Biologic Markers in Immunotoxicology,* by the National Research Council, Washington, D.C., National Academy Press, 1992.

- *What Your Doctor Won't Tell You,* by Jane Heimlich, New York, Harper/Collins, 1990.

- *The Other Medicines,* by Richard L. Grossman, Garden City, New York, Doubleday, 1985.

- *Drug-Induced Nutritional Deficiencies,* by Daphne E. Roe, second edition, Westport, Connecticut, AVI Publishing, 1985.

- *The Healing Herbs,* by Michael Castleman, Emmaus, Pennsylvania, Rodale Press, 1991.

- *The Great White Lie: How American's Hospitals Betray Our Trust and Endanger Our Lives,* by Walt Bogdanich, New York, Simon & Schuster, 1991.

- *Racketeering in Medicine: The Suppression of Alternatives,* by James P. Carter, MD, DrPH, Norfolk, Hampton Roads Publishing Company, 1992.

- *Medicine, Money & Morals: Physicians' Conflicts of Interest,* by Marc A. Rodwin, New York, Oxford University Press, 1993.

- *Alternative Medicine: The Definitive Guide,* by Burton Goldberg, Tiburon, California, Future Medicine Publishing, 1993.

- *Alternative Health Care Resources,* by Brett Jason Sinclair, West Nyack, New York, Parker Publishing, 1992.

- *Natural Health, Natural Medicine,* by Andrew Weil, MD, Boston, Houghton Mifflin, 1990.

- *Inconclusive by Design: Waste, Fraud, and Abuse in Federal Environmental Health Research,* by the Environmental Health Network and the National Toxics Campaign Fund, 1992; available from Jobs and Environment Campaign, 11689 Commonwealth Avenue, Boston, Massachusetts 02108; 616-232-0327.

- *10,289 Questionable Doctors;* individual state reports available for $15 each from Public Citizen, Publications Department, 2000 P Street NW, Suite 600, Washington, D.C. 20036.

- *Selected Bibliography: Chemicals and Health (1993),* compiled by Louise Kosta for the Human Ecology Action League, P.O. Box 49126, Atlanta, Georgia 30359.

- *The Townsend Letter for Doctors,* Jonathan Collin, MD, editor, 10 issues yearly, 911 Tyler Street, Port Townsend, Washington 98368-654l; 206-385-6021.

Organizations That May Help

- American Academy of Environmental Medicine, P.O. Box 16106, Denver, Colorado 80216; 303-622-9755.

- Practical Allergy Research Foundation (Doris Rapp, MD), P.O. Box 60, Buffalo, New York 14223-0060; 716-875-0398.

- Northeast Center for Environmental Medicine (Sherry A. Rogers, MD), P.O. Box 2716, Syracuse, New York 13220-2716; Dr. Rogers' books and newsletter are available from Prestige Publishing, P.O. Box 3161, Syracuse, New York, 13220; 1-800-846-ONUS.

- Commonweal Cancer Help Program, Box 316, Bolinas, California 94924; 415-868-0970.

- People's Medical Society, 462 Walnut Street, Allentown, Pennsylvania 18102; 215-770-1670.

- Planetree Health Information Service, 2040 Webster Street, San Francisco, California 94115; 415-923-3680.

- Foundation for Toxic-Free Dentistry, P.O. Box 608010, Orlando, Florida 32860-8010.

- Homeopathic Educational Services, 2124 Kittredge Street, Berkeley, California 94704; 415-649-0294.

- American Holistic Medical Association, 4101 Lake Boone Trail, Suite 201, Raleigh, North Carolina 27607-6518.

13

How Good Is Green: We the Endangered Species

MANY AMERICANS HAVE ALWAYS BEEN environmentalists, especially the very first Americans, whose attitudes are reflected in the words attributed to Chief Seattle, leader of the Suquamish Indians in the 1860s, who told his people that the president in Washington had sent word that he wishes to buy their land:

> But how can you buy or sell the sky? The land? The idea is strange to us. If we do not own the freshness of the air and the sparkle of the water, how can you buy them? . . . This we know: the Earth does not belong to us, we belong to the Earth. All things are connected like the blood that unites us all. We did not weave the web of life, we are merely a strand in it. Whatever we do to the web we do to ourselves.

Chief Seattle's ideas, however brilliantly expressed by writers then and now, did not make much headway with his land's purchasers until our own century. In 1908, President Theodore Roosevelt gave the country's increasing number of conservationists official standing by establishing the National Conservation Commission, headed by conservationist Gifford Pinchot. Protection of land, plants, animals, and other natural resources became government policy, at least in some parts of the country. The nineteenth-century preservationist writings of Henry David Thoreau and the beautiful bird drawings of John J. Audubon finally may have had some influence.

The conservationist tradition was carried on in the twentieth century by naturalist John Muir, who helped establish Yosemite National Park; by Ansel Adams's stunning nature photographs; by forester Aldo Leopold's *A Sand County Almanac*; by biologist Rachel Carson's *Silent Spring*; and by the writings of John McPhee, especially his *Encounters with the Archdruid*, a portrait of David Brower, probably our country's most ardent conservationist. Organizations dedicated to conserving wildlife and natural resources, such as the Wilderness Society, the Sierra Club, the World Wildlife Fund, the National Wildlife Federation, and the National Audubon Society, sprang up and became moderately affluent and influential.

But in the 1960s, with modern pollution increasingly obvious, the mood of the country changed, and with it, the terminology. "Conservationism" became "environmentalism." Instead of "conserve our natural resources," the watchword became "protect the environment; save the planet." Suddenly everyone was talking about "ecology," once only the name of a biology course that set students to wading in swamps for college credit. Public pressure at the time of Earth Day 1970 resulted in the establishment of a batch of government agencies designed to help, chief among them the EPA. David Brower, broadening his geographic scope, left the Sierra Club to found Friends of the Earth (he has since left that organization to work with an organization called Earth Island). Other new, more radical, more activist organizations sprouted alongside the old-line conservation groups: Greenpeace, the Natural Resources Defense Council, the Environmental Defense Fund, even several groups concerned about dangerous chemicals, such as the Environmental Research Foundation, Pesticide Action Network, the National Environmental Law Center, the National Coalition Against the Misuse of Pesticides, the Southwest Network for Environmental & Economic Justice, the National Toxics Campaign (now the Jobs and Environment Campaign), and the grass roots Citizen's Clearinghouse for Hazardous Wastes.

The Final Frontier

Yet something was—and still is—missing in the burgeoning movement for a better environment: human beings. Homo sapiens. Us. And the public health people. In all the concern for eagles, whales, spotted owls, wetlands, rain forests, wilderness areas, and coral reefs, where is the concern for human beings and their health? How can the EPA and environmental organizations assume that human beings can escape the fate of other species in this world? *Time*'s 1989 "Planet of the Year" issue, in thirty-one pages on the environment, made only one mention of human health effects from environmental degradation—and that from excess of sunlight, not from chemicals. From the mouth of a child, Zachary, the five-year-old son of EPA head Carol Browner, comes a telling statement: when asked if he knew what his mother does, he replied that she "saves trees, animals, rivers, lakes. And bananas."

So who is protecting the public health? An odd schizophrenia appears at work here, a schism, a split in thinking, a blurred focus. Presumably we protect the environment to protect ourselves, but it isn't put that way—and, more important, it isn't being done. Take the movement slogans: "The earth is under siege," "Restore health to the environment," "Water for life," "Leave me a green and peaceful planet," "Save endangered species" (not meaning humans), "Don't bungle the jungle," "No ocean dumping." All well-meaning, of course, but with misplaced emphasis. Yet to one discerning, if atypical, environment reporter, "the final frontier is what it all means to human health."

With a few notable exceptions, such as Greenpeace and the NRDC, the large, well-funded environmental/conservationist organizations have tended to ignore those who have suffered most from the widespread influx of toxic chemicals since World War II: children, the elderly, the poor and minorities, industrial workers, people in certain communities, people with EI/MCS, office workers in "sick buildings." Not even the name "environmental illness" gets the attention of the top environmental/conservationist groups, whose current donation incomes range from $15 million to $143 million. In contrast, the budget of the largest national organization of people with environmental illness, HEAL, has for some years been less than $100,000. Half a billion for the health of the planet; a pittance for the health of people. Half a billion is not enough to save the health of the planet; $100,000 is laughable when put beside the needs of thousands of human beings already injured by our toxic environment.

This is not to say that mainline environmental/conservationist organizations are not doing good things. They are, of course. But the focus is fuzzy. The vision is only peripheral. The most endangered species is us. Our delicate endocrine, nervous, and immune systems, developed to a high degree over millions of years and highly susceptible to external influences, have never before been put to the test of a chemical onslaught such as we are experiencing today. Whether we realize it or not, we are all slowly being poisoned in a process unique in human history.

Why this split? Curious it is that so few seem to make the connection—to notice the increasing number of news stories about environmentally ill factory workers, housewives, farmers, children. Bhopal was a die-off, just like that of the North Atlantic seals. "Mystery illnesses" often make headlines. Yet "endangered species" continue to be codified only as spotted owls and snail darters.

Part of the reason is historical. The mainline conservation organizations got their start before World War II, before untested chemicals began to be added to our indoor as well as outdoor environment. What we now see as concern for the planet may in fact be a guilt trip on the part of us humans, who are, as a group, the perpetrators of the planet's pollution. We who have fouled the nest are now worried about what's in the nest. Or perhaps it is a natural human concern for the small, the appealing, the voiceless, the defenseless, the inanimate. Who will speak for the endangered forests, the fouled waters, the oil-covered seals, the cormorants, the cranes, the golden-cheeked warbler if we humans do not?

We humans have poisoned them; we humans must clean up their habitat—so the thinking goes. We are the guilty ones, and we must learn to care for the animals and plants. They can't protect themselves, so we must protect them. But it's a "we-them," not an "all of us" mindset. Millions of humans are unprotected from the millions of tons of toxic chemicals yearly spewed into our air, water, and soil. We have little control over that, and little voice in our own well-being. We have more control over the products we buy, but either out of ignorance or because we are easily manipulated by advertising, we often select those that are not good for us.

So here's another reason for the split: our dependence on industry, on an industrial complex that yearly pushes us farther into uncharted chemical territory. More than a thousand new chemicals are added to the marketplace every year; most are untested for human health effects. Industry's fundamental interest is obvious—without profits it cannot exist. Environmentalism cuts into those profits, and despite its public face, industry does not like the intrusion.

Even the major environmental organizations, faced with dwindling private contributions, depend increasingly on industry support. And industry is often willing to oblige. In 1992, for example, industry support represented about 4 percent of the Audubon Society's $42 million budget, despite General Electric's withdrawal of support for Audubon's occasionally hard-hitting television series "World of Audubon." In 1993 the World Wildlife Fund received $2.5 million from Eastman Kodak, only one of many industrial donors to environmental organizations.

Alliances of natural antagonists like industry and environmentalists are uneasy for the participants and should be open to suspicion by the public. Industry pours millions of dollars not only into environmental organizations, but into advertising and public relations campaigns to give itself a good environmental face. Is it sincere? Waste Management, Inc., the huge disposal company convicted of price-fixing and environment-related violations, has donated hundreds of thousands of dollars to such groups as the National Wildlife Federation and the Nature Conservancy and spent more thousands on clever television spots showing butterflies hovering over its (actually leaking) landfills.

After years of secrecy, the Chemical Manufacturers Association in the early 1990s bought full-page ads saying "We want you to know." They want us to know what toxic chemicals they are putting into our air, ground, and water—now that the 1986 Right-to-Know Act has forced partial disclosure of these pollutants. They have set up a $50-million "Responsible Care" publicity program; call 1-800-624-4321, they say, and they'll let you know "what the chemical industry is doing to produce, transport, and handle chemicals more safely." They now have a Chemical Referral Center; call 1-800-262-8200, they say, if you have questions about chemicals on the labels of their products. (Many of these chemicals, of course, remain undisclosed as "trade secrets.") In *Chemecology*, the CMA's free magazine covering "health, safety, and the environment," Frank Popoff, CEO of Dow Chemical, candidly explained Responsible Care: "[It] is not a public relations campaign; it is our strategy for survival." *Chemecology*, another part of the CMA's strategy, has cute children on its cover, provides classroom tools for teachers, extols recycling, gives tips for preventing litter, and makes the chemical industry out to be a combination of Peter Rabbit and Smokey the Bear. Trust us, they say.

Some groups, like Greenpeace, do not solicit corporate donations for fear of hurting their credibility, but because of the economy, fear about jobs, and a widespread public opinion burnout on environmental matters, have suffered sharp declines in their finances. Riding high in 1991, highly visible Greenpeace saw its budget plummet from $58 million that year to $27 million in 1992, forcing the resignation of its director and the dismissal of twenty-five of its 235-member staff. For a decade Greenpeace had been expanding worldwide, with more than twenty-four offices planning daredevil exploits, building popularity, and exerting political influence. When West Germans were asked in a market survey "What do you admire most?" Greenpeace scored second to gold. But even activist Greenpeace has concentrated most of its efforts on plants and wildlife, sometimes at the expense of loggers' or hunters' livelihoods. As a result it has been accused of forcing people to choose between saving nature and saving human beings, meaning their jobs.

Actually, in the complex ecology of the modern world what's good for one occupation may be bad for another. For example, the Northwest salmon industry, a $1-billion employer of at least sixty thousand people, found its 1992 catch cut in half because of clearcutting by logging companies, a practice that destroys watersheds by significantly increasing runoff that clogs spawning pools and by removing shade that keeps the temperature-sensitive fish cool. Gulf of Mexico fishermen find their livelihood threatened by industrial discharges and farmers' fertilizers. If the eastern gulf is opened to oil and gas exploration, Florida's tourist industry will lose. One person's job gain is often another person's job loss.

But here again, the *health* of human beings is left out of the equation. If you aren't healthy, you may not be able to work at all. And environmentalism, whether embraced by Greenpeace or *Chemecology*, probably won't help here. The public health is not its concern.

The Public Health

What has happened to the public health professionals—the U.S. Public Health Service and the thirty-one-thousand-member American Public Health Association? Where have they been? Public-health consultant Earon Davis wrote in 1988 that "a serious mistake was made in the creation of the EPA when 'environmentalism' replaced (rather than augmented) 'public health' as the orientation of the federal and state regulatory programs. What should have been a partnership became a very unequal relationship. As a result, the entire environmental movement developed a severe case of 'grass-root rot,' from which it is only now beginning to recover." Davis believes that the unfortunate split between environment and health began around Earth Day 1970, when people quite rightly became concerned about what was happening to the environment but quite incorrectly assumed that taking care of the environment would take care of any public health problems.

It didn't work that way. Said Davis: "Little effort had been made to test chemicals in commerce—whether products, byproducts, pollutants, or contaminants—for chronic health effects. We were so upset about the endangerment of the bald eagle due to DDT that we didn't bother to read the rest of Rachel Carson's book—the chapters about human health effects. We didn't bother to network with occupational health professionals and industrial hygienists. We had lost touch with the orientation and the people of public health."

The result has been a health disaster for the chemically injured. In the late 1970s and early 1980s, wind of this possible public health problem reached Congress and influential scientists, and they began looking at the chemical scene. So now we have the 1976 Toxic Substances Control Act, the National Toxicology Program, the 1984 NRC report saying that few chemicals in commercial use have been tested for toxicity, the 1990 OTA neurotoxicity report, and, finally, two 1992 NRC reports, one calling for more research on environmental neurotoxicants and one calling for the investigation of multiple chemical sensitivities. More awareness, yes, but still no action to help the thousands with environment-related illnesses and the endangered millions. By 1994 the environmental health people and the public health people were beginning to communicate, though too often environmentalists are portrayed as pitting fish and trees against a third factor, economic health, as if a healthy environment always equals an unhealthy economy—which is by no means a certainty. Whatever the merits of this equation, public health deserves a place—actually the most important one—in it. The APHA's unanimously passed 1993 resolution calling for a phaseout of chlorine belatedly accords the organization some redemption for its past indifference.

Indeed, until the environmental movement, the government, and the medical and public health professionals take up the banner of human well-being, EI/MCS will remain an "orphan illness." Little research funding is expended on it, and few community resources are available to its sufferers. No charity balls are being held on their behalf. No celebrities hold press conferences on human neurotoxicity. Earth Day 1990's media blitz ignored human health. And though mass-media coverage of EI/MCS has increased in recent years, except for often-hard-to-get public or private disability payments there is little or no financial help available for those in need. Environment reporters, when reminded of EI/MCS, say "Oh?" and turn to something sexier, like toxic waste, recycling, oil spills, and other big-ticket items. It's still save the planet, not people.

The Wrong Answers

Let's take a look at just a few of the environmental movement's current favorite problems—and their problematic solutions. Saving energy gets a lot of attention. In the late 1980s articles began touting energy conservation not just for reducing energy costs, but for reducing the danger to the environment from home-generated carbon dioxide and CFC emissions. Home energy use, from furnaces, hot-water heaters, and stoves, was estimated to contribute more than one-fifth of the possibly global-warming emissions in the U.S. Other appliances, such as refrigerators and air conditioners, were thought to leak sizable amounts of CFCs. Proposed remedies: mandated high-efficiency home appliances and better insulation. But what about the health effects of recirculating natural-gas combustion products and other VOCs in tightly closed homes?

And of course, there's the new popularity of recyclng. Yet recycling sometimes is neither right nor economically sound. Kathy Evans, director of recycling in Berkeley, California, says, "Styrofoam recycling is a joke. It amounts to spending money to collect large quantities of a substance that's mostly air, spending more money and fossil fuel to take it someplace, spending more money to wash it, then spending more money to shape it into something else that's mostly air. That doesn't make any economic sense." Or health sense. In 1982 the EPA found the toxic chemical styrene in all of the human fat samples it analyzed, presumably the result of outgassing or leaching from polystyrene foam. Yet this important fact does not make its way into popular articles such as one in 1991 lamenting that nonbiodegradable polystyrene foam will remain in landfills for hundreds of years, with no mention that it will remain in our bodies the rest of our lives. Better than recycling would be a phasing-out of this persistent chemical entirely.

This is not to say that recycling is all bad, or worthless. It's probably better than incineration, or just dumping. But again, for toxic wastes, of which there are many, the ultimate solution is not recycling, but a reduction in the use of toxic substances by industry. According to Diane Brown, of the Illinois Public Interest Research Group, "The only way to address all the risks associated with toxic materials is to reduce and in some instances *eliminate their production and use.* By changing production processes, substituting safer raw materials or redesigning products, the quantity of toxic chemicals used to produce goods and services can be reduced or eliminated. This cuts risks from storage and transportation accidents, workplace exposure and *exposure from consumer products,* and reduces a company's toxic emissions and hazardous waste generation [emphasis added]." Waste recycling, says Northwestern University sociology professor Allan Schnaiberg, is too often a "'feel-good' effort that draws public attention away from deep-rooted environmental problems of industrialization, like the use of toxic chemicals."

Walking, bicycling, and jogging have for years been extolled as good for health and good for the environment. Americans by the millions, fashionably attired in brightly colored synthetics, have taken to streets and sidewalks to get their aerobic exercise in an environmentally benign way. True, they are not polluting, but what are the auto fumes surrounding them doing to their health? "There is no question that when you exercise, you are consuming more oxygen and are breathing deeper and are therefore taking in more of the environmental pollutants," says Dr. Bertram Carnow, University of Illinois pulmonologist and toxicologist. Chronic exposures like these can cause respiratory ailments and lung damage. Ozone created by the action of sunlight on auto exhaust can "grab onto protein and is destructive to it," Carnow warns. "There is also some concern that it may cause chromosomal changes and is carcinogenic." Not only do exhaust fumes endanger walkers, joggers, and bikers," says chemist Lou Marchi, "there's toxic 'road run-off' from such substances as motor oil, brake fluid, transmission fluid, anti-freeze, and windshield cleaner."

With indoor air pollution up to a hundred times worse than outdoor air pollution, exercising indoors may not be much better. Chemically sensitive people fare poorly in most "health" clubs, because of synthetic carpeting and glues, toxic cleaning products, perfumed and pesticide-containing soaps used in showers, regular (but unannounced) pesticide spraying by exterminators, and air "fresheners" bolted to walls and timed to spray toxic "masking fragrances" into the air. Thus contaminated, "health" clubs they are not.

Living the Green Life

One of the biggest trends in the recent environmental movement has been the "greening" of America. Starting in the late 1980s, environmentally conscientious consumers began to seek out "green" soap, "green" cotton, "green" toothpaste, "green" light bulbs, "green" paper, "green" furniture—and "green" stores to sell them to "green" consumers who have "green" careers. Green became the color of the 90s.

With this new consciousness—and fueled by the twentieth anniversary of Earth Day in 1990—came a seemingly endless stream of new books on the green life: *50 Simple Things You Can Do to Save the Earth; 50 More Simple Things You Can Do to Save the Earth; 50 Simple Things Your Business Can Do to Save the Earth; The Green Consumer Supermarket Guide; Shopping for a Better World; Shopping for a Better Environment; How Green Is My Home; Nontoxic, Natural & Earthwise* (the latter is the only one that pays much attention to chemical toxicity and human health). Buying green, like recycling, is here to make us feel good, even if, as biologist Barry Commoner points out, the tips "usually fail to address the deep complexities of environmental problems." Or of your health, one might add.

Experts disagree on whether the trend will last. As the media began to focus on the twentieth anniversary of the first Earth Day and "green" products began to appear, Syracuse University advertising professor John Philip Jones cautioned that "consumers will buy the best performing product. Only at the lunatic fringe will you get people who put environmental concerns first." But over a year later, Harvard University Business School professor Ray Goldberg predicted that "green products will be to the 1990s what 'lite' products were to the 1980s. The throwaway society is losing its momentum. The environment is a high priority for most shoppers." Indeed, a 1990 J. Walter Thompson "Greenwatch" poll found that 23 percent of American consumers were "greener-than-green" (willing to make many sacrifices for the environment), 59 percent were "green" (concerned but would make only some sacrifices), 15 percent were "light greens" (were concerned but not willing to make personal sacrifices), and only 3 percent were "un-greens" (unconcerned and uninterested).

Consumers today face a dizzying array of "environmentally correct" choices. The Environmental Defense Fund found in 1990 that more that 10 percent of new packaged goods in the nation carried some environmental claim, more than twice the 1989 figure. Can one believe labels like "environmentally friendly," "ozone-friendly," "recycled," and "recyclable"? How good are manufacturers' claims? Are there any standards?

The answer so far is unclear. There *has* been a movement to stan-
dardize and regulate "green" claims—to try to bring a little truth
and sense to all the hype. Two organizations certify products for environmental safety: Green Cross and Green Seal, the latter based on
Canada's EcoLogo and run by Denis Hayes, coordinator of Earth
Day 1970 and CEO of Earth Day 1990 (a significant change of
title?). The EPA has begun looking at label standardizing. And the
FTC has cited three companies for false green claims: Zipatone Inc.,
of Hillside, Illinois; American Enviro Products Inc., of Pacentia,
California; and Jerome Russell Cosmetics U.S.A., Inc., of North-
ridge, California. Local and state officials stepped in where the EPA
and FTC were reluctant to tread. In 1991 ten state attorneys general
issued "The Green Report," a guide for evaluating manufacturers'
overblown claims for packaging and aerosols and loose use of such
terms as "recyclable," "degradable," and "compostable." Also in
1991, the nation's second largest oil company, Mobil Corp., agreed
to pay six states $150,000 to settle charges that it made misleading
claims to consumers about the biodegradability of its trash bags—
said to be the first broad legal settlement between law enforcers and
industry stemming from so-called "green" claims. Finally, in 1992
the FTC issued new "green" advertising guidelines designed to prevent false or misleading use of such terms as "recyclable," degradable," and "environmentally friendly." How will this affect
business? According to Washington University business professor
Don Coursey, who sees business "greening" as it hears Americans
say they are willing to pay more for environmentally safe products,
even conservative economist Milton Friedman would say, "If they
can make money by doing this in the marketplace, that is fine."

So far, though, green is a murky hue. The average consumer has
good intentions, but hardly knows where to turn. The Dallas-based
National Center for Policy Analysis, a conservative think tank, con-
tends that most advice given to "green" consumers is wrong. Certainly, as a society, we need to look at all possible environmental
impacts—transportation, water use, energy use, animal testing, disposal, recyclability, renewability, and so on. But what has once
again been left out of most of this? What is missing? You guessed it.
Your health.

Green and Clean

Try substituting "health" for "environment" or "earth" or "planet" in a few phrases and see how the emphasis changes. "Environmentally safer" becomes "safer for my health." "Save the planet" becomes "save my health." "Shopping for a better environment" becomes "shopping for better health." "The earth is under siege" becomes "my health is under siege." "Save the seals" becomes "save the humans." "Not in my back yard" becomes "not in my body." The focus is different—and more accurate. The problem is closer to home. It is more urgent. It's no longer abstract, thousands of miles away, or even in your back yard. It's in your body. You don't want those toxic chemicals in your body fat. It's time to do something, to buy really safe products.

Let's look at one set of recommendations for "protecting the environment," published in an "issues that affect the earth" section of a local newspaper.

(1) "Compost your household vegetables." Fine, but for your own health, especially if you're going to put that compost on your garden, make those vegetables as pesticide-free as possible. You don't want to recycle poisons.

(2) "Take paper bags to the grocery store to reuse." Be aware that some stores use bags that have been sprayed with pesticides; use your own untreated cotton-mesh or canvas bags.

(3) "Stop using disposable razors." OK. Just take care to use nontoxic, unscented shaving cream.

(4) "Avoid buying products packaged in plastic; glass can be recycled." Good advice, especially so because plastic leaches toxic chemicals into the liquids you drink or put on your skin.

(5) "Buy tissue and paper towels made from recycled paper." Even recycled paper may outgas formaldehyde; try to buy formaldehyde-free products.

(6) "Conserve water when you flush your toilet." More important for your health is not to use any toxic deodorizers or bowl cleaners; use pumice on a stick (available from catalogs), baking soda, vinegar, or borax. Invest a few dollars in Annie Berthold-Bond's indispensable *Clean & Green* (as an EI/MCS sufferer, she knows what she's talking about).

(7) "Buy energy-efficient, compact fluorescent light bulbs." But be aware that research on the adverse health effects of fluorescent bulbs exists.

(8) "Set up a clothes line outdoors." Fine, but be sure to use non-toxic detergents and fabric softeners (available from catalogs and health food stores).

(9) "Install a set-back thermostat to cut your home heating costs." But what are you heating with? Combustion by-products can make you sick. And have you tightened your house, also to reduce heating costs? If so, be sure you are not circulating poisoned air.

(10) "Recycle used motor oil." If you do it yourself, protect yourself from inhaling fumes by wearing an adequate mask. Petrochemicals are the chief villain in this scenario.

Now the instructions are more complete—not perfect, but they no longer leave out health. Once health enters the picture, the focus is clearer, and decisions become easier. Once you get used to making purchases with your and your family's health in mind, "green" does become "clean." Often health and environment needs coincide; sometimes they do not, at least at present, and they will not until our society's way of doing things changes. As long as we continue to rely on cars that pollute, exercising near their exhausts is not wise. As long as industry continues to use toxic chemicals in its products instead of researching safe substitutes, we are all in danger.

Living with Less

Our attitudes may need to change in other ways. Ours is notoriously a materialistic, affluent society. We don't feel happy unless we have things, but are the things making us happy? Paul Wachtel, author of *The Poverty of Affluence*, thinks not. The things we buy, he believes, are only a substitute for the sense of community shattered by our profit-oriented, growth-oriented economy. Also, the things we buy are putting stress on the global environment and, we now know, affecting our health. We need to re-examine our priorities and lifestyles and move toward a safer, healthier, more fulfilling society.

Harvard economist Juliet Schor, in her book *The Overworked American: The Unexpected Decline of Leisure*, explores the trend toward longer hours on the job and greater pressure on workers to produce—and to buy. Americans, she says, are trapped in the "insidious cycle of work-and-spend'—the 'shop till you drop'" syndrome satirized by the T-shirt saying "born to shop." Emphasizing ownership, Americans buy many things they don't want, need, or have time to enjoy. Instead of enjoying them, she says, "they watch television, which tells them to go out and buy more things." U.S. advertising expenditures went from $12 billion in 1960 to $125 billion in 1991, the latter amount not even including promotional mail. The average American is now exposed to an unbelievable three thousand advertising messages a day, each of which reinforces the idea, according to former FTC chair Michael Pertschuk, that "the way to solve all of life's problems is to look for a product—to look for something that's in the marketplace to deal with it."

Just before the first Earth Day, advertising executive Jerry Mander addressed the environmental consequences of unbridled advertising in an article published in *The Environmental Handbook: Prepared for the First National Environmental Teach-In.* He advocated less emphasis on acquisition and material wealth and "beginning now, national preparation toward a no-growth economy." Toward that end, he argued, advertising should be merely a matter of informing the public that, say, "The new Fords are in" or asking "Is this trip necessary?" If you watch television, you know how far he got with that suggestion. Twenty years later, Pertschuk was still trying. On camera, no less, he made the following heretical statement: "There ought to be ads that say, 'You've got a headache? Go upstairs, lie down, take a nap.' Most headaches will pass without ever taking anything. You don't always have to solve your problems by taking something."

Thus, to the three environmental Rs—reduce, reuse, recycle—should be added one more: resist. Don't look at ads; if you can't avoid them, remember not to believe them. Do your own research on products. By trial and error, find what's safest and best for you. And, as University of Illinois industrial design professor William

Becker advised his packaging design students, ask yourself, "Is this really needed?" This gewgaw, this extra wrapping . . . or even the product itself.

Chemically injured people have found themselves going back to the products of the 1930s, those used before literally millions of new chemicals were synthesized. Bon Ami and borax and washing soda worked fine for millions of Americans. The 1930s also brought the little poem: Use it up, wear it out; make it do, or do without. Most Americans lived by words that sound, to many in the 1990s, ancient, foreign, bizarre.

But even today some people are choosing a simpler lifestyle. "We're seeing a strong trend toward downscaling or returning to the simple life," said psychologist Ross Goldstein, of the marketing firm Generation Insights, in 1991. "Baby Boomers are finding material possessions didn't give them the satisfaction they expected. It doesn't mean people won't buy [nice cars and VCRs], but they won't raise [this] to a religious quest again."

Thoreau's most famous dictum was "Simplicity, simplicity, simplicity!" Debra Lynn Dadd, the once chemically sensitive author of the influential books *Nontoxic & Natural* and *The Nontoxic Home*, explained her own journey to simplicity in her last book, *Nontoxic, Natural & Earthwise*: "I began to live simply for two reasons. When I realized that every virgin product I buy costs a piece of Nature, I wanted to respect life by taking as little of it as possible. Also, when I discovered that I spent most of my waking hours working, for the sole purpose of making payments on my credit cards and on my house (which I had to buy to store all the things I wasn't using anyway), I decided that the effort needed to maintain all my material goods wasn't worth the sacrifices I was making in other areas of my life. By the time I sold everything I really didn't need, everything I owned fit in an eight-by-ten food-storage locker and two suitcases. I don't miss any of the things I no longer have, and simple living feels so good that even though I buy new things, I continue to look for ways to reduce even further the amount of material goods I own. My life now actually is one of higher quality, even though there is less quantity."

How can *we* begin to simplify? Where do we start? In the first issue of her newsletter *The Earthwise Consumer*, Dadd gave what has to be the most complete instruction possible: "When you make a purchase, choose products that are nontoxic and nonpolluting, natural, renewable and sustainable, organically grown or wild-crafted, compassionate to animals, recycled, energy-efficient, packaged responsibly, reusable or recyclable, biodegradable, and provided by companies with socially conscious business practices." Even with her book in hand, it's a big order—complicated and overwhelming.

Can you do it? In 1990 the American Psychological Association took a realistic point of view: "It is clear that an increasing number of Americans have some knowledge about risky . . . health behaviors. Despite that knowledge, long-term patterns of behavior still account for as much as 50 percent of mortality from the ten leading causes of death in the U.S., and seven out of ten leading causes of death in this country are in large part behaviorally determined and can be significantly reduced through changes in behavior. These statistics suggest that personal health behavior change is not as easy as it might seem."

What Don Marquis said in 1935 is just as true now. The *New York Sun* columnist induced archy, his typewriter hopping cockroach, to write the following words (archy wrote his masterpieces at night, on Marquis's typewriter, but could only land on one key at a time, hence the lack of capitals): "america was once a paradise of timberland and stream but it is dying because of the greed and money lust of a thousand little kings who slashed the timber all to hell and would not be controlled and changed the climate and stole the rainfall from posterity and it won't be long till everything is desert from the alleghenies to the rockies the deserts are coming the deserts are spreading the springs and streams are drying up one day the mississippi itself will be a bed of sand ants and scorpions and centipedes shall inherit the earth . . . it won't be long now it won't be long till earth is barren as the moon and sapless as a mumbled bone . . . dear boss I relay this information without any fear that humanity will take warning and reform signed archy."

In other words, even when you know that something is bad for the environment or bad for you, you may not do anything about it. We are all fallible human beings, we procrastinate, we deny reality, we think "It won't happen to me," "I won't get sick from these things," "The government will take care of everything." In the case of our own health, adverse health effects often are not immediate; damage may show up slowly or years later. "The changes are often subtle and subclinical, and months or years can elapse between exposure to a neurotoxicant and the appearance of dysfunction and disease," said the NRC in its 1992 report *Environmental Neurotoxicology.* "For the future, one of the major challenges for neurotoxicology will be to use insight from clinical medicine, epidemiology, and toxicology to design effective systems for the prevention of neurotoxic disease in the American public." Unfortunately, it's a little like locking the barn door after our health has been stolen.

Living a Better Life

One person who literally opens his barn door almost every day is Wendell Berry, a former English professor who left the groves of academe in the mid-1960s for those of a farm in Kentucky, where he had grown up. In between plowing, harvesting, and doing the chores, he writes books embodying the perception that "there is no longer any honest way to deny that a way of living that our leaders continue to praise is destroying all that our country is, and all the best that it means." According to *New Yorker* writer Bill McKibben, Berry believes that "we face an agricultural crisis, and that it is a part of a moral, philosophical, and social crisis that demands that we change our lives."

Our way of life, Berry says, is built on the avoidance of physical labor, to the detriment of our environment and our health. Indeed, we seem to see evidence of this everywhere today: in the escalators we ride instead of climbing stairs; in the cars we drive for a few blocks instead of walking; in the lawn-care workers with noisy gasoline-powered machines strapped to their backs, venting noxious fumes into the environment and their own lungs; how many of them go home sick at night?

The way of living that Berry prefers is that of the Kentucky hill country where he grew up. As described in his collection of essays *What Are People For?*, the people who lived there "were poor, as country people have often been, but they had each other, they had their local economy in which they helped each other, they had each other's comfort when they needed it, and they had their stories, their history together in that place. To have everything but money is to have much." Berry also admires the Amish for their lack of reliance on debt and government subsidies; for their use of horses rather than tractors, which forces farmers to pay more attention to the contours of the fields and thus reduces soil erosion; and for their use of crop rotation, rather than petroleum-based fertilizers, to renew the soil.

To Berry, physical work can provide a profound satisfaction. Writing of the hard work involved in hand harvesting, he says that for himself and "for most of the men and women who have been my companions in this work, it has not been drudgery. None of us would say that we take pleasure in all of it all of the time, but we do take pleasure in it, and sometimes the pleasure can be intense and clear. Some of my dearest memories come from these times of hardest work. . . . Neighbors work together; they are together all day every day for weeks. The quiet of the work is not much interrupted by machine noises, and so there is much talk. . . . There is much laughter; because of the unrelenting difficulty of the work, everything funny or amusing is relished. . . . Ultimately, in the argument about work and how it should be done, one has only one's pleasure to offer."

We can't all become farmers again, of course. What does Berry suggest? Where possible, a life of economic self-sufficiency, so common before this century, so uncommon now. Careful husbanding of resources, soils managed to prevent erosion, and forests managed for continuous yields. Small enterprises, with greater value placed on careful work and craftsmanship than on quantity. A shift to organic produce and an avoidance of unnecessary packaging. But above all, a change of attitudes and a vision, a sense of how things *could* be in our daily lives. To McKibben, what this means is that we need to "live in real places, not in the generalized lobbies that modern houses often are. We need to be at home in our bodies, too—not in the 'useless, weak' husks that we drag daily to the fluorescently cheerful 'health club,' but a body that each day knows the 'elemental pleasures of eating and drinking and resting, of being dry while it is raining, of getting dry after getting wet, of getting warm again after getting cold, of cooling off after getting hot.' Of being tired at sundown, and at life's end feeling 'a great weariness . . . like the lesser weariness that comes with day's end—a weariness that had been earned and was therefore accepted.' "

How far most of us have come from these simple pleasures. Can we ever return? All of us can. Many of us must.

Economic Growth

But what if we all did this, you object anxiously at this point. What would happen to our economy? Our jobs? Wouldn't our economy collapse? Doesn't our economy need to keep growing?

Never fear. Just remember archy. Sixty years ago he said that we wouldn't take warning and reform, and he was right. And it won't happen now. Only a relatively few people will read this book. Still fewer will put any of these recommendations into practice. Change *will* come about, however, slowly and gradually, as those few who choose change live differently and buy less. The things they do buy will support small businesses, like Tom's of Maine, Seventh Generation, and Heart of Vermont, that are already producing or selling safer, healthier, less toxic, and less environmentally damaging products. Some of these products may carry high prices, but consider the costs to society and to your health if you opt for the cheaper, polluting, more-toxic products. Practice what environmentalist Hazel Henderson calls a "buycott." Forget your worries about the nation's economy; focus on improving your health instead: for you, *that* is the bottom line.

Actually, in 1992 a Roper survey indicated that "Americans are not willing to trade off environmental protection for economic development, despite the weak economy." The economy will doubtless continue to grow, despite these trends and despite the warnings about the effects of uncontrolled growth that are found in such books as the 1972 *The Limits to Growth* and its 1992 sequel, *Beyond the Limits to Growth: Confronting Global Collapse, Envisioning a Sustainable Future*. The former book presented computer models of five factors affecting growth on our planet—population, agricultural production, natural resources, industrial production, and pollution. What their models indicated was that uncontrolled or exponential growth in one or more of these areas would soon bring society perilously close to its limits. Banned in the Soviet Union, panned by oil corporations, and investigated by former President Richard Nixon's staff, *Limits to Growth* sold nine million copies in twenty-nine languages. More optimistic, *Beyond the Limits* says that "given some of the technologies and institutions invented in [the last twenty years] . . . a sustainable society is still technically and economically possible. . . . The transition to [one] requires a careful balance between long-term and short-term goals and an emphasis on sufficiency, equity, and quality of life rather than on quantity of output. It requires more than productivity and more than technology; it also requires maturity, compassion, and wisdom." We have yet to see how right either of these forecasts is.

Again McKibben: "As citizens we demand lower taxes, instead of devoting ourselves to figuring out how to share the world's greatest concentration of wealth with an increasingly poor nation and world. Suspicious of real change, and of more work and less luxury, we place our faith in frequent incantations about unceasing economic growth and technological expansion, even though our logic tells us they are as unlikely as endless growth in the food supply and our scientific instruments tell us they are starting to harm our planet as surely as poor farming erodes our soils."

More important, they are harming our health. For all his perceptiveness, Wendell Berry has not stumbled on what may ultimately be the strongest argument yet for changing our lives: whatever we do to the web we do to ourselves.

* * * *

To Find Out More

- *The Poverty of Affluence: A Psychological Portrait of the American Way of Life*, by Paul L. Wachtel, New York, Free Press, 1983.

- *The Overworked American: The Unexpected Decline of Leisure*, by Juliet Schor, New York, Basic Books (Harper/Collins), 1991.

- *The Limits to Growth, A Report for the Club of Rome's Project on the Predicament of Mankind*, by Donella H. Meadows, Dennis L. Meadows, Jørgen Randers, and William W. Behrens III, New York, Universe Books, 1972.

- *Beyond the Limits to Growth: Confronting Global Collapse, Envisioning a Sustainable Future*, by Donella H. Meadows, Dennis L. Meadows, and Jørgen Randers, Post Mills, Vermont, Chelsea Green, 1992.

- *What Are People For?*, by Wendell Berry, San Francisco, North Point Press, 1990.

- *The Hidden Wound*, by Wendell Berry, Boston, Houghton Mifflin, 1970.

- *The Unsettling of America: Culture and Agriculture*, by Wendell Berry, San Francisco, Sierra Club, 1977.

- *The Good Life: Helen and Scott Nearing's Sixty Years of Self-Sufficient Living*, by Scott and Helen Nearing, Schocken, 1954. *Loving and Leaving the Good Life*, by Helen Nearing, Post Mills, Vermont, Chelsea Green, 1992.

- *A Fierce Green Fire: The American Environmental Movement*, by Philip Shabecoff, New York, Hill & Wang, 1993.

- *Forcing the Spring: The Transformation of the American Environmental Movement*, by Robert Gottlieb, Washington D.C., Island Press, 1993.

- *Deeper Shades of Green: The Rise of Blue-Collar and Minority Environmentalism in America*, by Jim Schwab, San Francisco, Sierra Club, 1994.

- "Trust Us, Don't Track Us," U.S. Public Interest Research Group, 215 Pennsylvania Avenue SE, Washington, D.C. 20003-1155; 202-546-9707.

14

Riders on the Earth Together

I N THE LATE 1940s Dr. Theron Randolph made an important discovery: he observed in one of his patients a distinct relationship between fossil-fuel-based chemicals and illness. As he began to see more and more patients with similarly caused illnesses, he became concerned and began publishing his observations, ending up with three books and several hundred articles on susceptibility to chemicals. Unfortunately, much of the attention he received was negative. Had he been able to send out Paul Revere, or had George Washington been on hand to mobilize the troops, we might not be in the planetary and human predicament we are in today.

In the twentieth century, modern science has flourished, expanded, and even exploded far beyond the expectations of its early proponents. Aided by modern technology, it has synthesized millions of new chemicals, crisscrossed much of the world with electric power lines, developed highly sophisticated electronic systems, and built atomic bombs and nuclear plants. It has released a powerful genie from its bottle, with the full consequences as yet unknown.

One consequence in the U.S. was an unprecedented prosperity as industry returned to peacetime production after World War II. Thousands of veterans went to college under the G.I. Bill of Rights, many of them studying chemistry and other sciences. To shelter them and their growing families, housing developments sprang up across our landscape. The auto industry boomed, and along with it other petroleum-based industries, such as the pharmaceutical, pesticide, cosmetics, clothing, cleaning product, and food industries. Chemists were busy discovering all the exciting new things that could be made from the world's vast reserves of oil. We became a disposable society, using products only briefly before discarding them. Demand was high, and supply seemingly unlimited. Americans were said to be richer and better off than kings and queens in the past.

But a dark side began to appear. City dwellers were coughing, rivers were filled with dead and dying fish, cows' milk was found to contain radioactive strontium 90 (later, mothers' milk was found to contain PCBs), garbage was increasingly hard to dispose of, and dying robins appeared on well-kept suburban lawns. In 1962 Rachel Carson published *Silent Spring*—and Dr. Randolph published *Human Ecology and Susceptibility to the Chemical Environment*. Though Carson's book was a bestseller (Randolph's was not), the chemical revolution continued unabated. Carson wrote that "the new chemicals come from our laboratories in an endless stream; almost five hundred annually find their way into actual use in the U.S. alone. The figure is staggering and its implications are not easily grasped—five hundred new chemicals to which the bodies of men and animals are required somehow to adapt each year, chemicals totally outside the limits of biologic experience." By 1991, five hundred a year had become a thousand a year, and Dr. Randolph had treated close to nine thousand chemically sensitive patients and trained dozens of other doctors to recognize and treat this profoundly life-altering condition.

Damage to Us All

Yes, the genie is out of the bottle. The tiny wisp of modern chemicals emerging from chemists' laboratories before World War II has become a giant plume blanketing our earth and filling our homes and workplaces. Anyone with an eye and a nose and without a vested interest to protect cannot help being aware of what has happened. And there is no way we can put the genie back in the bottle. DDT, PCBs, CFCs, plutonium 239 (with a half-life of twenty-four thousand years), and many, many other toxic chemicals are here to stay, riders on the earth with us.

This is not to say that some such chemicals did not exist before World War II. They did. And they were undoubtedly making some people sick then: in 1925 Dr. Alice Hamilton, of the Harvard Medical School, published *Industrial Poisons in the United States*. Even as the petrochemical era dawned in the early 1940s, annual U.S. production of synthetic organic chemicals was about one billion pounds. But by the 1980s that production stood at over four hundred billion pounds. The overwhelming majority of these industrial chemicals, Dr. Epstein reminds us, has never been adequately, if at all, tested for long-term toxic, carcinogenic, mutagenic, and teratogenic effects. In what he calls a "runaway chemical technology," we are now paying the price with our health, some of us more than others . . . so far.

"Us" includes animals, our fellow riders on the earth, and the most visible victims of the plume. "Animals are good indicators for what we are doing to our environment, particularly high-order predators, who eat what you or I eat," said Samuel Sadove, research director of the Okeanos Ocean Research Foundation. "It raises questions about our environment." (It also raises the question of why such spokespersons say "environment" instead of "health.")

Indeed, animal victims abound in our times, and sometimes in our back yards, especially the watery ones (according to the Worldwatch Institute's "State of the World 1993," water bodies are increasingly polluted). A "mystery illness" among harbor seals led investigators to speculate about damage to their immune systems from PCBs: many distressed seals picked up on Long Island had a low count of infection-fighting white blood cells, similar to the low count of white blood cells reported in rats and other laboratory animals fed PCBs. Scientists suspect that viral infection die-offs of Mediterranean dolphins may have been caused by immune-system vulnerability, itself possibly caused by manmade pollutants; at any rate, high levels of toxic PCBs are often found in carcasses.

Half a century after the chemical revolution began, dead whales washed ashore from the St. Lawrence River were found to have very high levels of more than thirty hazardous chemicals, including DDT, PCBs, Mirex, mercury, cadmium, and polycyclic aromatic hydrocarbons (PAHs) similar to those found in cigarettes and regarded as carcinogenic. Most apparently died from septicemia, which killed them because their immune systems failed—a kind of animal AIDS. Roger Payne, of the Whale Conservation Institute, has found mounting evidence that the slow accumulation of toxic substances in whales is beginning to wreak havoc with their immune systems, cause birth defects, and seriously threaten their fragile existence.

Not only immune systems, but reproductive systems are at risk—in both animals and humans. In an event that has sent ominous ripples through the scientific community, an international group of twenty-one scientists, meeting in July 1991 at the Wingspread Conference Center, in Racine, Wisconsin, reviewed animal studies made over the preceding decade and arrived at a chilling consensus: "We are certain of the following," they said. "A large number of man-made chemicals that have been released into the environment, as well as a few natural ones, have the potential to disrupt the endocrine system of animals, including humans. Among these are the persistent, bioaccumulative, organohalogen compounds that include some pesticides (fungicides, herbicides, and insecticides) and industrial chemicals, other synthetic products, and some metals." Furthermore, continued this historic statement, "Many wildlife populations are already affected by these compounds. The impacts include thyroid dysfunction in birds and fish; decreased fertility in birds, fish, shellfish, and mammals; decreased hatching success in birds, fish, and turtles; gross birth deformities in birds, fish, and turtles; metabolic abnormalities in birds, fish, and mammals; behavioral abnormalities in birds; demasculinization and feminization of male fish, birds, and mammals; defeminization and masculinization of female fish and birds; and compromised immune systems in birds and mammals (mammals, you will recall from grade school, include all creatures that suckle their young).

The scientists estimated "with confidence" that "experimental results are being seen at the low end of current environmental concentrations." One study, led by Richard E. Peterson of the Environmental Toxicology Center of the University of Wisconsin, found that with male rats exposed to TCDD (the most toxic of the chemical compounds known as dioxins) before and after birth, "the consequences of TCDD exposure extended into adulthood: sex organ weights were decreased, spermatogenesis was impaired, regulation of luteinizing hormone (LH) secretion was feminized, and sexual behavior was both demasculinized and feminized." Another study found that when the estrogenic pesticide DDT was added to gull eggs, the male hatchlings had feminized sex organs; in effect they had been "chemically castrated." Researchers have discovered that the males of the Florida panther, a species now down to fifty or so surviving animals, have both reproductive abnormalities and unusual steroid hormone ratios. In 1989 mercury, a reproductive toxin, was found in "astronomical" levels in the body of a female panther found dead near the Everglades National Park.

In the October 1993 issue of the journal of the National Institute of Environmental Health Sciences, Theo Colborn, Frederick S. vom Saal, and Ana M. Soto summarize the available data on endocrine-disrupting chemicals in wildlife and humans: forty-five chemicals or classes of chemicals have been reported to cause changes in reproductive or hormone systems, thirty-five of them pesticides, the rest industrial chemicals such as mercury. Especially interesting to people with EI/MCS, Soto has found that even small amounts of such chemicals add up. By taking ten estrogenic chemicals and combining each of them at one-tenth of their effective dose, she says, "you now have an effective dose."

In other words, we tinker with our environment at peril to our own reproductive systems and our sexuality. The findings of scientists trying to explain the rise of breast cancer suggest that "an unintended side effect of industrialization is an environment that bathes its inhabitants in a sea of estrogenic agents," according to *Science News.* "Some of these agents, such as pesticides and ingredients in plastics, mimic the hormone estrogen in their effects on the body. Others, such as magnetic fields and certain combustion by-products, can boost the concentration of estrogens circulating in the bloodstream. And . . . factors that increase a woman's lifetime exposure to estrogen, such as early puberty and late menopause, are among the leading known risk factors for breast cancer."

However, our concentration on cancer as a possible consequence of pollution is obscuring other effects. Dr. Barry Johnson, of the ATSDR, has criticized the almost exclusive focus on cancer as the major "end point" of pollution: "We find ourselves in this situation because we've given disproportionate attention to the study of cancer as the only risk from environmental hazards because people are frightened by it, and they can understand it. Many of us are hopeful that the testing programs for these chemicals can become much more holistic." Perhaps a holistic approach would even include EI/MCS.

Hopeful they may be, but "chemical-by-chemical research isn't going to give us the answers we need," said William Facemire, of U.S. Fish and Wildlife Research, speaking at a 1992 World Wildlife Fund symposium on endocrine disrupters in the environment. Unwilling to wait, in early 1994 Facemire issued a prohibition on the use of estrogenic chemicals—principally pesticides—in all federal wildlife refuges in the southeastern U.S. Others at the symposium, mostly government regulators and industry representatives, argued, predictably, for just such research. But according to Mary O'Brien, staff scientist with Environmental Alliance Worldwide, this would be a "decades-long process of incorporating endocrine disruption into the chemical-by-chemical risk assessment process that each year examines less than a hundredth of one percent of the chemicals used by industry, and that is literally incapable of considering the cumulative developmental impacts of the array of endocrine disrupters to which you and [all living things] are being exposed."

Scientists like those at the Wingspread conference have yet to concern themselves with EI/MCS as another effect of environmental chemicals. But referring to the chemicals causing developmental damage to animals, World Wildlife Fund scientist Theo Colborn (considered by some the Rachel Carson of the 1990s) has said, "We'll never be able to come up with a risk model to protect us from these chemicals. The problem is too complex. So what's the answer? Don't release any more." That would be welcome news indeed for the chemically injured.

Around the World

Meanwhile, health damage continues worldwide, to humans as well as to other species, though most reports cover only outdoor pollution. Consider the following:

- Fallout from the 1986 Chernobyl nuclear power plant fire has undermined the health of thousands of Byelorrussians, who suffer increasingly from anemia, gastritis, thyroid cancer, tuberculosis, susceptibility to other infections. While some Western radiation experts attribute these effects to stress, others say they recall the "atom bomb sickness" experienced by Hiroshima and Nagasaki survivors in the 1950s, including weakened immune systems and heightened susceptibilities to infections.

- Residents of Katowice, Poland, where the Communists built a ring of factories and mines, are finding a generation of children deformed, retarded, or debilitated by the toxic stew spewed by the industrial belt. Other consequences suffered by the children are lingering colds, piercing headaches, learning disabilities, and nervous disorders.

- In Mexico City, schools are closed during pollution alerts, booths sell oxygen in parks and malls, and officials ban cars in the city's center and consider using enormous fans to blow away the pollution. Approximately 11 percent of the 55.3 million Mexicans over fifteen years of age suffer from migraines, according to a 1992 study.

- "State of the World 1992," the Worldwatch Institute's annual report, cited an *American Journal of Public Health* study showing that thousands of children in the Los Angeles area have permanent lung damage from pollution by the age of ten.

- The *British Medical Journal* notes the 50 percent drop in sperm count worldwide, the threefold to fourfold increase in testicular cancer in the past forty years, and the twofold to fourfold increase in birth defects of the male reproductive system in the same period; and *The Lancet* wonders whether such phenomena can be traced to the exposure of males to estrogens or estrogen-mimicking substances in the womb. Boys in Taiwan exposed to PCBs while in their mothers' wombs and male alligators exposed to pesticides in Florida have developed smaller-than-normal penises.

Can we really think that these illnesses are connected to the new-chemical plume blanketing the earth? Scientific proof, in the form of randomized, double-blind, controlled studies of the human health effects of the (by now) more than seventy thousand new chemicals in our environment, plus their interactions and decay products, does not exist and probably never will—too expensive, too complicated, too short-range (many effects may not occur for years). Only long-range epidemiological studies have even a shot at providing a partial answer: either formal epidemiology, or finally paying attention to the mounting number of "anecdotes" from people worldwide—including those who suffer from EI/MCS—who have successfully connected their symptoms with chemical exposures.

Around the Planet: Far Out

Daily we hear more about two other twentieth-century phenomena: global warming and a damaged ozone layer, both with implications for human health or even human existence. *Time* magazine's January 1989 "Planet of the Year" issue cited four major threats to the earth's environment: overpopulation, waste, extinction (meaning to *Time*, of course, plants and animals, not people), and global warming, result of the trapping of carbon dioxide and other greenhouse gases by the earth's atmosphere.

For years the scientific community has seesawed on global warming—how much, how ominous, does it even exist? Obvious biases, an anti-environmental backlash in the mass media, and an unusually cold 1993–94 winter in the U.S. complicate the issue. Yet the NAS and the world-wide insurance industry are taking global warming seriously, according to Peter Montague, who says that there are two undisputed facts about global warming: greenhouse gases do trap heat close to the earth; and human activities are creating more and more greenhouse gases. The possibilities are there, making skittish insurance companies cancel policies in coastal areas. As the NAS says, "In essence, we are conducting an uncontrolled experiment with the planet."

Time did not consider ozone depletion a major threat. Is it? And is it connected with EI/MCS? With little dispute, it can be said that the ozone layer is a thin stratospheric skin currently getting thinner. (Ozone, a form of oxygen, is a substance we want up there but not down here, where it is a smog component dangerous to human beings, especially those with respiratory problems.) Chlorofluorocarbons (CFCs), the chief culprits in ozone depletion, were first synthesized around 1930 and quickly became "miracle" industrial chemicals. Thought to be nontoxic to human beings, they became widely used in refrigerators, air conditioners, packaging, and many other products, and as propellants in aerosol containers. But in 1974 a University of California scientist, Sherwood Rowland, discovered that CFCs break down in the upper atmosphere, with each liberated chlorine atom capable of destroying up to a hundred thousand ozone molecules. This news prompted comedian Lily Tomlin to wonder why we were "sacrificing the ozone layer for the convenience of Pam, a nonstick cooking spray" and the U.S. government to ban the use of CFCs in aerosol sprays in 1978.

The first known hole in the earth's ozone layer, over Antarctica, was discovered in 1985 by British scientist Joe Farman. Since then, human earth-riders have been trying to cope with the implications of this surprising and unprecedented threat to their vehicle. By 1990 the U.S. and fifty-five other nations had agreed to end the production and use of CFCs, halons, and carbon tetrachloride (now known to eat ozone) by the year 2000 and of another ozone-depleter, methyl chloroform, by 2005. And in 1992, after NASA scientists warned that "an ozone hole stretching from northern New England to northern Europe could form during the next two months," President Bush announced a plan to speed the phaseout from the year 2000 to the end of 1995. Said Al Gore, "It took an ozone hole over Kennebunkport [Maine] to get his attention."

In fact, the great ozone hole predicted by NASA did not appear; in October 1993, however, scientists observed a record ozone low over Antarctica, the lowest recorded anywhere in the world. And according to a May 1992 UN report, by the year 2000 the ozone layer is expected to be depleted by as much as 10 percent during the summer in temperate regions, which would produce a 26 percent increase in the most common forms of skin cancer. Discovering the same year that the ozone was vanishing faster than predicted, ninety-three nations agreed to speed up the phasing out of ozone-destroying chemicals, targeting methyl chloroform for 1996, nine years earlier than before. Meanwhile, these chemicals continue to float upward.

According to recent research, worldwide emissions of two CFCs—CFC-11 and CFC-12—are growing at only 1 percent, down from 5 percent in the 1980s. But don't expect the ozone layer to return to normal for a century, the researchers say. Another estimate came from the normally cautious 145,000-member American Chemical Society, rebuking the *Washington Post* for an article minimizing the dangers from ozone depletion: "Scientists actively involved in ozone research are convinced the problem of ozone depletion is real and will continue for decades to come. . . . To the working atmospheric science community, such ignorance of twenty years of intense research, coupled with the constant repetition of misrepresentations and half-truths, is frustrating and insulting."

Another effort by earth-riders to cope with contamination of their vehicle—and yours—began with wanting to know more about the chemicals in toxic waste dumps, and uncovered along the way a particularly potent agent of destruction for both the ozone layer and human beings. In 1986 Congress asked the ATSDR to prepare "toxicological profiles" for the 250 chemicals most commonly found in such dumps. The result is a remarkable series of well-written, well-researched, easy-to-read reports that go far beyond the concerns of the people living near toxic waste dumps. The profile of 1,1,1-trichloroethane, also known as methyl chloroform, extensively documents the reality that what is hurting the ozone layer up there is also hurting us down here. In a calm, matter-of-fact way, the profile brings you from the stratosphere right back down to your living-room and your workplace. Dubbed "Public Enemy No. 1,1,1" by the NRDC, methyl chloroform is found in some 140 commonly used but often toxic consumer products, from cosmetics to correction fluid, shoe polish to stain repellent; it is also the highest-volume ozone-depletion chemical. A bad actor, that one. For a copy of the 215-page profile for 1,1,1-trichloroethane and for a list of other profiles, contact the National Technical Information Service, 5285 Port Royal Road, Springfield, Virginia 22161; 1-800-336-4700 or 703-487-4650 (NTIS order number PB/91/180463/ AS).

So there you have it. A genie from a bottle, a wisp that promised a better, easier life for all of us, has instead become a giant plume poisoning some of us. Methyl chloroform, CFCs, carbon tetrachloride are but a few toxic chemicals among many: they are obviously not something to fool around with. Bad for the ozone layer, bad for our health.

Ecology, Not Economics

For years society has had two ways to handle environmental assaults: either "we don't know what effect this has, so let's go on using it" or "we don't know what effect this has, so let's stop using it." As the evidence accumulates, however, and it becomes increasingly harder to justify the first route, some promising earth-riders have warned against complacency. Listen to a few:

- "Better sign the papers while [the planet] is still willing to make a deal"— paleontologist Stephen Jay Gould.

- "If you don't put something in the ecology, it's not there"—ecologist Barry Commoner's fifth law of ecology. (Add this to his other four "laws": "Everything is connected to everything else," "Everything must go somewhere," "Nature knows best," and "There is no such thing as a free lunch.")

- "Know that you're an adult in your own right and that your leaders aren't your leaders—you're their leaders. Do your own investigation, work out yourself what's the truth. Never accept anything at face value. Know that you often get lied to by media, by the corporations, by the advertising, by your politicians"— Australian pediatrician and environmental activist Helen Caldicott.

- "Human inventiveness has created problems because human judgment and humanity's ability to deal with the consequence of its creations lag behind its ability to create"—Robert Ornstein and biologist Paul Ehrlich, who wonder whether we are like the frog immersed in water that is being slowly heated. Unable to sense the lethal change, it sits there until it dies.

- "Man is a strange animal. He doesn't like to read the handwriting on the wall until his back is up against it"—Adlai Stevenson, twice a presidential candidate.

- "Conserve brains first, else all may be lost"—Dr. Kaye Kilburn, of the University of Southern California. He cites two recent

findings: that living or working near oil refining, chemical manufacturing, and waste disposal has impaired critical brain functions and that some people exposed to plastics, epoxys,
pesticides, disinfectants, and solvents, particularly in tight buildings, have developed mentally debilitating illnesses and chemical
encephalopathies.

Once again, though, the emphasis is on saving the planet. Maybe
the good folk working toward a healthier planet would get farther if
they stressed the connection between the global environment and
what is happening to our health, right now, right here. Most of us,
however good our intentions about saving the planet, pay more attention to something affecting our health. Yet even when the health
effects of our twentieth-century dependence on toxic chemicals are
brought home to us, we often find it hard to pay heed. In the words
of Susan Cooper, NCAMP staff ecologist, "Many human cultures
have tried to set themselves apart from nature, above nature, have
striven to believe that they can poison the world around them without harming themselves. But we are part of the same ecosystem.
When the animals around us are sick and dying, how can we believe
that we can walk unharmed? When we poison the Earth, we poison
our own flesh and blood and air. We have become addicted to [the
use of] toxic substances, and like addicts we continue to deny our
own illness. Those of us who can see the symptoms . . . must all
strive to break this habit—nobody ever said it was easy."

Daily our society urges us to buy the goods we produce, whether
they are good for us or not. Nobel prizes are given to economists,
not ecologists. They are also given to the chemists, physicists, and
physicians who make stunning breakthroughs, not to the ecologists
and physicians who try to put the broken pieces together, who try to
understand what effects these and other discoveries are having on
the fabric of our planet and our lives. "Economics" and "ecology,"
two twentieth-century sciences, have common roots in "eco," from
the Greek word for "house." Though both concern "behavior of in-
tricate, interdependent systems of enormous diversity, natural and
manmade," economics has taken this century's spotlight, with ecology lagging behind, reacting but not controlling. The bottom line
decides. But in the words of environmentalist David Brower, conventional economists make two crucial mistakes: they view the

Earth's resources as being provided free of charge, and they don't take the future into account.

Yet, though we worship economic growth, we may also be changing. In 1992 a group of business leaders, including the heads of Chevron Oil, Mitsubishi, Dow Chemical, and Du Pont, published a remarkable book, *Changing Course: A Global Business Perspective on Development and the Environment.* Together, they asserted that "sustainable development will obviously require more than pollution prevention and tinkering with environmental regulations. Given that ordinary people—consumers, business people, farmers—are the real day-to-day environmental decision-makers, it requires political and economic systems based on the effective participation of all members of society in decision making. It requires that environmental considerations become a part of the decision-making processes of all government agencies, all business enterprises, and in fact all people. . . . This can only be achieved by a break with 'business as usual' mentalities and conventional wisdom, which sideline environment and human concerns." Important, startling words: do they really mean them? Later that year, ministers of thirteen European countries agreed in principle to eliminate all discharges and emissions of chemicals that are toxic, persistent, and likely to accumulate in the food chain. In 1993 the International Joint Commission overseeing the Great Lakes concluded that persistent toxic substances are too dangerous to the biosphere and to humans to permit their release in any quantity.

Such changes cannot come too soon. As Herman E. Daly, a World Bank senior economist, has said, "Further growth has become destructive of community, the environment, and the common good. If the media could help economists and politicians to see that, or at least to entertain the possibility that such a thing might be true, they will have rendered a service far greater than all the reporting of statistics on GNP growth, Dow Jones indexes, and junk bond prices from now until the end of time."

The Bottom Line

This, then, is the sad story of what we as a species have done to the small and blue and beautiful planet we inhabit. But the real bottom line is your health and that of those you love. Your health *has* been affected, whether you know it or not, by the twentieth-century's chemicals, many of which you cannot avoid. The situation *is* grim, but by no means hopeless. Once you are aware of what's around you and in you, there is much you can do to detoxify your body, your home, your workplace, and your way of life. The people with diagnosed EI/MCS, those whose stories you have read, are a warning of what has happened to our environment and a warning of what could happen to you. Take heed. Examine carefully the products you buy. Go with the American Public Health Association's latest advice: regard chemicals as harmful until proven safe. And find a health practitioner who can help you detoxify; some practitioners are aware of both the need and the process.

The popular press has sometimes termed EI/MCS "rare" or "mysterious." Given the evidence, the only mystery is why it is still considered rare. Actually, there is another mystery—why the large national environmental organizations mostly ignore environmental illness. They use their million-dollar budgets to protect trees, whales, dolphins, spotted owls, and other endangered species, while environmental illness organizations are small, underfunded, and staffed by volunteers. They seem not to realize that humans are also not only endangered, but falling ill in their midst. Because most doctors have not been trained to look for environmental causes, chemical injury to our bodies is either misunderstood or overlooked.

What can you and I do? On national and local levels, we must all work for the ultimate goal: *pollution prevention*, in the form of *toxics use reduction* or *source reduction*. This means the reduction of toxic chemicals at their source—industry. All chemicals should be fully tested for human health effects before they can be put into any product. What isn't made or isn't used can't hurt us. Impossible? Not according to ecologist Barry Commoner: "Nearly every petrochemical product is a *substitute* for some preexisting product made of natural materials such as wood, cotton, or paper, or of common materials such as metal and glass. Hence, many current petrochemical products could readily be replaced by [products using] one of these older and more ecologically sound materials. Unique, irreplaceable petrochemical products, such as pharmaceuticals or videotape, represent only a very small fraction of the total output, so that substitution could sharply reduce the output of hazardous petrochemical products and the wastes generated by manufacturing them." If no toxics are used or produced in the manufacturing process, none will come out— either in the product or in the waste. NO TOXICS IN = NO TOXICS OUT.

Good advice. But it will take time: don't wait up. Take heed now, for the sake of your own health. Recognize the effects, subtle and not so subtle, that modern chemicals are having on your health, and take steps to be healthier. What you do to help yourself will also help the earth on which we all ride together.

* * * *

If You Still Want to Know More

- *World Watch* magazine and the yearly "State of the World" publication, available through the Worldwatch Institute, 1776 Massachusetts Avenue NW, Washington, DC 20036.

- *New World New Mind: Moving Toward Conscious Evolution*, by Robert Ornstein and Paul Ehrlich, New York, Doubleday, 1989.

- *If You Love This Planet: A Plan to Heal the Earth*, by Helen Caldicott, MD, New York, Norton, 1992.

- *Changing Course: A Global Business Perspective on Development and the Environment*, by Stephen Schmidheiny and the Business Council for Sustainable Development, Cambridge, Massachusetts, MIT Press, 1992.

For Information and Action

- For information on toxicological profiles, contact Division of Toxicology, Agency for Toxic Substances and Disease Registry, 1600 Clifton Road, Mail Stop E-29, Atlanta, Georgia 30333; 404-639-0730.

- For copies of toxicological profiles, contact the National Technical Information Service, 5285 Port Royal Road, Springfield, Virginia 22161; 1-800-336-4700 or 703-487-4650.

- For a copy of *A Citizen's Toxic Waste Audit Manual*, by Ben Gordon and Peter Montague, May 1989, contact Greenpeace U.S.A., 1436 U Street NW, Washington, D.C. 20009; 202-462-1177.

- For a copy of "Developmental Effects of Endocrine-Disrupting Chemicals in Wildlife and Humans," by Theo Colborn, Frederick S. vom Saal, and Ana M. Soto, *Environmental Health Perspectives*, October 1993, send a stamped (with 52 cents postage), self-addressed envelope to the Environmental Research Foundation, P.O. Box 5036, Annapolis, Maryland 21403-7036.

- To locate and access TRI data, call EPA's Toxics Release Inventory User Support Service at 202-260-1531.

- To obtain documents, call EPA's EPCRA Hotline, 1-800-535-0202 or 703-920-9877.

- To contact the Working Group on Community Right-to-Know, call 202-546-9707.

- To contact the Right-to-Know Computer Network (RTK NET), call 202-234-8494.

- To find out about the On-Line Computer Database (TOXNET), call 301-496-1131.

Afterword

Who Is Most to Blame

IT IS HARD TO REALIZE what is going on and not ask yourself who is to blame. In the early 1970s I accepted Pogo's charming if facile answer: "We have met the enemy and he is us." Then and now, we Americans litter, smoke, drive cars, rely on bug bombs, use more than our share of the world's resources, and create mountains of smelly garbage. Postwar affluence made us conspicuous consumers. Our lifestyle was polluting our nation.

But after I learned that in the process I had been chemically injured, Pogo's answer was not enough. I did not know that all these toxic chemicals had been accumulating in my blood and body fat, silently and insidiously. No one had told me, no one had asked me if I wanted them there. Who had requested my informed consent? Where was the consent form? The cause lay deeper than "us." Or was it just some of us?

Is the person who buys a toxic detergent or soap to blame? Or is the person who wrote the advertising copy . . . or who produced the TV commercial that induced the consumer to buy it? Or the salesperson who sold it? Or the CEO of the company that manufactured it? Or the board of directors or the stockholders of the company? Or the scientist who first synthesized the toxic chemical used in the product? Or the EPA, for not banning it? Or Congress, for not passing laws requiring strict testing before such products can be produced and marketed? Or environmentalists, for concentrating on forests and animals? Or doctors, for not being more aware of environmental hazards? Or medical schools, for not being receptive to new ideas? Pogo's answer seemed even less adequate. I took a closer look.

Every Earth Day brings out a flood of ecospeak: Save the Earth! Save the planet! Searching for causality, writers probe below the surface. Kirkpatrick Sale, writing "The Trouble with Earth Day" for the *Nation*, April 30, 1990:

> The Earth Day organizers . . . seem totally blind to the elemental ecological truth that, at bottom, the modern industrial economy is antithetical to ecological harmony: or, as [writer] Jeremy Seabrook has put it, "If it had been the purpose of human activity on earth to bring the planet to the edge of ruin, no more efficient mechanism could have been invented than the market economy."

Gary Cohen, writing "It's Too Easy Being Green," for the Summer 1990 *Toxic Times*, newsletter of the National Toxics Coalition:

> Earth Day offered little political analysis, no vision of how corporate America has manipulated consumer demand, how corporate interests have gradually shaped our addiction to products containing a wide array of environmentally destructive chemicals, how American companies went from producing one billion pounds of toxic chemicals in 1940 to over 220 billion in 1987. Earth Day failed to educate people about the limited range of choices consumers really have, and how industry, especially the automotive, petrochemical, and paper industries, bear more responsibility than the rest of us. Earth Day organizers, in their efforts to be inclusive and broad-based, missed a momentous opportunity to educate millions of people about the real causes of the environmental crisis: the chemical invasion of our society and the lack of democratic decision making in the production (and disposal) of goods.

These writers' blaming the system got me a little closer, though none of them seemed aware of what any of this has done to human health. And what lies behind the system?

One striking instance of damage to an American's health moved me still closer to an answer. In 1990, as a result of careful detective work, a twenty-three-year-old woman, Fawna Wright, received a $3.75 million out-of-court settlement for the leukemia she had apparently contracted from being exposed as a newborn to a toxic chemical used in laundering diapers in the hospital where she was born. The chemical, pentachlorophenol, was used in the laundry additive Loxene to prevent mildew. The number of babies and others exposed in this and other hospitals is unknown. Though the chemical was taken off the market in 1967, it is still used as a pesticide and wood preservative. Wright's lawyer, Robert Bogard, of St. Louis, uncovered documents dating back to 1955 indicating that Wyandotte Chemicals Corp, now BASF Corporation, sold the chemical despite receiving explicit information that it could be harmful to humans.

From this example I arrived at a partial answer to the question of who is most to blame: greed and ignorance. Not necessarily "who," but "what." The company's greed, the hospital's ignorance. One's fault was willful, deliberate; the other's not. One cause is rooted in human character, the other in society's misplaced priorities. The latter we can do something about, but greed? Can greed ever be controlled, much less eradicated from the human psyche?

The prospect does not look good. With the recent revelations of government-sponsored nuclear radiation research on unsuspecting human beings, some scientists have been speaking up. About unscrupulous researchers, nuclear biologist Dr. John Gofman says, "Some scientists will say the earth is flat; I guarantee I'll produce them. Anything you want that flies in the face of reality, just increase my checkbook a little and I'll find you scientists who say it's true." About the dangers from nuclear radiation, occupational health scientist Dr. Thomas Mancuso says, "There is no decent word to describe the magnitude of the public health tragedy that has been unfolding and will continue to unfold, I'm sorry to say, for so many decades and hundreds of years, I'm sorry, sorry to say." And I was sorry to hear.

The Library of Congress's Research Service reports that its most requested quotation is one from a 1977 speech by former Vice President Hubert H. Humphrey: "It was once said that the moral test of government is how that government treats those who are in the dawn of life, the children; those who are in the twilight of life, the elderly; and those who are in the shadows of life—the sick, the needy, and the handicapped." Who is reading those words? And who is paying attention to them? For these questions I have no answer.

Appendix

An EPA Epiphany

This poignant personal history, by an EPA employee, is printed here in its entirety.

Prior to Illness

I am 26 years old. I have a BA in Reclamation and Spanish from Frostburg State University and a Master of Environmental Studies from Yale University. I began working at EPA in July 1987. I enjoyed my work very much; it was challenging and interesting. I had a great deal of responsibility and found that rewarding. I was also fortunate enough to work with people whose company I enjoyed. Thinking about my future was exciting. I was also very active, had a great social life and excellent health.

When I Became Ill

In February and March 1988, I started to experience health problems, such as unusual fatigue, amenorrhea, abnormal acne, nausea, headache, burning eyes, runny nose, sore throat, diarrhea, dizziness, clumsiness, memory lapses, irritability, and difficulty concentrating. These symptoms coincided with progressive renovations on my floor, but I didn't associate the two.

My symptoms continued and I often felt mentally dull and overwhelmed by the type of work I had completed successfully before. I also found that I always felt better in the evenings, in the early morning, and on weekends—when I was not at work.

We moved to a newly renovated office on Monday, March 28. The chemical odor was very strong and I began to feel awful. All my symptoms grew worse and I became more disoriented and confused. I began to realize that my problems were related to the materials used in the renovations, as with people who are often affected by fresh paint fumes. On Friday I began to feel worse than ever and literally could not perform my duties. That afternoon I ended up sitting at my desk, eyes and nose running, arms and legs numb, throat closing up, gasping for breath, and barely able to speak or move. Someone happened by, and I gestured for help. I was helped outside and we encountered my boss, whose only question was, "Are you reacting to that stuff?" After reaching the outdoors and sitting for a few minutes, I began to feel better. Over the weekend my muscles ached, I felt weak, and I slept a lot. On Monday, my boss advised me to avoid the new office until the fumes had dissipated. I worked in the library and other parts of the building, but still felt poorly. On Thursday, April 7, I arrived at work feeling fine. Ninety minutes later I was helped outside again. The nurse was summoned and told me not to go back inside. She sent me to the hospital. Of course, by the time I saw a doctor, I was feeling much better. He found nothing wrong except that I was slightly "out of it."

The doctor referred me to an occupational health specialist, who advised me not to return to Waterside Mall until the "environment is more clearly defined." That was just the beginning of my visits to doctors and my medical bills. I've seen other occupational health specialists, an allergist, a gynecologist, a neurologist, my general practitioner, and a clinical ecologist. I have also researched this medical problem extensively and discussed it with many people. The diagnosis? I have multiple chemical sensitivities resulting from an exposure to something at work. The treatment? Avoid the source of the problem and other irritants. There is not much else I can do, except eliminate as many sources of irritation as possible.

Since My Illness Began

I have been working at home. In fact, I have spent the majority of time at home. At first I tried working in other buildings, where we have additional offices, contractors, training classes, etc. I always ended up reacting to something and leaving very ill. My exposure to the renovation materials at EPA caused me to become sensitive, or allergic, to many other substances, some of which I can identify, others I cannot. For example, I cannot tolerate natural gas and I have to avoid all buildings where gas is used so that I don't become ill. I have just purchased a home and had to renovate so that it is completely electric. I feel ill at gas stations, stores, department stores, office buildings, others' homes, restaurants, malls, etc. Some places make me react worse than others, but there are only a few safe havens where I can spend an entire day without experiencing some adverse symptoms. Some reactions are caused by things like cleaning products, building materials, carpets, paints, and finishes and preservatives on new products. Most buildings are so energy-efficient that all sorts of irritants have built up and are not dispersed with enough fresh air. The most frustrating reactions are those that I have in such buildings, where I don't know exactly what is causing the problem, and those that I have outside, caused by construction, exhaust, air pollution. Even my skin is extremely sensitive to sunlight now! Before this problem at EPA, I didn't even have hay fever and my only allergy was to poison ivy.

The Present

Now I spend most of my time at home. I try to use nontoxic products and avoid irritants and problem places. I become ill on the Metro and on buses, and I have no car, so I am restricted by transportation as well as by problem places. My social life is not as satisfying and I do not feel as healthy as I used to. I also do not feel as mentally sharp and find it difficult to concentrate on mental tasks. My memory is not as good.

My career has suffered. I am working at home. I was due for a promotion in August 1988, but my boss said that my situation made me lose it. I simply cannot work as effectively at home as I could at the office. Since I can hardly go anywhere, it's hard to find another job. Now, when I think about my career future, it's not exciting. It's scary.

The Players: Who's Who and What's What

AAEM   American Academy of Environmental Medicine

ADA   Americans with Disabilities Act

ALA   American Lung Association

AMA   American Medical Association

APHA   American Public Health Association

ASF   Americans for Safe Food

ASHRAE   American Society of Heating, Refrigerating, and Air-Conditioning Engineers

ATSDR   Agency for Toxic Substances and Disease Registry, part of the Public Health Service

CCHW   Citizen's Clearinghouse for Hazardous Wastes

CDC   Centers for Disease Control and Prevention

CERCLA   Comprehensive Environmental Response, Compensation, and Liability Act

CFC   chlorofluorocarbon

CFS   chronic fatigue syndrome

CIIN   Chemical Injury Information Network

CMA   Chemical Manufacturers Association

CPSC   Consumer Product Safety Commission

CSPI	Center for Science in the Public Interest
DDT	dichlorodiphenyltrichloroethane
DREDF	Disability Rights Education and Defense Fund
EEOC	Equal Employment Opportunity Commission
EI/MCS	environmental illness/multiple chemical sensitivities
EMF	electromagnetic field
EPA	Environmental Protection Agency
ERF	Environmental Research Foundation
FDA	Food and Drug Administration
FIFRA	Federal Insecticide, Fungicide, and Rodenticide Act
FTC	Federal Trade Commission
GAO	General Accounting Office, Congress's chief investigative arm
HEAL	Human Ecology Action League
HHS	Health and Human Services
HUD	Housing and Urban Development
IPM	integrated pest management
JAMA	Journal of the American Medical Association
JEC	Jobs and Environment Campaign, formerly the National Toxics Campaign
MCS	multiple chemical sensitivities
MSDS	Material Safety Data Sheet
NAS	National Academy of Sciences
NASA	National Aeronautics and Space Administration
NCAMP	National Coalition Against the Misuse of Pesticides
NCAP	Northwest Coalition for Alternatives to Pesticides
NCEHS	National Center for Environmental Health Strategies
NCHS	National Center for Health Statistics
NCI	National Cancer Institute

NEJM	New England Journal of Medicine
NHATS	National Human Adipose Tissue Survey
NIH	National Institutes of Health
NIOSH	National Institute for Occupational Safety and Health
NLEA	Nutrition Labeling and Education Act
NOHA	Nutrition for Optimal Health Association
NPL	National Priorities List
NRC	National Research Council, NAS's research arm
NRDC	Natural Resources Defense Council
NTC	National Toxics Campaign, now the Jobs and Environment Campaign
NTP	National Toxicology Program, part of Health and Human Services
NYCAP	New York Coalition for Alternatives to Pesticides
OMB	Office of Management and Budget, in the White House
OPPTS	Office of Pollution Prevention and Toxic Substances
organic	(1) carbon-containing, as in organic chemistry (2) grown without synthetic or other toxic chemical pesticides
OSHA	Occupational Safety and Health Administration
OTA	Office of Technology Assessment, Congress's research arm
outgassing	giving off gas molecules trapped in substances, especially synthetics
PAH	polycyclic aromatic hydrocarbons
PCB	polychlorinated biphenyl
PCHRG	Public Citizen Health Research Group
PEL	permissible exposure limit
PET scan	positron emission tomography scan

PVC	polyvinyl chloride
RACHEL	remote access chemical hazards electronic library
SAB	Science Advisory Board, an advisory arm of the EPA
SBS	sick building syndrome
SPECT scan	single photon emission computed tomography scan
SSA	Social Security Administration
SVTC	Silicon Valley Toxics Coalition
TCE	trichloroethylene
TEAM	Toxics Exposure Assessment Methodology
TRI	Toxics Release Inventory
TSCA	Toxic Substances Control Act
USDA	United States Department of Agriculture
USPIRG	United States Public Interest Research Group
VOC	volatile organic compound
WHO	World Health Organization

Notes

Page | **Chapter 1**

32   Iris R. Bell et al., "Self-reported Illness from Chemical Odors in Young Adults without Clinical Syndromes or Occupational Exposures," *Archives of Environmental Health*, January/February 1993, pp. 6–13.

32   Iris R. Bell et al., "Possible Time-Dependent Sensitization to Xenobiotics: Self-reported Illness from Chemical Odors, Foods, and Opiate Drugs in an Older Adult Population," *Archives of Environmental Health*, September/October 1993, pp. 315–27.

34   Grace E. Ziem, "Multiple Chemical Sensitivity: Treatment and Followup with Avoidance and Control of Chemical Exposures," *Toxicology and Industrial Health*, Vol. 8, No. 4, 1992.

34   Emily Soloff, "Environment is toxic for some," *Life Extra* (a Pulitzer-Lerner Community Newspaper), week of May 28, 1988.

35   David Beach, "Learning to deal with chemical sensitivity," *In These Times*, August 2–29, 1989.

35   Alan S. Levin and Merla Zellerbach, *The Type 1/Type 2 Allergy Relief Program*, Los Angeles, Jeremy P. Tarcher, 1983, p. 72.

36   Susan Kissir, "Environmental Illness: When everything around you makes you sick," *Bestways*, April 1990.

39   Robert Schaeffer, "Car Sick: Automobiles Ad Nauseam," *Greenpeace Magazine*, May/June 1990.

39   Samuel S. Epstein, "If Rachel Carson Were Writing Today: Silent Spring in Retrospect, *Environmental Law Reporter* 17:10182, June 1987.

40   Bruce Ames, *Science* 221:1256–64, September 23, 1983; "Diet link to cancer 'small,'" *Chicago Sun-Times*, February 20, 1990.

40   Ruth Adams, letter to the editor of *Chemecology*, November 1991.

42   Melvyn R. Werbach, *Third Line Medicine: Modern Treatment for*

Persistent Symptoms, New York, Routledge & Kegan Paul, 1986, pp. 2–7.

43   Institute of Medicine, *Role of the Primary Care Physician in Occupational and Environmental Medicine*, Washington, D.C., National Academy Press, 1988, p.x.

44   Sharon Feldman, "Rheumatoid Arthritis: Patient Follow-up After Hospitalization in a Comprehensive Environmental Control Unit," *Clinical Ecology*, Vol. VI, No. 3, p. 94, 1989.

45   Nicholas A. Ashford and Claudia S. Miller, *Chemical Exposures: Low Levels and High Stakes*, New York, Van Nostrand Reinhold, 1991, p. 30.

46   Theron G. Randolph and Pauline Harding, "The Greening of Medicine," unpublished work.

46   "They Eat Lion Meat," *Newsweek*, August 20, 1990.

46   *Chicago Sun-Times*, February 24, 1981.

47   *Chicago Sun-Times*, June 6, 1979.

47   *Chicago Tribune*, December 29, 1986.

48   Kathleen Matusik, "Man's building project will let wife come home," *Michigan City (Indiana) News Dispatch*, November 24, 1989.

49   Linda Joy, "Woman thinks of home as a safe house: Toxic world drives woman to safety," *Frederick (Maryland) Post*, July 30, 1990; NBC-TV interview, October 28, 1990.

50   Peter Montague, *RACHEL'S Hazardous Waste News #149*, October 3, 1989.

50   The EarthWorks Group, *50 Simple Things You Can Do to Save the Earth*, Berkeley, California, Earthworks Press, 1989.

50   *RACHEL'S Hazardous Waste News*, October 3, 1989.

50   Arthur J. Barsky, "The Paradox of Health," *New England Journal of Medicine*, February 18, 1988.

51   Mark R. Cullen, editor, *Workers with Multiple Chemical Sensitivities*, Vol. 2, No. 4, *Occupational Medicine: State of the Art Reviews*. Philadelphia, Hanley & Belfus, 1987.

52   U.S. Congress, Office of Technology Assessment, *Neurotoxicity: Identifying and Controlling Poisons of the Nervous System*, OTA-BA-436, Washington, D.C., U.S. Government Printing Office, April 1990, p. 6.

52   Geoffrey Cowley and Rebecca Crandall, "Bad Water, Faulty Genes: Closing in on the causes of Parkinson's disease," *Newsweek*, September 3, 1990.

52   *Neurotoxicity*, April 1990, pp. 54–55; National Research Council, *Environmental Neurotoxicology*, Washington, D.C., National Academy Press, 1992, p. 15.

52   "Sharp increase found in childhood asthma," *Chicago Tribune*, October 8, 1992.

52   Lawrence K. Altman, "Rise in Asthma Deaths Is Tied to Ignorance of Many Physicians," *New York Times*, May 4, 1993.

52   *Chicago Tribune*, February 2, 1989.

53   Marcia Barinaga, "Better Data Needed on Sensitivity Syndrome," *Science*, March 29, 1991.

53   *American Journal of Psychiatry*, August 1987; as reported in *The Reactor*, November/December, 1987.

53   Elisabeth Carlsen et al., "Evidence for decreasing quality of semen during the past 50 years," *British Medical Journal*, 305:609–13, 1992.

53   Reading about this astonishing drop in worldwide fertility inspired British mystery writer P.D. James to write *The Children of Men*. Set in 2021, her novel describes a world into which no children had been born after 1995 and in which the characters struggle to cope with the problems of an aging population and a dying species.

53   Bill Lambrecht, "Pesticides take toll on Third-World health, ecology," *San Antonio Express-News*, December 5, 1993.

54   Richard W. Martin and Charles Becker, "Headaches from Chemical Exposure," *Headache*, November/December 1993, pp. 555–59.

54   *Des Moines Register*, Summer 1989; as cited in *The Human Ecologist*, Spring 1990.

Chapter 2

59   Lance A. Wallace, "Project Summary: The Total Exposure Assessment Methodology (TEAM) Study," U.S. Environmental Protection Agency, EPA/600/S6–87/002, September 1987.

59   Rick McGuire, "Can't Hide from Pollution Indoors," *Medical Tribune*, January 7, 1987.

60   Mike Toner, "Home Serves Up 'Cocktail of Pesticides,'" *Atlanta Journal/Atlanta Constitution*, September 27, 1988.

60   "Comparing Risks and Setting Environmental Priorities: Overview of Three Regional Projects (PM-220)," U.S. Environmental Protection Agency's Office of Policy, Planning, and Evaluation, 1989.

61   In spring 1989 EPA's Region V office, for example, had only one out of approximately a thousand employees handling indoor air pollution, and that less than full time.

61   "Caution: An Ill Wind May Be Blowing in Your Office, Warns Building Doctor Gray Robertson," *People*, February 20, 1989.

61   Lynne Durham, "Preventive Actions Could Save Building Owners from SBS Lawsuits," *Indoor Air Review*, March 1992.

61   Dan Fagin, "Sick Buildings, Sick People," Long Island *Newsday*, November 15–17, 1992; from the National Safety Council's *Environment Writer*, December 1992.

62   "Indoor pollution greatest hazard?," *Los Angeles Times*, reprinted in the *Lincoln (Nebraska) Star*, December 27, 1989.

62   "Building Green," Audubon videotape, 1993.

63   "Indoor pollution greatest hazard?," *Los Angeles Times*; reprinted in the *Lincoln (Nebraska) Star*, December 27, 1989.

64   Sonia L. Nazario, "Children Become Centerpiece of Efforts to Set

Tighter Restrictions on Pollutants," *Wall Street Journal*, October 15, 1990.

65 Casey Bukro, "This living lab is a survivalist's dream," *Chicago Tribune*, October 27, 1988.

66 Stevenson Swanson, "Chicago-area firms top list of Great Lakes polluters, group says," *Chicago Tribune*, April 2, 1992.

66 "Great Lakes spills exceed 5,000," *Chicago Tribune*, April 20, 1990.

66 "Lake called safe despite Gary waste," *Chicago Tribune*, October 2, 1989.

66 Casey Bukro, "Toxic signs on rise in Great Lakes," *Chicago Tribune*, September 18, 1988.

66 Stevenson Swanson, "Great Lakes pollution persists," *Chicago Tribune*, October 12, 1989.

67 Stevenson Swanson, "Great Lakes still unhealthy, experts say," *Chicago Tribune*, February 27, 1991.

67 Stevenson Swanson, "DDT, PCBs still lurk in Lake Michigan waters," *Chicago Tribune*, November 23, 1992.

69 Barry Commoner, talk given at Northeastern Illinois University, Chicago, Illinois, April 6, 1989.

70 Casey Bukro, "20 years later, Earth Day's legacy lingers," *Chicago Tribune*, April 16, 1990.

70 Casey Bukro, "Ecologists find success in own back yards," *Chicago Tribune*, April 17, 1990.

70 Keith Schneider, "For Communities, Knowledge of Polluters Is Power," *New York Times*, March 24, 1991.

71 Barry Commoner, *Making Peace with the Planet*, New York, Pantheon, 1990, p. 52.

71 Merrill Goozner, "Clearing the air on workers' asthma," *Chicago Tribune*, March 3, 1991.

71 G. L. Waldbott, *Health Effects of Environmental Pollutants*, St. Louis, C.V. Mosby Company, 1973; as reported in *Indoor Air Pollution and Housing Technology*, August 1983.

71 D'Vera Cohn, "Letting the Feds Get Away with What Business Never Could," *Washington Post National Weekly Edition*, June 5–11, 1989.

72 Office of Pollution Prevention and Toxic Substances, U.S. Environmental Protection Agency, *1991 Toxics Release Inventory: Public Data Release*, EPA 745-R-93–003, May 1993, p. 11.

72 "Air Pollution: A Few Hints of Progress Noted, But Many Challenges, Questions Remain," *Journal of the American Medical Association*, August 7, 1991.

72 Charles Weschler et al., "Ozone Radiation Levels Reaching Danger Points," *Indoor Pollution Law Report*, November 1989.

72 "Study links pollutants, early death," *Chicago Tribune*, May 17, 1993.

73 "Citizens Question Reported Reductions," *Working Notes on Community Right-to-Know*, May 1992.

73   "EPA to Continue Human Monitoring Program," *Foundation for Advancements in Science and Education Reports*, Spring 1988.

74   Nicholas A. Ashford and Claudia S. Miller, *Chemical Exposures: Low Levels and High Stakes*, New York, Van Nostrand Reinhold, 1991.

74   Peter Montague, *RACHEL's Hazardous Waste News* #292, July 1, 1992.

75   Hilary R. French, "You Are What You Breathe," *World Watch*, May-June 1990.

75   Stevenson Swanson, "Chicago's air getting cleaner, but . . . ," *Chicago Tribune*, March 6, 1991.

75   J. E. Ferrell, "Saving clean air from its last gasp," *Chicago Tribune*, May 27, 1990.

76   Bukro, April 16, 1990.

76   William Greider, *Who Will Tell the People: The Betrayal of American Democracy*, New York, Simon & Schuster, 1992, p. 29.

76   Greider, pp. 116–17.

77   Sara Terry, "Drinking Water Comes to a Boil," *New York Times*, September 26, 1993.

77   Ruth Pe Palileo, "Lung group to sue EPA over air dust," *Chicago Tribune*, July 17, 1993.

78   Peter Montague, *RACHEL'S Hazardous Waste News* #215, January 9, 1991.

79   Jeff Bailey, "Fading Garbage Crisis Leaves Incinerators Competing for Trash," *Wall Street Journal*, August 11, 1993.

79   Michael Weisskopf, "The Supermanagement of Superfund," *Washington Post National Weekly Edition*, August 5–11, 1991.

79   Keith Schneider, "New View Calls Environmental Policy Misguided," *New York Times*, March 21, 1993; from *Chemecology*, May 1993.

79   Bukro, April 17, 1990.

80   Michael Silverstein, "Bush's Polluter Protectionism Isn't Pro-Business," *Wall Street Journal*, May 28, 1992; as cited by Peter Montague, *RACHEL's Hazardous Waste News* #293, July 8, 1992.

80   Barry Commoner, "Free Markets Can't Control Pollution," *New Patriot*, June 30, 1990.

80   John Holusha, "Hutchinson No Longer Holds Its Nose," *New York Times*, February 3, 1991; Stevenson Swanson, "Business cleans up on pollution," *Chicago Tribune*, April 18, 1990.

81   U.S. General Accounting Office, "Advantages of and Barriers to Reducing the Use of Toxic Chemicals," GAO/RCED-92–212, June 1992.

81   Fen Montaigne, "When pollution is an inside job," *Chicago Tribune*, April 5, 1987.

82   L.S. Sheldon et al., "Indoor Air Quality in Public Buildings; Project Summary," Volumes I and II, U.S. Environmental Protection Agency, EPA/600/S6–88/009a and 009b, September 1988.

82   "Indoor Air Facts No. 4: Sick Buildings," U.S. Environmental Protection Agency, July 1988.

82 "Indoor Air Facts No. 6: Report to Congress on Indoor Air Quality," U.S. Environmental Protection Agency, August 1989.

84 J. Brundage et al., "Building-Associated Risk of Febrile Acute Respiratory Disease in Army Trainees," *Journal of the American Medical Association*, 259:2108–12, 1988.

85 Steven L. Taylor, "NIOSH Deluged by Sick Building Complaints," *Indoor Air Review*, October 1993; "Florida Courthouse Plagued by SBS Undergoes Renovation," *Indoor Air Review*, August 1993.

85 Janet Fox, "Indoor Pollution and Health," *Piedmont Airlines Magazine*, September 1988.

85 "Indoor Air Facts No. 3: Ventilation and Air Quality in Offices," U.S. Environmental Protection Agency, February 1988.

86 R. Menzies et al., "The Effect of Varying Levels of Outdoor-Air Supply on the Symptoms of Sick Building Syndrome," *New England Journal of Medicine*, 328:821–27, 1993.

86 Janet Raloff, "EPA: Paper products pose no risk of dioxin," *Science News*, February 18, 1989.

86 Paul Galloway, "Breathe (a bit) easier," *Chicago Tribune*, April 11, 1989.

87 Earon S. Davis, "Chemicals, risk, and the public," *Chicago Tribune*, April 29, 1989.

87 Joel Brinkley, "Animal Tests as Risk Clues: The Best Data May Fall Short," *New York Times*, March 23, 1993.

88 "ACS views of toxic substances, patent issues," *Chemical and Engineering News*, August 31, 1992.

88 U.S. Congress, Office of Technology Assessment, *Neurotoxicity: Identifying and Controlling Poisons of the Nervous System*, OTA-BA-436, Washington, D.C., U.S. Government Printing Office, April 1990.

88 Peter Montague, *RACHEL'S Hazardous Waste News #187*, June 27, 1990.

89 Galloway, April 11, 1989.

89 Eric Mann, "Environmentalism in the Corporate Climate," *Tikkun*, March/April 1990.

89 Jeanne Gutin, "At Our Peril: The False Promise of Risk Assessment," *Greenpeace Magazine*, March/April 1991.

89 Keith Schneider, "How a Rebellion Over Environmental Rules Grew From a Patch of Weeds," *New York Times*, March 24, 1993; for a critique of the OMB's statistical method, see *RACHEL's Hazardous Waste News #379*, March 3, 1994.

89 Joe Thornton, "Risking Democracy," *Greenpeace Magazine*, March/April 1991.

89 William Neikirk, *Chicago Tribune*, April 15, 1989.

90 Philip Shabecoff, "Tax Proposed on Products and Activities That Harm Environment," *New York Times*, February 10, 1991.

90 *RACHEL'S Hazardous Waste News*, June 27, 1990.

91 Such lists, subject to frequent revision, occasionally appear in the Federal Register. The ARC used "Food Use Pesticides with Evidence

of Carcinogenicity," *Federal Register*, Vol. 53, No. 202, pp. 41, 119, October 19, 1988.

91   "I Want You to Adopt a Chemical," folder from the Agricultural Resources Center, Carrboro, North Carolina, 1990.

91   Gutin, March/April 1991.

93   Most modern products and processes are either "solvent"-based, meaning that they contain or use solvents (like xylene) other than water (examples: oil-based paints; "dry" cleaning) or are water-based (examples: latex paints; your washing machine).

Chapter 3

100   Frank Hutchins, "Chemicals take toll on woman: Outside world fraught with risks," *Charleston (West Virginia) Daily Mail*, January 12, 1990.

101   Michael Townsend, "Harpswell woman and son fight obscure environmental illness," *Brunswick (Maine) Times-Record*, July 28, 1989.

102   W. Alfred Mukatis, "Chemical sensitivity," letter to the editor, *Chemical & Engineering News*, June 4, 1990.

102   Stephen K. Hall, "The worker with chemical hypersensitivity syndrome," *Pollution Engineering*, February 1989.

103   William Greider, *Who Will Tell the People: The Betrayal of American Democracy*, New York, Simon & Schuster, 1992, p. 119.

103   Howard Wolinsky, "71,000 deaths a year linked to job disease," *Chicago Sun-Times*, September 1, 1990.

103   Margo Harakas, "The Endangered," *Boca Raton (Florida) Sun-Sentinel*, May 23, 1989.

104   David Moberg, "Work Kills," *Chicago Reader*, January 31, 1992.

104   U.S. Congress, Office of Technology Assessment, *Neurotoxicity: Identifying and Controlling Poisons of the Nervous System*, OTA-BA-436, Washington, D.C., U.S. Government Printing Office, April 1990, p. 3.

105   Merrill Goozner, "Job diseases remain a major cause of death," *Chicago Tribune*, August 31, 1990.

105   "Health Hazards in the Arts and Crafts," based on a talk by Bertram W. Carnow, April 19, 1974, published in *Chicago: Hazards in the Arts*, 1974.

105   National Research Council, "Toxicity Testing: Strategies to Determine Needs and Priorities," Washington, D.C., National Academy Press, 1984.

105   Harakas, May 23, 1989.

105   U.S. General Accounting Office, "Toxic Substances: EPA's Chemical Testing Program Has Made Little Progress," GAO/RCED-90–112, April 1990, p. 4.

105   National Research Council, *Environmental Neurotoxicology*, Washington, D.C., National Academy Press, 1992.

106   Nicholas A. Ashford and Claudia S. Miller, *Chemical Exposures:*

Low Levels and High Stakes, New York, Van Nostrand Reinhold, 1991, p. 65.

106 Greider, 1992, pp. 121–22.

107 *Neurotoxicity*, April 1990, pp. 9, 296.

107 Kathy Anderson, "Toxics and Learning Disabilities: Putting Two and Two Together," *Not Man Apart*, May-June 1986; see also W. K. Anger, "Neurobehavioral Testing of Chemicals: Impact on Recommended Standards, " *Neurobehavioral Toxicology and Teratology* 6:147–43, 1984.

107 Christopher M. Ryan, Lisa A. Morrow, and Michael Hodgson, "Cacosmia and Neurobehavioral Dysfunction Associated with Occupational Exposure to Mixtures of Organic Solvents," *American Journal of Psychiatry* 145:11, November 1988.

107 Janette D. Sherman, *Chemical Exposure and Disease*, New York, Van Nostrand Reinhold, 1988, pp. 53, 73, 102, 105.

109 Tina Adler, *American Psychological Association Monitor*, May 1989.

109 U.S. Congress, Office of Technology Assessment, "Preventing Illness and Injury in the Workplace," OTA-H-256, Washington, D.C., 1985, pp. 3–5; as cited by Sherman, 1988, p. 2.

109 Abba Terr, "Clinical Ecology in the Workplace," *Journal of Occupational Medicine* 31:257–61, 1989.

109 Peter Montague, *RACHEL's Hazardous Waste News* #266, January 1, 1992.

110 Dorothy Nelkin and Michael S. Brown, *Workers at Risk: Voices from the Workplace*, University of Chicago Press, 1984, p. *xiv.*

110 Kaye H. Kilburn, "Evidence That the Human Nervous System Is Most Sensitive to Environmental Toxins," in *Approach to a Consensus for the Basis of Regulation of Environmental Chemicals*, editors Joseph C. Arcos, Mary F. Argus, and Yin-tak Woo, Special Issue of *Environmental Carcinogenesis Reviews: Part C of Journal of Environmental Science and Health*, Vol. C8, No. 2, New York, Marcel Dekker, 1990–91.

110 Marla Donato, "Environmental poverty law takes root," *Chicago Tribune*, September 29, 1992.

110 Mike McAndrew, "Workers Sue Waste Firm over Toxic Fumes," *Syracuse (New York) Post-Standard*, March 2, 1990.

111 D.L. Smith Jr., "Mental effects of mercury poisoning," *Southern Medical Journal* 71:904–5, 1978.

111 C. Ngim et al., "Neurobehavioral Effects of Elemental Mercury in Dentists," *British Journal of Industrial Medicine*, Vol. 49, No. 11, November 1992.

111 T.A.Cook and P.O. Yates, "Fatal mercury intoxication in dental surgery assistant," *British Dental Journal* 127:553–55, l969.

111 "Editor: This is only a test," *Journal of the California Dental Association* 12:37, 1984.

111 Ronald Finn, "Organic Solvent Sensitivity," *Clinical Ecology*, Vol. V, No. 4, 1987/88.

112 T.J. Howard, "Clearing the Air," *Chicago Tribune*, July 25, 1993.

112   Jessica Seigel, "OSHA: Masks worn in fumes death unsafe," *Chicago Tribune*, February 9, 1989.

112   Debra Lynn Dadd, *Nontoxic & Natural: How to Avoid Dangerous Everyday Products and Buy or Make Safe Ones*, Los Angeles, Jeremy P. Tarcher, 1984, p. 178.

113   "Breathing easier in the hospital," *Modern Healthcare*, May 19, 1989.

113   "Allergic reactions on rise from using latex items, doctors say," *Chicago Tribune*, December 8, 1993.

113   "Allergy to latex can threaten life," *Chicago Tribune*, December 8, 1991.

113   Gordon P. Baker, "Hazardous Chemicals in the Workplace," *The Human Ecologist*, Summer 1990.

114   Finn, 1987/88.

114   P. Moszczynxki, "Organic solvents and T lymphocytes," *Lancet* I:1464–65, 1982; as cited by Finn, 1987/88.

114   Frederick Hargreave, Jerry Dolovich, and Stephanie Griffiths, *Living with Asthma*, Toronto, Canada, Hume Medical Information Services, 1990; as cited in *Air Currents*, May/June 1991.

114   Karin Winegar, "Home Remedies: Designers, health experts search for nontoxic building materials," *Minneapolis Star Tribune*, September 3, 1989.

114   Greider, 1992, p. 121.

114   Leslie Eimas, "Worry at the Workplace," *Syracuse (New York) Herald American*, October 27, 1991.

115   Peter Schaffer, "An Overdose of Progress: Chemical Sensitivity Spreading," *Syracuse (New York) Post-Standard*, March 14, 1989.

115   "Rare Neurological Disease Linked to Toxin Exposure," *Psychiatric News*, November 20, 1987.

115   Robert Reinhold, "When Life Is Toxic," *New York Times Magazine*, September 16, 1990.

116   Gary Dorsey, "The Poison Factory," *Hartford Courant Northeast Magazine*, June 14, 1987.

117   "Job-Related Murder Convictions of 3 Executives Are Overturned," *New York Times*, January 22, 1990; Harold Henderson, "Murder in the Air," *Chicago Reader*, June 15, 1990.

117   Matt O'Connor, "A setback for defense in toxic case," *Chicago Tribune*, February 14, 1991.

117   Gordon P. Baker, "Aerospace Workers Syndrome: A Disease of Our Advanced Technology," *The Human Ecologist*, Winter 1989.

118   Diana Hembree and Sarah Henry, "Mystery disease strikes high-tech workers," *Chicago Sun-Times*, December 7, 1986.

118   Jane A. Lipscomb et al., "Pregnancy Outcomes in Women Potentially Exposed to Occupational Solvents and Women Working in the Electronics Industry," *Journal of Occupational Medicine*, 33: 597–604, 1991.

118   Mark Upfal, "Liver Enzymes among Microelectronic Equipment Maintenance Technicians," *Journal of Occupational Medicine*, April 1992.

119 "Buyer links ills, Gulf War," *South Bend Tribune*, June 10, 1993.

119 Warren E. Leary, "High Dioxin Levels Linked to Cancer," *New York Times*, January 24, 1991.

119 Vicki Monks, "See No Evil," *American Journalism Review*, June 30, 1992.

120 R. Menzies et al., "The Effect of Varying Levels of Outdoor-Air Supply on the Symptoms of Sick Building Syndrome," *New England Journal of Medicine*, 328:821–7, 1993.

120 "Can a building really make you sick?," *University of California at Berkeley Wellness Letter*, July 1991.

120 Steve Kerch, "Sick of your job? Maybe it's the office," *Chicago Tribune*, June 5, 1992.

121 Charles Piller and Michael Castleman, "Is your office making you sick?," *Redbook*, April 1990.

121 Steve Kerch, "Buildings can make you sick," *Chicago Tribune*, July 22, 1990.

121 Melanie Menagh, "In Our Time: A Green, Well-Lighted Place," *Omni*, March 1991.

121 Schaffer, March 14, 1989.

122 Casey Bukro, "Incinerator adds to EPA woes: 'Solution' for toxic waste is now part of the problem," *Chicago Tribune*, December 12, 1990.

122 Environmental and Occupational Health Sciences Institute, "Health Effects of Exposure to Toxic Wastes," *INFOletter*, Volume 4, Number 2, 1990.

123 Ed Pope, "Cancer linked to deadly diet of 'smoke eaters,'" *Chicago Tribune*, January 5, 1992.

123 A. Mutti et al., "Nephropathies and Exposure to Perchloroethylene in Dry-Cleaners," *Lancet*, July 25, 1992.

124 Greider, 1992, pp. 120–21.

124 James Warren, "Top OSHA scientists join chorus of criticism," *Chicago Tribune*, April 20, 1988.

125 Public Citizen publication #999, January 23, 1985.

125 Barry I. Castleman and Grace Ziem, "Corporate Influence on Threshold Limit Values," *American Journal of Industrial Medicine*, 13:531–59, 1988.

125 David Moberg, "In the Nation: Work," *In These Times*, May 3–9, 1989.

126 David Moberg, "Oversight of workplace hazards," *In These Times*, April 25-May 1, 1990.

Chapter 4

133 *Garbage*, March/April 1990, p.16.

135 J. Linn Allen, "Builder becomes pollution-buster," *Chicago Tribune*, November 7, 1987.

135 John R. Hughes, "Allergy Free in Ottawa: A house for a chemically sensitive family," *Fine Homebuilding*, April/May 1988, pp. 70–73.

136   Sally Falk, "Safe house wards off environmental illness," *Chicago Tribune*, June 10, 1989.

136   Lew Sichelman, "Author coughs up several home-related maladies," *Ft. Myers (Florida) News Press*, June 15, 1990.

136   John Bower, "Cellulose Insulation, Handle with Care: If at All," *Environ*, No. 11, 1991.

136   Sichelman, June 15, 1990.

137   Patricia Prijatel, "Breathing easy: Building a healthier house is easier and cheaper than you might think," *Better Homes and Gardens*, Summer 1993.

137   Patricia Leigh Brown, "A 'Healthy House' That's High in Style But Low in Chemicals," *New York Times*, April 19, 1990.

138   Miriam Horn, "Designing in hues of green," *U.S. News & World Report*, February 25, 1991.

138   Michael D. Lemonick, "Architecture Goes Green," *Time*, April 5, 1993.

138   Karin Winegar, "Home Remedies: Designers, health experts search for nontoxic building materials," *Minneapolis Star Tribune*, September 3, 1989.

139   John N. Ott, *Health and Light*, New York, Simon & Schuster (Pocket Books), 1973, p. 83.

139   John Banta, "Full Spectrum Light," *The Reactor*, Winter 1989–1990.

140   William J. Rea, "Indoor Air Pollution," *The Human Ecologist*, Summer 1990.

141   Larry S. Finley, "'Home-icide'—indoor pollution assault," *Chicago Sun-Times*, March 22, 1981.

142   "Mercury in some paint a threat, report warns," *Chicago Tribune*, October 18, 1990.

142   "Indoor Air Pollution," *Consumer Reports*, October 1985.

143   Marshall Mandell and Lynn Waller Scanlon, *Dr. Mandell's 5-Day Allergy Relief System*, New York, Thomas Y. Crowell, 1979; as cited in Theron G. Randolph and Ralph W. Moss, *An Alternative Approach to Allergies*, New York, Harper & Row, 1989.

143   Deborah Branscum, "Washington Rethinks ELF Emissions," *MacWorld*, December 1990.

143   "Study links cancer in kids, electric appliances," *Chicago Tribune*, February 10, 1991.

143   George E. Shambaugh, *Shambaugh Medical Research Institute Newsletter* 26, Fall 1990.

144   Bill Sanders, "Field Trip," *Green Alternatives*, July/August 1993.

144   Doug Turetsky, "Making a Killing off Children," *In These Times*, Oct./Nov. 5, 1991.

144   Jon Hilkevitch, "A punch in the breadbasket," *Chicago Tribune*, September 21, 1990.

145   Michael Tackett, "Farmers' Catch-22: Safe wells or high yields with chemicals," *Chicago Tribune*, March 4, 1980.

145   David Steinman, "We Are All Sick: Low-level poisoning from toxic

chemicals in the environment affects nearly everybody living in Los Angeles," *Los Angeles Reader*, September 1, 1989.

145   Sara Terry, "Drinking Water Comes to a Boil," *New York Times*, September 16, 1993.

146   Casey Bukro, "Milwaukee aim: Curb lake toxins," *Chicago Tribune*, September 7, 1990.

146   Terry, September 26, 1993.

146   "Toxic Euphemisms—Number 2: Air 'Fresheners,'" *Rachel Carson Council Newsletter*, November 1990.

147   R.H. Lawson, "Is there an air freshener syndrome?," *Bristol Medico-chirurgical Journal* 10–13, 1985.

147   Mary Lamielle, "Do Disinfectants Do the Job?," *The Delicate Balance*, Fall/Winter 1990/1991.

147   U.S. General Accounting Office, "Disinfectants: Concerns Over the Integrity of EPA's Data Bases," GAO/RCED-90–232, September 21, 1990.

147   Anthony R. Wood, "Environmental movement pampers diaper service's growth," *Chicago Tribune*, April 30, 1990.

147   David Evans, "U.S. has to upgrade gear for dealing with chemical arms," *Chicago Tribune*, September 21, 1990.

148   "Carpets as reservoirs of PAH-lution," *Science News*, July 10, 1993.

148   J. Raloff, "Home carpets: Shoeing in toxic pollution," *Science News*, August 11, 1990.

149   Herbert Kohl, "Screen Test," *Nation*, September 3, 1990.

150   Sandy Rovner, "Beware of Biting Insects That Don't Buzz Off," *Washington Post Health*, May 8, 1990.

150   "Christmas tree growers try environmental tack," *Chicago Tribune*, November 23, 1990.

151   From "Home for the Holidays: Avoiding Toxic Consumer Products," a report by the National Environmental Law Center, Winter 1992.

151   Jeanne F. Neath and Paula D. Dotter, "The Search for Nontoxic 100% Cotton, *East/West*, September 1988.

152   Eve M. Kahn, "Natural Bedding: Counting on Sheep or Milkweed," *New York Times*, March 28, 1991.

152   "The Hazards of Chlorine Bleaching," *ESP (Environmentally Sound Paper) News*, published by Conservatree Paper Company, March 1991.

153   "Toward a Chlorine-free Pulp and Paper Industry," *Greenpeace Action*, a fact sheet received in 1990.

153   NIOSH, "Current Intelligence Bulletin 39: Glycol Ethers," May 2, 1983.

157   Thad Godish, "Indoor Air Quality Notes: Residential Formaldehyde Control," Department of Natural Resources, Ball State University, Summer 1986.

Chapter 5

170 Truman Temple, "On the Cutting Edge," *EPA Journal,* October 1980.

171 *Arizona Republic,* June 1988.

172 Myra Cypser, editor, *Indoor Air News: A Monthly Newsletter on EPA's Indoor Air,* August 31, 1991.

173 J.William Hirzy, "The Other Voice from EPA: The Role of the Headquarters Professionals' Union," *Environmental Law Reporter,* February 1990.

173 Daniel Grossman, *In These Times,* June 22-July 5, 1988.

174 Leonard Schachter, "Carpet Related Health Complaints," U.S. Consumer Product Safety Commission, July 1990.

175 Hirzy, February 1990.

175 *Arizona Republic,* June 1988.

175 Bob Bretschneider, *Pioneer Press,* February 8, 1990.

176 Linda Lee Davidoff, *Amicus Journal,* Winter 1989.

177 Yvonne Daley, "Emissions from carpets spur concern in Vermont, *Boston Sunday Globe,* August 23, 1992.

177 "Toddlers with Heart Attacks," *Harvard Medical School Health Letter,* February 1990.

177 *Science News,* July 10, 1993.

179 Gretchen Biggs, "Interview with Earon Davis," *RE-SOURCES,* Vol. 7, #2, 1988.

179 *Federal Register,* Vol. 55, No. 79, April 24, 1990.

179 On December 23, 1993, five EPA employees were awarded $950,000 for respiratory and neurological disorders; similar cases are pending.

179 Cypser, August 31, 1991.

180 Stevenson Swanson, "Firm in bind over EPA foot-dragging," *Chicago Tribune,* March 5, 1990.

180 Executive Summary, "The Carpet Policy Dialogue: Compendium Report," September 27, 1991; available for $66 from the National Technical Information Service, 5285 Port Royal Road, Springfield, VA 22261, by requesting PB 92–115005.

181 "Carpet-Related Industry Finds No Evidence Linking 4-PC with Health Problems," *Indoor Air Review,* April 1993.

181 "EPA finds no link between carpet, illness," *Chicago Tribune,* June 12, 1993.

182 Cindy Duehring, "Hazardous Chemicals in Carpet," *Informed Consent,* Jan/Feb 1994.

182 Steven Taylor, "Media Reports Spur Further Demands for EPA Probe of Carpet-Health Hazard Link," *Indoor Air Review,* December 1992.

182 "Industry agrees to put warning labels on carpet," *USA Today,* November 16, 1993.

183 Steven Taylor, "Carpet Industry Announces New Consumer IAQ Label Program," *Indoor Air Review,* December 1993.

184   Mary Oetzel, "School Districts Pay a High Price for Carpeting," unpublished research, 1992.

184   Cindy Duehring, "Carpet Concerns. Part 1: EPA Stalls and Industry Hedges While Consumers Remain at Risk," *Informed Consent*, Nov/Dec 1993; Bill Sanders, "Carpet Guard: Protecting Yourself from Your Carpet," *Green Alternatives*, October/November 1993.

Chapter 6

187   Report #175, Tariff Commission Reports, 1951; *Predicasts Basebook*, November 1989. Since 1966, particleboard production has increased nearly fourfold. In 1990 formaldehyde use in the U.S. was projected to grow by 3 percent a year by 1994. Formaldehyde is also produced by plants, animals (including humans), and all types of combustion, such as auto exhaust, cigarette smoke, gas stoves, and incinerators. "Our bodies produce it as a necessary metabolite to sustain the life process," says the Formaldehyde Institute. "We could hardly live without it or without exposure to it."

188   "Economics" and "Formaldehyde," Formaldehyde Institute, 1986.

188   "Health," Formaldehyde Institute, 1986.

188   National Safety Council *Environment Writer*, September 1992.

188   "Formaldehyde: Determination of Significant Risk," *Federal Register*, Vol. 49, No. 101, May 23, 1984, pp. 21872–74.

189   EPA Science Advisory Board, "An SAB Report: Formaldehyde Risk Assessment Update," EPA-SAB-EHC-92–021, September 1992.

189   *Federal Register*, May 23, 1984, pp. 21873–94.

190   As cited by Mary Lamielle in *The Delicate Balance*, Fall/Winter 1989.

190   Jonathan M. Samet, Marian C. Marbury, and John D. Spengler, "State of Art: Health Effects and Sources of Indoor Air Pollution. Part II," *American Review of Respiratory Diseases 1988*, 137: 221–42.

190   Tracy Freedman, "Warning: Staying at Home Can Be Dangerous to Your Health," *Common Cause*, June 1982.

190   Jack Thrasher and Alan Broughton, *The Poisoning of Our Homes and Workplaces*, Santa Ana, California, Seadora, Inc., 1989, p. 6.

191   Thad Godish, "Indoor Air Quality Notes: Formaldehyde—Our Homes and Health," Ball State University Indoor Air Quality Research Laboratory, Summer 1989.

191   Kaye H. Kilburn, "Formaldehyde Impairs Memory, Equilibrium, and Dexterity in Histology Technicians," *Archives of Environmental Health*, 42(2):117–20, 1987.

191   Lamielle, Fall/Winter 1989.

191   Jack D. Thrasher, Roberta Madison, Alan Broughton, and Zane Gard, "Building-Related Illness and Antibodies to Albumin Conjugates of Formaldehyde, Toluene Diisocyanate, and Trimellitic Anhydride," *American Journal of Industrial Medicine* 15:187–95, 1989; Jack D. Thrasher, Alan Broughton, and Roberta Madison, "Immune

Activation and Autoantibodies in Humans with Long-Term Inhalation Exposure to Formaldehyde," *Archives of Environmental Health*, July/August 1990; Alan Broughton, Jack D. Thrasher, and Roberta Madison, "Biological Monitoring of Indoor Air Pollution: A Novel Approach," paper presented at Indoor Air '90, The 5th International Conference on Indoor Air Quality and Climate, Toronto, Canada, July 29-August 3, 1990.

191   Thrasher and Broughton, *The Poisoning of Our Homes and Workplaces*, 1989, p. 10.

192   Frank James, "Taking vertigo for a spin," *Chicago Tribune*, June 17, 1981.

192   Fred Pierce, "County Sued over Inmate-Made Desks," *Syracuse (New York) Post-Standard*, March 24, 1990.

193   Irwin Arieff, "Experts brainstorm about headaches," *Chicago Sun-Times*, July 1, 1991.

193   Irene Wilkenfeld, "Formaldehyde: A Dangerous Chemical," *The Human Ecologist*, Winter 1989.

194   "Urea Formaldehyde Foam Insulation," Illinois Department of Public Health, Division of Environmental Health, May 1990.

195   "Reaction," *Inkblots* (published by the Toronto branch of the Human Ecology Foundation of Canada), August 1982.

195   Peter Fossel, "Sick-Home Blues," *Harrowsmith*, September/October, 1987.

196   Debbie Goldberg, "Houses That Hurt," *Wall Street Journal*, May 19, 1989.

196   Karin Winegar, "Home Remedies: Designers, health experts search for nontoxic building materials," *Minneapolis Star Tribune*, September 3, 1989.

196   Thad Godish, "Indoor Air Quality Notes: Residential Formaldehyde Control," Ball State University Indoor Air Quality Research Laboratory, Summer 1986.

196   Godish, Summer 1989.

196   *Federal Register*, May 23, 1984, p. 21892.

197   "Formaldehyde," Indoor Air Pollution Fact Sheet, American Lung Association, August 1986.

200   Godish, Summer 1989.

Chapter 7

205   Barbara Reynolds, "'Cide means 'kill'; that's exactly what pesticides do," *USA Today*, April 22, 1991.

206   In 1991 Japanese physicians, having observed caddies with chronic symptoms, called for a ban on golf course pesticide use. In the U.S., breast cancer was dignosed in four women golf professionals in the years 1990–91.

206   John E. Davies, "Changing Profile of Pesticide Poisoning," *New England Journal of Medicine*, March 26, 1987, pp. 807–08. In India in the 1980s, with tragic irony, at least thirty-five desperate farmers

impoverished by buying pesticides to which local insects had developed resistance committed suicide, many using the very pesticide that had failed them.

207   U.S. General Accounting Office, "Pesticides: EPA's Formidable Task to Assess and Regulate Their Risks," GAO/RCED-86-125, April 1986, p. 10.

207   U.S. General Accounting Office, "Nonagricultural Pesticides: Risks and Regulation," GAO/RCED-86-97, April 1986, p. 8.

208   Beth Hanson, "Spoiled Soil," *Amicus Journal*, Summer 1989.

208   Marian Burros, "New Urgency Fuels Effort To Improve Safety of Food," *New York Times*, May 7, 1990.

208   Ward Worthy, "Pesticides, nitrates found in U.S. wells," *Chemical & Engineering News*, May 6, 1991.

208   Paul Gionet-Caine, "Progress cited in water quality: Runoff pollution from farms, parking lots, lawns a threat," *Chicago Tribune*, June 15, 1991.

208   Quoted by Barbara Mullarkey in *NutriVoice: a Health-Watch Newsletter*, Fall 1989-Winter 1990.

209   "Broad Scan Analysis of the FY82 National Human Adipose Tissue Survey Specimens," Volume 1 (Executive Summary), U.S.Environmental Protection Agency and Office of Toxic Substances, EPA-560–5-86–035, December 1986.

209   Joe Thornton, *Chlorine, Human Health and the Environment: The Breast Cancer Warning*, Washington, D.C., Greenpeace, 1993.

209   "Chlordane: Gone, But Not Forgotten," *Health & Environment Digest*, a publication of the Freshwater Foundation, December 1988.

210   "Pesticide Hazards: Public Citizen's Action Guide," February 1988.

210   C. Shannon Stokes and Kathy D. Brace, "Agricultural Chemical Use and Cancer Mortality in Selected Rural Counties in the U.S.A.," *Journal of Rural Studies*, Vol. 4, No. 3, 1988, pp. 239–47.

210   James R. Davis et al., "Family Pesticide Use in the Home, Garden, Orchard, and Yard," *Archives of Environmental Contamination and Toxicology*, Vol. 22, 1992, pp. 260–66; James R. Davis et al., "Family Pesticide Use and Childhood Brain Cancer," op cit., Vol. 24, 1993, pp. 87–92; and Lynn A. Gloeckler Ries et al., *Cancer Statistics Review 1973–1988*, Bethesda, Maryland, National Cancer Institute, 1991, p. II.32.

210   "Updates," *Health & Environment Digest*, a publication of the Freshwater Foundation, May 1989.

210   Sharon Begley, Mary Hager, and Judy Howard, "Dangers in the Vegetable Patch," *Newsweek*, January 30, 1989.

211   "Herbicide gets EPA's approval, with limits," *Chicago Tribune*, December 17, 1987.

211   Sonia L. Nazario, "EPA Under Fire for Pesticide Standards," *Wall Street Journal*, February 17, 1989.

211   Frank Falck Jr. et al., "Pesticides and Polychlorinated Biphenyl Residues in Human Breast Lipids and Their Relation to Breast Cancer, *Archives of Environmental Health*, Vol. 47, No. 2, March/April 1992, pp. 142–46.

212 Mary S. Wolff et al., "Blood Levels of Organochlorine Residues and Risk of Breast Cancer," *Journal of the National Cancer Institute*, Vol. 85, No. 8, April 21, 1993, pp. 648–52.

212 J.B. Westin, "Carcinogens in Israeli milk: a study in regulatory failure," *International Journal of Health Services*, Vol. 23, no. 3, 1993, pp. 497–517.

212 From the "editors' summary" of an article by Samuel S. Epstein and Shirley Briggs, "If Rachel Carson Were Writing Today: Silent Spring in Retrospect," *Environmental Law Reporter*, June 1987.

213 George W. Ware, *Pesticides: Theory and Application*, San Francisco, W.H. Freeman and Company, 1983, p. 151.

213 Bambi Batts Young, "Neurotoxicity of Pesticides," *Journal of Pesticide Reform*, Summer 1986.

213 "Manifestations of organophosphate insecticide poisoning," information provided in one-page handout from EPA Region VI, First International Building, 1201 Elm Street, Dallas, Texas 75270.

213 James E. Cone and Thomas A. Sult, "Acquired intolerance to solvents following pesticide/solvent exposure in a building: A new group of workers at risk for multiple chemical sensitivities," *Toxicology and Industrial Health*, Vol. 8, No. 4, July-August 1992.

214 William J. Rea, Joel R. Butler, John L. Laseter, and Ildefonso R. DeLeon, "Pesticides & brain-function changes in a controlled environment," *Clinical Ecology*, Summer 1984.

214 Warren P. Porter, Department of Zoology and Environmental Toxicology, University of Wisconsin (Madison), telephone conversation with Marjorie Fisher, March 5, 1991, reported in the *League of Women Voters/Lake Michigan Inter-league Group (LMILG) Spring Newsletter*, April 1991.

214 Tina Adler, "Pesticides' long-term effects get a closer look from EPA," *American Psychological Association Monitor*, December 1992.

215 "16 Million Americans Are Sensitive to Pesticides," press release from Serammune Physicians Lab, 11100 Sunrise Valley Drive, Reston, Virginia 22091, 1990.

215 William Legro, "Under Siege," *Organic Gardening*, April 1988.

216 G. Tyler Miller Jr., *Environmental Science*, third edition, Belmont, California, Wadsworth, 1991, pp. 313–17; as cited in *RACHEL'S Hazardous Waste News #240*, July 3, 1991.

216 U.S. Department of Agriculture, U.S. Environmental Protection Agency, National Research Council, as cited in the *Hartford Courant*, May 27, 1987.

216 Hendrik Hertzberg, "Summer's Blood," *Time*, August 10, 1992.

216 Obituary in the *Chicago Tribune*, September 21, 1990.

217 John B. Clark, "Notes from an Organic Farmer," *The Human Ecologist*, Spring 1990.

217 Daniel P. Jones, "Environmental fears, economic interests" *Hartford Courant*, May 27, 1987.

217 "Spokesman sees safer pesticides in industry's future," *Hartford Courant*, May 25, 1987.

218   Russell Clemings, "Pesticide probes questioned: Critics charge state's agriculture department is biased," *Fresno (California) Bee*, September 21, 1986.

218   "Governor Lowry bans pesticide," *VOICE* (a publication of Washington State's chemically disabled workers), Fall 1993.

219   Jo Sandin, "Years of pain: Family haunted by herbicide's lasting effects," *Milwaukee Journal*, May 3, 1990.

220   Gary Wisby, "Mosquitoes: Spring has stung," *Chicago Sun-Times*, May 5, 1991.

220   Samuel S. Epstein, talk in Glencoe, Illinois, sponsored by the League of Women Voters, April 24, 1991.

221   Grace Lichtenstein, "They're Poisoning Our Children," *Woman's Day*, November 27, 1990.

221   Patrick Quillin, *Safe Eating*, New York, M. Evans, 1990.

222   Bernadette Jorgensen, as told to Barbara Yost, "I'm Allergic to My Family," *Redbook*, April 1987.

223   U.S. Environmental Protection Agency, Office of Pesticide Programs, "Pesticide Industry Sales and Usage: 1990 and 1991 Market Estimates," H-7503W, Fall 1992.

223   Kirstie Alley, on NBC's "A Clearer Look," July 9, 1991.

223   Donella Meadows, "People Who Pay the Price of Our Dependency on Chemicals," *Plainfield (Connecticut) Valley News*, August 19, 1989.

224   Frank Edward Allen, "As Issue of Fertilizer Safety Takes Root, Firm's Feisty Commercials Burn Rivals," *Wall Street Journal*, April 26, 1991.

224   John Skow, "Can Lawns Be Justified?," *Time*, June 3, 1991.

224   Kathryne V. Sagan, "Poison in Your Backyard: The Pesticide Scandal," *Family Circle*, April 2, 1991.

225   Lorens Tronêt, "Housecalls to Main Street: Doctoring the Nation's Lawns with Chemicals," *Not Man Apart*, May-June 1986.

226   Jessica Seigel, "Opponents of lawn-care pesticides are proliferating," *Chicago Tribune*, April 18, 1990.

226   Janette Sherman, *Chemical Exposures and Disease*, New York, Van Nostrand Reinhold, 1988, p. 195.

227   Robert Abrams, "Lawn Care Pesticides Alert," New York State Department of Law, June 1989.

228   Porter, March 5, 1991.

228   Coralie R. Clement and Theo Colborn, "Herbicides and Fungicides: A Perspective on Potential Human Exposure," in *Chemically-Induced Alterations in Sexual and Functional Development: The Wildlife/Human Connection, Volume XXI, Advances in Modern Environmental Toxicology*, M.A. Mehlman, series editor, Princeton, New Jersey, Princeton Scientific Publishing Co., 1992.

229   W. Joseph Campbell, "Pesticides still sow unknown perils," *Hartford Courant*, May 24, 1987.

229   "Nonagricultural Pesticides: Risks and Regulation," April 1986, p. 35.

229   Office of the Inspector General, U.S. Environmental Protection

Agency, "Report of Audit: Labeling of Pesticides," September 30, 1992, p. ii, 31, 36, 39, 40.

229   U.S. General Accounting Office, "Lawn Care Pesticides: Risks Remain Uncertain While Prohibited Safety Claims Continue," GAO/RCED-90–134, March 1990.

230   Office of the Inspector General, September 30, 1992, p. 46.

230   Louis Marchi, "Secret 'Inert' Ingredients Compound Pesticide Toxicities," *The Human Ecologist*, Spring 1990.

230   Robert Abrams, "The Secret Hazards of Pesticides: Inert Ingredients," New York State Department of Law, June 1991; Frank Baird, president of a Philadelphia-area EI/MCS support group, has described an incident in which a salesman used a sophisticated device (called a capillary gas chromatograph/computerized mass spectrometer) to tell the owner of a chemical company exactly which chemicals had been used in the manufacture of one of the company's products. Thus, says Baird, "Any corporation which is curious about what is in a competitor's product can easily find out, if they don't already know. The only remaining reason for trade secrets is to prevent consumers from knowing."

231   Interview by Paul Orum in *Working Notes on Community Right-to-Know*, December 1990.

231   Stevenson Swanson and Linda P. Campbell, "U.S. Supreme Court OKs local restrictions on use of pesticides," *Chicago Tribune*, June 22, 1991.

232   Barbara Mullarkey, "A young hero speaks out in pesticide wars," *Wednesday Journal*, April 18, 1990.

232   Anastasia Toufexis, "Coming a Cropper: Du Pont faces charges it sold a tainted pesticide," *Time*, August 9, 1993.

232   "Iowa Supreme Court Refuses to Adopt Rule Requiring Epidemiological Evidence on Cause," *Occupational Safety & Health Reporter*, June 16, 1993.

233   Legro, April 1988.

233   W. Joseph Campbell and Daniel P. Jones, "Report highlights system's failures to identify tainted food," *Hartford Courant*, May 26, 1987.

Chapter 8

243   Bob L. Smith, "Organic foods vs. Supermarket Foods: Element Levels," *Journal of Applied Nutrition*, Vol. 45, No. 1, 1993.

243   Anne Mendelson, "Nutribabble," *Nation*, June 17, 1991.

244   "Problem: Contaminated Food," *Safe-Food Gazette*, March 1987.

244   "Extra-Label Drug Use Bills Draw Response," *Safe Food Action*, published by Americans for Safe Food, Autumn 1992.

244   Beatrice Trum Hunter, "Foodborne Disease: A Needless Epidemic," *NOHA (Nutrition for Optimal Health Association) NEWS*, Spring 1988.

245   Bruce Ingersoll, "Dairy Dilemma: Milk Is Found Tainted with a

Range of Drugs Farmers Give Cattle," *Wall Street Journal*, December 29, 1989.

246 Michael Woods, "Studies Show Public Fear of Pesticides Unfounded," *Chemecology*, July/August 1991.

246 U.S. Congress, Office of Technology Assessment, *Neurotoxicity: Identifying and Controlling Poisons of the Nervous System*, OTA-BA-36, Washington, D.C., U.S. Government Printing Office, April 1990, p. 50.

246 Rick Hind and Jim Baek, *Presumed Innocent: A Report on 69 Cancer-Causing Pesticides Allowed in Our Food*, U.S. Public Interest Research Group, 1990.

246 "Problem: Contaminated Food," March 1987.

246 Bill Lambrecht, "Despite government inspections, tainted food pouring into the U.S.," *San Antonio Express-News* (Scripps Howard Service), December 5, 1993.

246 Samuel S. Epstein and Jay Feldman, "'Negligible Risk' Is Still Much Too Great," *Los Angeles Times*, November 16, 1989.

247 David Steinman, *Diet for a Poisoned Planet*, New York, Harmony Books, 1990, p.26.

247 Steven Pratt, "Ruckus a la mode: *Diet for a Poisoned Planet* leaves some health officials with a bad taste," *Chicago Tribune*, November 1, 1990.

247 *Neurotoxicity*, April 1990, pp. 237–38.

247 "Problem: Contaminated Food," March 1987.

247 *Neurotoxicity*, April 1990, pp. 315–19.

249 "FDA Findings," *NutriVoice: A Health-Watch Newsletter*, Barbara Mullarkey, editor, Spring 1989.

250 "Reactions to NutraSweet Probed by Scientists," *Rodale's Allergy Relief*, May 1987.

250 Theodore E. TePas, "Trick or Treat?," *NOHA NEWS*, Fall 1990.

250 "Dyes in Your Food," from Public Citizen Health Research Group *Health Letter*, March/April 1985; in *Eating Clean2: Overcoming Food Hazards*, Center for Study of Responsive Law (undated); available from Eating Clean, P.O. Box 19367, Washington, D.C. 20036.

251 "FDA bans some uses of red additive," *Chicago Tribune*, January 30, 1990.

251 "Chemists Concoct New Taste Sensations," *Chemecology*, published by the Chemical Manufacturers Association, December 1990-January 1991.

251 Terry Kinney, "Supper secrets," *Chicago Tribune*, June 27, 1991.

252 George R. Schwartz, *In Bad Taste: the MSG Syndrome*, Santa Fe, New Mexico, HealthPress, 1988, pp. 2, 13, 25.

253 Donna Jacobs, "Campaign to uncover 'hidden' MSG," *Pioneer Press*, July 25, 1991.

254 "Problem: Contaminated Food," March 1987; also Beatrice Trum Hunter, "Non-Toxic Living: Unmasking Hidden Hazards," The Green Earth Lecture Series, Chicago, April 23, 1987.

254 Robert Cross, "Debate rages over the urethane, sulfite content of alcohol," *Chicago Tribune*, January 21, 1988.

255 "FDA Concerned about Contamination of Oil during Shipping," *Food Chemical News*, October 5, 1987.

256 James Wallace, "Lax truck checks charged: Whistle-blowers point finger at food firms," *Seattle Post-Intelligencer*, September 22, 1989.

258 Peter Montague, *RACHEL's Hazardous Waste News #356*, September 23, 1993.

258 "FDA needs more clout, panel finds," *Chicago Tribune*, May 16, 1991.

259 Glen Elsasser, "Food debate," *Chicago Tribune*, June 13, 1991.

259 Michael L. Millenson, "New FDA commissioner: Change not just 'idle talk,'" *Chicago Tribune*, May 24, 1991.

259 Marian Burros, "Eating Well," *New York Times*, November 6, 1991.

260 Bruce Ingersoll, "U.S. Is Ready to Limit What Food Processors Can Claim on Labels," *Wall Street Journal*, November 6, 1991.

260 Nancy Ryan and Linda M. Harrington, "FDA offers new rules on food labels, claims," *Chicago Tribune*, November 7, 1991.

260 Jan Schakowsky, "Buyers need data on chemicals," *Pioneer Press*, May 23, 1991.

261 Wade Roush, "Who Decides About Biotech?," *Technology Review*, July 1991.

261 Samuel S. Epstein, "Growth Hormones Would Endanger Milk," *Los Angeles Times*, July 27, 1989; letter to David Kessler, February 14, 1994; "A Needless New Risk of Breast Cancer," *L.A. Times*, March 20, 1994.

261 Pat Dailey, "Savior or folly, irradiation heads for a showdown," *Chicago Tribune*, January 13, 1994.

262 "'Pyramid' points to healthy diet," *Chicago Tribune*, April 29, 1992.

262 "A Pyramid Topples at the USDA," *Consumer Reports*, October 1991.

263 John Robbins, *A Diet for a New America*, Walpole, New Hampshire, Stillpoint Publishing, 1987, pp. 149–50.

263 Leo Galland, *Superimmunity for Kids*, New York, E.P. Dutton, 1988.

264 Joseph D. Beasley and Jerry J. Swift, *The Kellogg Report: The Impact of Nutrition, Environment & Lifestyle on the Health of Americans*, Amityville, New York, The Institute of Health Policy & Practice, 1989; now published as *The Betrayal of Health: The Impact of Nutrition, Environment, and Lifestyle on Illness in America*, New York, Times Books, 1991.

264 Joseph D. Beasley and Jerry Swift, as cited in "Our Optimal Nutrient Needs: What Are They and Can We Meet Them?," *NOHA News*, Spring 1990.

264 Jean Mayer, *A Diet for Living*, New York, David McKay Company, 1975.

265 Beatrice Trum Hunter, *The Sugar Trap and How to Avoid It*, Boston, Houghton Mifflin Company, 1982.

265 Beatrice Trum Hunter, "Food Health Claims: Fact vs. Fiction," *Consumers' Research*, May 1991.

266 About fish, a word of caution: both salt-and fresh-water fish have picked up toxic chemicals from the water they live in and from the food chain; and mislabeling, fish-market misinformation, and lax government inspection allow us to buy and consume contaminated fish. Furthermore, the Environmental Defense Fund has charged that an EPA survey of toxic chemicals in fish tissue "vastly underestimates human health risks from eating contaminated fish." Frustrated fish lovers can get some useful clues from David Steinman's *Diet for a Poisoned Planet*.

266 "Migraine Headaches and Food," interview of Dr. Jean Monro by Marjorie Hurt Jones, reported in *NOHA News*, Spring 1989.

267 Alan R. Gaby, "Food Allergy as a Cause of Chronic Illness," *Nutrition Connection*, Baltimore, Maryland, Consumers for Nutrition Action, 1989.

267 "Vary Those Veggies to Beat Pesticides," *New York Times*, July 12, 1993.

267 Michael Hirsley, "The Cave Menu," *Chicago Tribune*, May 13, 1987.

267 Working at the Land Institute in Salina, Kansas, agricultural researcher Wes Jackson would like to see our petroleum-based, wheat-corn-and-soy monoculture gradually replaced by a high-yield system of "polyculture perennials"—a mixture of plants that do not need to be started from seed every year and doused with expensive, wasteful, dangerous pesticides.

268 Michael A. Crawford and Sheilagh Crawford, *What We Eat Today*, London, Neville Spearman, 1972.

269 Bernard Rimland, "Nutrition, Behavior, and the Nutritional Supplement Controversy," talk to NOHA April 3, 1989; reported in *NOHA News*, Fall 1989.

269 "Vitamin, good diet help delay onset of AIDS," *Chicago Tribune*, September 5, 1993.

269 "Vitamins halt Cuban mystery epidemic," *Chicago Tribune*, September 30, 1993.

269 Jon Van, "'A carrot a day,' vitamin E found to cut heart risk," *Chicago Tribune*, November 14, 1991.

269 Meir J. Stampfer et al., "Vitamin E consumption and the risk of coronary disease in women," *New England Journal of Medicine*, May 20, 1993, pp. 1444–49; Eric R. Rimm, "Vitamin E consumption and the risk of coronary heart disease in men," *New England Journal of Medicine*, May 20, 1993, pp. 1450–66.

269 "Research boosts vitamins," *Chicago Tribune*, September 15, 1993.

269 "The Supplement Story: Can Vitamins Help?," *Consumer Reports*, January 1992.

270 Doug Levy, "Group urges pills to boost vitamin benefits," *USA Today*, March 4, 1994.

271 Jon Carroll, "The FDA offers protection from things that are good for us," *Boulder Daily Camera*, August 12, 1993.

271 "Americans Found Retreating From Healthy Eating Habits," *New York Times*, March 14, 1993.

Chapter 9

278 Doretta Zemp, "Scents of Trouble; For the Sensitive, Fragrances Can Trigger Problems," *Los Angeles Times*, September 18, 1991.

278 "Potential Health Hazards of Cosmetic Products," Hearings before the Subcommittee on Regulation and Business Opportunities of the Committee on Small Business, House of Representatives, Serial No. 100–67, Washington, D.C., U.S. Government Printing Office, 1989, p.2.

278 National Research Council, *Toxicity Testing: Strategies to Determine Needs and Priorities*, Washington, D.C., National Academy Press, 1984.

278 "Neurotoxins: At Home and the Workplace: Report to the Committee on Science and Technology, U.S. House of Representatives," Washington, D.C., U.S. Government Printing Office, 1989, pp. 1,2,5 and 6.

280 Peter S. Spencer, Monica C. Bischoff-Fenton, Oscar M. Moreno, Donald L. Opdyke, and Richard A. Ford, "Neurotoxic Properties of Musk Ambrette," *Toxicology and Applied Pharmacology* 75: 571–75, 1984.

280 D.L. Opdyke, editor, *Monographs on Fragrance Raw Materials*, published by the Research Institute for Fragrance Raw Materials, New York, Pergamon Press, 1979.

280 Transcript of first session of hearings before the Subcommittee on Investigations and Oversight, Serial 99–68, October 8 and 9, 1985, p. 18.

280 Peter S. Spencer and Monica C. Bischoff, "Skin as a Route of Entry for Neurotoxic Substances," in *Dermatoxicology*, third edition, Francis N. Marzulli and Howard I. Maibach, editors, Washington, D.C., Hemisphere Publishing, 1984.

281 Mary Lamielle, *The Delicate Balance*, Vol. 4, Nos. 3–4, 1991.

282 Opdyke, 1979.

282 Ronald S. Fenn, "Aroma Chemical Usage Trends in Modern Perfumery," *Perfumer & Flavorist*, March/April 1989.

282 Sherry Rogers, "Introduction to the Detoxication System: Part I," *20th Century Living*, reprinted in the Rocky Mountain Environmental Health Association newsletter, November-December 1991.

282 Reported by the Candida Research and Information Foundation (CRIF), 1991.

283 David W. Dunlap, "Sensitive Topic: Fighting Ads That Hit You in the Nose," *New York Times*, December 6, 1989.

283 Zemp, September 18, 1991.

284 Chang Shim and M. Henry Williams Jr., "Effect of Odors in Asthma," *American Journal of Medicine* 80:18–22, January 1986.

284 Zemp, September 18, 1991.

284 Rick Hampson, "Big stink raised over 'scent strips' in fragrance ads," *Arizona Republic*, August 26, 1990.

285 Amy Pagnozzi, "Get a whiff of this one," *New York Post*, June 8, 1989.

285 Paul Z. Bedoukian, "Perfumery and Flavor Materials: Bedoukian's 45th Annual Review," *Perfumer & Flavorist*, May/June 1989.

286 Laurie M. Grossman, "The Smell of Chanel May Be No. 2 Issue After Cigarettes," *Wall Street Journal*, May 13, 1993.

286 In 1989 one reader, "Choking," complained to "Dear Abby" about her coughing, wheezing, and severe headaches after receiving a scented *TV Guide*. A response to "Choking" brought the Human Ecology Action League (HEAL) more than four thousand responses from people affected by skunk mail and other scent exposures. Senator Connor's response to "Choking" brought him over a hundred letters, one saying "it almost feels like I've been exposed to toxic waste." According to a survey of 750 people done by D.J. Olson Market Research, the biggest headache for airline passengers is sitting next to a perfumed person.

286 Joanne Lipman, "Some Turn Up Their Noses At Magazine," *Wall Street Journal*, December 6, 1989.

287 Timothy Kalich, "What's in a Smell? The perfumes industry is now mainly a American one, and it has a problem or two," *Atlantic*, October 1987.

287 Anne B. Fisher, "Mark Laracy's Obsession," *Inc. Magazine*, May 1988.

287 Ralph Nader, "Introduction," *Being Beautiful*, Center for the Study of Responsive Law, 1986.

288 "Report to the [FDA] Commissioner in Response to January 5, 1989, Letter from the Honorable Ron Wyden Regarding Consumer Complaints of Adverse Effects Allegedly Caused by Cosmetic Products," from the FDA's Center for Food Safety and Applied Nutrition, unsigned.

288 Zemp, September 18, 1991.

288 Letter from Heinz J. Eiermann, dated November 21, 1989. Can we really avoid fragrances, as Eiermann suggests? Your nose tells you part of the answer. A 1990 survey by the Opinion Research Corporation tells you more: that American women now spend more than $2.5 million annually on fragrances, and more than 80 percent of the women polled said that they regularly use perfume or cologne, and apply it more than once daily. And men are fast catching up with women. A 1990 Gallup poll found that 89 percent of American men used after-shave or cologne at least once in the previous six months, that fully 50 percent use it five or more times a week, and that 33 percent use the stuff every day, often in "huge" amounts. Manufacturers, sensing a trend, have begun to follow the introduction of new perfumes for women by men's versions of the same scent—Passion for Women followed by the heavier, more "masculine" Passion for Men.

288 Letter from Janine E. Loosley, dated November 22, 1993.

289   Zemp, September 18, 1991.

289   Barbara MacKay, "Eau de wonders of the nose," *Chicago Tribune*, December 9, 1990.

289   Sandra Blakeslee, "Pinpointing the Pathway of Smell," *New York Times*, October 4, 1988.

289   William Mullen, "In the realm of the senses," *Chicago Tribune*, October 7, 1990.

290   Blakeslee, October 4, 1988.

291   William Booth, "The Sweet Smell of Success May Be Piped-in Peppermint," *Washington Post*, February 20, 1991.

291   Alix M. Freedman, "Search Is on for Emotion-Eliciting Scents," *Wall Street Journal*, October 13, 1988.

291   "Researchers Follow Their Noses to Ways of Improving Performance," *Chemecology*, April 1991.

291   "Air fresheners too foul, so firm shut," *Chicago Tribune*, March 13, 1990.

292   Beth Ann Krier, "Health seekers use common scents: Understanding nose-how of aromatherapy," *Chicago Sun-Times*, July 23, 1991.

292   Jon Anderson, "Perfume 'doc' detects the smell of excess," *Chicago Tribune*, March 21, 1991.

293   Grossman, May 13, 1993.

293   Katherine Bishop, "In a Bastion of Civil Liberties, a Yearning to Banish the Publicly Fragrant," *New York Times*, September 12, 1991.

293   Connie Lauerman, "Makeover: Environmental concern is changing the cosmetics industry," *Chicago Sun-Times*, April 28, 1991.

294   Jenifer Joyce, "Scent Suits May Be the Newest Tort Category," *Indoor Pollution Law Report*, November 1991.

294   "Dear Abby," *Chicago Tribune*, November 21, 1989.

295   Joyce, November 1991.

295   *Chicago Tribune*, January 14, 1987.

Chapter 10

299   Ken and Jan Nolley, "Of Heredity and Environment: Parenting Chemically Sensitive Children," *Journal of Pesticide Reform*, Summer 1986.

300   "Pesticides imprison me, boy tells senators," *Chicago Tribune*, March 29, 1990.

301   "So thoroughly has the age of poisons become established that [people] may walk into a store and, without questions being asked, buy substances of far greater death-dealing power than the medicinal drug for which [they] may be required to sign a 'poison book' in the pharmacy next door. A few minutes' research in any supermarket is enough to alarm the most stouthearted customers—provided, that is, [they have] even a rudimentary knowledge of the chemicals presented for [their] choice." These words were written more than thirty years ago by Rachel Carson, in her still-classic *Silent Spring*.

301 U.S. Congress, Office of Technology Assessment, *Neurotoxicity: Identifying and Controlling Poisons of the Nervous System*, OTA-BA-436, Washington, D.C., U.S. Government Printing Office, April 1990, pp. 4, 5, 8.

301 Beverly Paigen, "Children and Toxic Chemicals," *Journal of Pesticide Reform*, Summer 1986.

301 "Fetuses found exposed to asbestos," *Chicago Tribune*, April 12, 1992.

302 "Town links rare cancer, coal factory," *Chicago Tribune*, January 19, 1990.

303 Peter Korn, "The Persisting Poison," *Nation*, April 8, 1991; retired U.S. Admiral Elmo R. Zumwalt, Jr., believes that Agent Orange not only killed his soldier son but caused his grandson's learning disabilities.

303 Allan Bruckheim, *Chicago Tribune*, March 11, 1990.

304 John Elkington, *The Poisoned Womb: Human Reproduction in a Polluted World*, New York, Viking Penguin, 1985, pp. 48–49.

304 W.E. Daniell and T.L. Vaughan, "Paternal employment in solvent-related occupations and adverse pregnancy outcomes," *British Journal of Industrial Medicine* 45:193–97, 1988; "Study: Dads' smoke, kids' health tied," *Chicago Tribune*, January 24, 1991; Devra Lee Davis, "Fathers and Fetuses," *New York Times*, March 1, 1991; "Dads' Jobs Are Linked to Birth-Defect Risks," *Wall Street Journal*, December 11, 1991; Peter Montague, "Popular solvent, TCE, seems to cause serious birth defects in animals, humans," *RACHEL's Hazardous Waste News #267*, January 8, 1992; Peter Montague, "Male reproductive system is harmed by toxic exposures, causing birth defects, sterility," *RACHEL's Hazardous Waste News #321*, January 20, 1992.

304 Alan R. Gaby, "Decline in male fertility," *Townsend Letter for Doctors*, January 1993.

305 Edo D. Pellizzari et al., "Purgeable Organic Compounds in Mother's Milk," *Bulletin of Environmental Contamination and Toxicology*, Vol. 28, 1982; Walter J. Rogan et al., "Pollutants in Breast Milk," *New England Journal of Medicine*, Vol. 302, June 26, 1980; as cited in *RACHEL's Hazardous Waste News #193*, August 8, 1990.

305 Peter Schaffer, "Diagnosis Divides Doctors," *Syracuse (New York) Post-Dispatch*, March 15, 1989.

305 "Some baby products carry chemical risk," *Chicago Tribune*, November 24, 1991.

306 Paigen, Summer 1986.

306 Frederick W. Immerman and John L. Shaum, *Nonoccupational Pesticide Exposure Study (NOPES)*, EPA/600/S3–90/003, April 1990.

307 Peter Montague, *RACHEL's Hazardous Waste News #294*, July 15, 1992.

307 *Chicago Tribune*, December 21, 1990.

307 Peter Montague, *RACHEL's Hazardous Waste News #214*, January 3, 1991.

307 Kathy Anderson, "Toxics and Learning Disabilities: Putting Two

and Two Together," *Not Man Apart*, May-June 1986; David Bellinger et al., "Longitudinal Analyses of Prenatal and Postnatal Lead Exposure and Early Cognitive Development," *New England Journal of Medicine*, Vol. 316, No. 17, April 23, 1987.

308 *Dental & Health Facts: Foundation for Toxic-Free Dentistry Special Edition*, 1990.

308 Rebecca Bascom, *Chemical Hypersensitivity Syndrome Study*, prepared for the the State of Maryland Department of the Environment, March 1989.

309 Small and his wife, Barbara, started tutoring their daughter, Carolyn, at home after she developed frequent headaches when starting seventh grade in an Ontario school. The entire Small family is chemically sensitive; in *Sunnyhill: The Health Story of the 80s*, you can read the story of their return to health and of the beautiful new house and research center that they have built with safe, nontoxic building materials.

310 Don Knudson, "Toxic Chemicals: The Other Drug War," *The Lutheran*, November 8, 1989; also Don and Eline Knudson, "Managing High School and College with Chemical Sensitivities," *The Human Ecologist*, Fall 1990.

310 Anita Smith, "EI: When the world becomes hostile to staying healthy," *Benton Harbor/St. Joseph (Michigan) Herald-Palladium*, June 10, 1990.

311 Irene Wilkenfeld, letter to the editor, *South Bend (Indiana) Tribune*, June 26, 1990.

311 "Contaminated Classrooms," *Public Citizen*, September/October 1990.

311 Ellen Flax, "Pesticides in Schools: Focus Shifting From Indifference to Concern," *Education Week*, Vol. VII, No. 30, April 20, 1988.

312 Julie Accola, "A Look at IPM in One Arizona School," *The Human Ecologist*, Fall 1993.

313 First evidence of the threat from emfs came with physicist Louise Young's 1973 book *Power Over People*, which described the futile struggle of Ohio farmers to stop the construction of high-voltage lines over their property and warned of the dangers of living and working near high-voltage transmission lines.

313 Paul Brodeur, "Department of Amplification," *New Yorker*, November 19, 1990.

313 Peter Nye, "Grassroots Movement Seeks to Ground Electro-Magnetic Fields," *Public Citizen*, January/February 1994.

313 Sonia L. Nazario, "Children Become Centerpiece of Efforts to Set Tighter Restrictions on Pollutants," *Wall Street Journal*, October 15, 1990.

314 *Neurotoxicity*, April 1990, p. 8.

314 *American Association of Retired Persons Bulletin*, Washington, D.C., January 1991.

314 *Neurotoxicity*, April 1990, p. 9.

315 Sue Chastain, "The accidental addict: Are you hooked on your prescriptions?," *Modern Maturity*, February/March 1992.

315 Forrest G. Hester, director of Pharmacy Services, Memorial Medical Center, Springfield, Illinois, letter to the editor, *Chicago Tribune*, January 11, 1981.

315 *American Association of Retired Persons Bulletin*, January 1991.

316 Personal communication, 1993.

316 Debra Lynn Dadd, *Nontoxic & Natural: How to Avoid Dangerous Everyday Products and Buy or Make Safe Ones*, Los Angeles, Jeremy P. Tarcher, 1984, pp. 178–79.

317 Samuel S. Epstein, "The Chemical Jungle," *Multinational Monitor*, May 1989.

318 *Everyone's Backyard*, published by Citizen's Clearinghouse for Hazardous Waste, November/December 1993.

Chapter 11

323 Judith Berns, "An Interview with Dr. Randolph," *The Human Ecologist*, Fall 1989.

324 Julie Martoccio, "Ecological illness gaining official recognition," *Arlington Heights (Illinois) Daily Herald*, March 10, 1989.

324 Linda Davidoff, "Multiple Chemical Sensitivities: Research on Psychiatric/Psychosocial Issues," presented at the annual meeting of the APHA, November 13, 1991, and "Models of Multiple Chemical Sensitivity Syndrome: Using Empirical Data (Especially Interview Data) to Focus Investigations," presented at a workshop sponsored by the Association of Occupational and Environmental Clinics, September 21, 1991; as cited in AGES, Marie Laurin, editor, September 1993.

326 James M. Miller, "Workers' Compensation in New York State: This part of the 'safety net' could strangle you," *The Human Ecologist*, Winter 1990.

327 Merrill Goozner, "Proving job-related ills difficult, costly," *Chicago Tribune*, September 3, 1990.

329 David Halbrook, "Plea For Help: Workers' comp little recourse for MCS victims," *Longmont (Colorado) Times-Call*, July 8, 1991.

330 "Multiple Chemical Sensitivity," videotape by Greg Allen and Rudy Gallardo, 1993.

330 G. Heuser, A. Vojdani, and S. Heuser, "Diagnostic Markers of Multiple Chemical Sensitivity," *Multiple Chemical Sensitivities: Addendum to Biologic Markers in Immunotoxicology*, Washington, D.C., National Academy Press, 1992, pp. 117–38.

330 Lisa Morrow, Stuart R. Steinhauer, and Michael J. Hodgson, "Delay in P300 Latency in Patients with Organic Solvent Exposure," *Archives of Neurology* 49:315–20, 1992.

330 Thomas Callender, Lisa Morrow, Kodanallur Subramanian, Dan Duhon, and Mona Ristovv, "Three-Dimensional Brain Metabolic Imaging in Patients with Toxic Encephalopathy," *Environmental Research* 60:295–319, 1993.

330 Aristo Vojdani, Mamdooh Ghoneum, and Nachman Brautbar, "Im-

mune Alteration Associated with Exposure to Toxic Chemicals," *Toxicology and Industrial Health*, Vol. 8, No. 5, 1992; as cited in Cindy Duehring's "Environment Access Profiles."

330 Grace Ziem, talk presented at the Annual Meeting of the American Public Health Association, Washington, D.C., November 10, 1992.

331 U.S. Congress, Office of Technology Assessment,"Identifying and Controlling Immunotoxic Substances—Background Paper," OTA-BP-BA-75, Washington, D.C., U.S. Government Printing Office, April 1991, pp. 71–72.

331 "Analysis of Workers' Compensation Laws," U.S. Chamber of Commerce, p. viii, 1990 (as cited by Dr. John W. Ellis at the October 1990 meeting of the American Academy of Environmental Medicine).

332 Jerry Borrell, "Technology and Science Policy in the Late Twentieth Century: ELF Emissions," *MacWorld*, December 1990, p. 28.

332 "APA Files Amicus Brief in Neurotoxic Poisoning Court Case," *Psychological Science Agenda*, April/May 1991.

333 "Flight attendants sue tobacco firms," *Chicago Tribune*, November 1, 1991.

333 Michael Schroeder, "Did Westinghouse Keep Mum on PCBs?," *Business Week*, August 12, 1991; as cited in the National Safety Council's *Environment Writer*, September 1991.

334 Earon S. Davis and Mary Lamielle, "MCS New to Law, Medicine," *Indoor Pollution Law Report*, January 1992.

334 "Firm loses suit over dioxin leak," *Chicago Tribune*, February 2, 1992.

334 Patricia Kelsey, "'See You in Court' Say New Sick Building Victims," *Air Conditioning, Heating, and Refrigeration News*, December 5, 1988; reprinted in *The Reactor*, September-October 1989.

335 Constance Holden, "Science in Court," *Science*, March 1989.

335 Jon Van, "Ruling on 'junk science' may affect jury awards," *Chicago Tribune*, July 6, 1993.

336 Benjamin Weiser, "Salt Road's Covenant of Silence with Xerox: A secret settlement keeps health hazards from being made public," *Washington Post National Weekly Edition*, April 2, 1989.

337 Letter from HUD Assistant Secretary Timothy L. Coyle to Senator Frank R. Lautenberg, received October 26, 1990.

339 Letter to *The Reactor*, September-October 1989.

339 "Pesticide Use Violates Civil Rights," *Pesticides and You*, October 1990.

340 Raymond Cartwright, "Protecting Your Right to a Toxic-Free Home," *Pesticides and You*, June 1992.

340 Mario Donato and Stevenson Swanson, "Almost all-female army fighting city hall in suburban war on pesticides." *Chicago Tribune*, February 2, 1982.

340 "Drivers petition for safe buses," *The Reactor*, September-October 1989.

341 "Breathing easier in the hospital," *Modern Healthcare*, May 19, 1989.

341 ABC's "20/20," March 13, 1992.

341 Richard Price, "Nightmare on the border: Many blame toxic waste from Mexico," *USA Today*, October 27, 1993.

341 Phil Brown, "Popular Epidemiology: Community Response to Toxic Waste-Induced Disease in Woburn, Massachusetts," *Science, Technology, & Human Values*, Vol. 12, pp. 78–85, Summer/Fall 1987.

342 Jorge Casuso, "Black Tuesday for Big Green backers," *Chicago Tribune*, November 11, 1990.

342 Jim McNeill, "Getting a few things clear in L.A.," *In These Times*, January 22–28, 1992.

342 Susan Zeidler, "Environment is right to catch more polluters," *Chicago Tribune*, February 11, 1990.

343 "Firm Pleads Guilty in EPA Toxics Case," *San Francisco Chronicle*, August 27, 1991.

344 David Lapp, "A suite-crime bill worth emulating," *Chicago Tribune*, November 1, 1990.

344 "Indoor Pollution Can Pose Serious Threat," *Martinez (California) News Gazette*, November 21, 1991.

345 Marla Donato, "Pollution is the crime, ecocops are the cure," *Chicago Tribune*, January 2, 1991.

345 Carol Rose, "Duo tracks environmental crime for criminal prosecution," *Des Moines Register*, December 11, 1989.

345 Timothy Egan, "On his beat, 'Styro-Cop' looks for violators of plastic foam law," *Chicago Tribune*, May 10, 1990.

346 Report of the National Council on Disability, 800 Independence Avenue SW, Suite 814, Washington, D.C. 20591.

348 Thomas R. Bergerud and Joel Rodney, *Milwaukee Journal*, February 15, 1993.

349 Garrett De Bell, *The Environmental Handbook: Prepared for the First National Environmental Teach-in*, editor Garrett De Bell, New York, Ballantine, 1970, p. xiii.

350 J. William Hirzy, "The Other Voice from EPA: The Role of the Headquarters Professionals' Union," *Environmental Law Reporter*, February 1990.

350 "Daughter Raps Reagan," *Chicago Tribune*, April 19, 1990.

350 Peter Montague, *RACHEL'S Hazardous Waste News #315*, December 9, 1992.

351 Linnet Myers, "Crying foul: the bittersweet business of exposing corruption on the job," *Chicago Tribune*, March 2, 1989; from Myron and Penina Glazer, *The Whistle-Blowers: Exposing Corruption in Government & Industry*, New York, Basic Books, 1989.

352 William Sanjour, "Why EPA Is Like It Is," a talk to the Coalition for Health Concern, Kenlake, Kentucky, November 17, 1990; Sanjour's most cynical observations: "No one in EPA ever got sent to jail, or lost his or her job, or suffered any setback in his or her career for failing to do what the law required him or her to do and for which he or she was being paid; lots of people have ruined their careers in EPA by trying to do what the law required them to do and for which they were being paid."

353 William Sanjour, "Why EPA Is Like It Is and What Can Be Done About It," Annapolis, Environmental Research Foundation, 1992.

353 Adapted, with permission, from Susan Molloy's "Declaration of Rights for the Environmentally Hypersensitive."

354 Helen Moore, "The Nuisance Factor," *Prairie Street Companion*, December 1986.

Chapter 12

358 Joseph D. Beasley and Jerry J. Swift, *The Kellogg Report: The Impact of Nutrition, Environment, & Lifestyle on the Health of Americans*, Amityville, New York, The Institute of Health Policy and Practice, 1989; also published as *The Betrayal of Health: The Impact of Nutrition, Environment, and Lifestyle on Illness in America*, New York, Times Books, 1991.

361 Office of Technology Assessment, "Assessing the Efficacy and Safety of Medical Technologies," September 1978, pp. 4,7.

361 Michael L. Millenson, "Many medical procedures may be unneeded," *Chicago Tribune*, March 21, 1991.

361 "9,479 Questionable Doctors," Public Citizen Health Research Group *Health Letter*, July 1991.

361 "Malpractice: A Straw Man," *Consumer Reports*, July 1992.

361 Jon Van, "Doctors prescribe some white lies, new study reports," *Chicago Tribune*, May 26, 1989.

362 "Drug Alert," Public Citizen Health Research Group *Health Letter*, September 1990.

363 Sue Chastain, "Calling the shots: More parents are demanding the right to pick and choose the vaccinations their children receive," *Chicago Tribune*, May 19, 1991.

364 "Upjohn says it will sue critic of Halcion," *Chicago Tribune*, January 21, 1992.

364 "Updates," Public Citizen Health Research Group *Health Letter*, March 1991.

364 Michael L. Millenson, "Consumer concerns put focus on FDA safety reviews," *Chicago Tribune*, January 26, 1992.

364 "Researchers give high marks to new asthma, hay fever drugs," *Chicago Tribune*, January 26, 1992.

365 Frank Edward Allen, "One Man's Suffering Spurs Doctors to Probe Pesticide Drug Link," *Wall Street Journal*, October 14, 1991.

365 "Chronic Use of Pain Relievers Can Cause Kidney Failure and Cancer," Public Citizen Health Research Group *Health Letter*, March 1991.

367 "Inexpensive pills may be arthritis elixir," *Chicago Tribune*, July 11, 1991.

367 "More Than One Million Implants Need to be Replaced Annually: Better Pre-Market Testing Needed," Public Citizen Health Research Group *Health Letter*, May 1991.

368   Herbert Burkholz, "A Shot in the Arm for the F.D.A.," *New York Times Magazine*, June 30, 1991.

368   "FDA Drags Its Feet on Enforcing Medical Device Reporting Violations," Public Citizen Health Research Group *Health Letter*, October 1989.

369   "When Safety Is Secret," *Public Citizen*, January/February 1991.

370   Jane Meredith Adams, "Victim of silicone breast implants wants value placed on women's lives," *Chicago Tribune*, February 9, 1992.

370   "Implant impact," *Chicago Tribune*, February 23, 1992.

370   "Questions about Silicone Gel Breast Implants," Public Citizen Health Research Group *Health Letter*, March 1992.

371   R.M. Goldblum et al., "Antibodies to silicone elastomers and reactions to ventriculoperitoneal shunts," *Lancet* 340:510–13, 1992.

371   David F. Horrobin, "The Philosophical Basis of Peer Review and the Suppression of Innovation," *Journal of the American Medical Association*, March 9, 1990, pp. 1438–41.

372   Beasley and Swift, 1989.

373   Karen Wright, "Going by the Numbers," *New York Times Magazine*, December 15, 1991.

373   Barbara Graham, "Exploring the 'other medicines,'" *Chicago Sun-Times*, April 23, 1991.

373   Steven T. Taylor and Morton Mintz, "A Word From Your Friendly Drug Co.," *Nation*, October 21, 1991.

374   Donna Shaw, "Abuse alleged in drug marketing to doctors," *Chicago Tribune*, January 2, 1991.

376   "New Drug Company Bribes for Doctors," Public Citizen Health Research Group *Health Letter*, January 1991.

376   Carla Atkinson and John Geiger, "Just Say No? When Drug Companies Make Offers Doctors Can't Refuse," Public Citizen Health Research Group *Health Letter*, March/April, 1991.

376   "Drug repackaging companies a presciption for controversy," *Chicago Tribune*, June 12, 1989.

376   "Medicine's rewards irk Americans, survey says," *Chicago Tribune*, March 31, 1993.

377   "Miracle Drugs or Media Drugs?" *Consumer Reports*, March 1992.

378   Adriane Fugh-Berman, "The Case for 'Natural Medicine,'" *Nation*, September 6/13, 1993.

379   "Study looks at unproven cancer care," *Chicago Tribune*, April 25, 1991.

379   Tom Peters, "Ounce of caring can lessen health industry woes," *Chicago Tribune*, November 9, 1992.

379   Madeline Drexler, "Hostile Environment," *Boston Globe Magazine*, November 1989.

380   James L. Bryant, letter to the editor, *New England Journal of Medicine*, October 17, 1991, pp. 1171–72.

381   Earon S. Davis, letter to the editor, *Resident and Staff Physician*, July 1990.

382   Richard L. Doty et al., "Olfactory Sensitivity, Nasal Resistance, and Autonomic Function in Patients with Multiple Chemical Sensitivi-

ties," *Archives of Otolaryngology and Head and Neck Surgery* 114:1422–27, December 1988.

382   Christopher M. Ryan, Lisa A. Morrow, and Michael Hodgson, "Cacosmia and Neurobehavioral Dysfunction Associated with Occupational Exposure to Mixtures of Organic Solvents," *American Journal of Psychiatry* 145(11):1442–45, November 1988.

382   William J. Meggs and Crawford H. Cleveland Jr., "Rhinolaryngoscopic Examination of Patients with the Multiple Chemical Sensitivity Syndrome," *Archives of Environmental Health*, January/February 1993.

383   Iris R. Bell, Claudia S. Miller, and Gary E. Schwartz, "An Olfactory-Limbic Model of Multiple Chemical Sensitivity Syndrome: Possible Relationships to Kindling and Affective Spectrum Disorders," *Biological Psychiatry* 32:218–42, 1992.

383   Marco Kaltofen, letter to the editor, *Chemical & Engineering News*, September 24, 1990.

384   Mistaken therapies like these have led jokesters to describe the triple blind test developed since those times: "The participants don't know what they're taking. The nurses don't know what they're giving. And the investigators don't know what they're doing." A good example is a Finnish study of 612 men treated for high blood pressure and elevated cholesterol by a combination of diet and drugs. After fifteen years, cardiac deaths were 2.4 times higher in the "prevention" group than in the controls. Deaths from all causes, including accidents and suicides, were 45 percent higher in the "prevention" group. This study, which *should* have been stopped sooner than it was, indicates that even controlled studies are a slow, flawed way of arriving at some truths.

384   C. Everett Koop, *Koop: The Memoirs of America's Family Doctor*, New York, Random House, 1991, p. 190.

385   Associated Press, as cited in *The Daily Northwestern*, May 22, 1987.

385   Ronald Kotulak, "Mind pollution: Scientists fear modern life may be poisoning the psyche," *Chicago Tribune*, May 13, 1988.

385   Paul Galloway, "Dr. Detective: Physician's books clue readers in to neurological mysteries," *Chicago Tribune*, June 20, 1990.

385   Nicholas A. Ashford, "New Scientific Evidence and Public Health Imperatives," *New England Journal of Medicine*, April 23, 1987.

385   M.S. Marion and M.J. Cevette, "Tinnitus," *Mayo Clinic Proceedings* 6:614–20, 1991; as cited in Public Citizen Health Research Group *Health Letter*, September 1991.

386   David R. Francis, "Why the medical bill keeps growing," *Christian Science Monitor*, November 18, 1991.

387   Richard J. Sagall, "Speaking My Mind—Medical School Secrets," *Pediatrics for Parents*, September 1991.

388   Beasley and Swift, 1989, p. 84.

Chapter 13

393 Susan Jeffers, *Brother Eagle, Sister Sky*, New York, Dial Books, 1991.

395 *Chicago Tribune*, June 20, 1993.

395 Casey Bukro, "Toxic signs on rise in Great Lakes," *Chicago Tribune*, September 18, 1988.

398 "Responsible Care: A Public Commitment," *Chemecology*, October 1992.

399 Earon S. Davis, "Environmentalism and Public Health after the Reagan Era: Finding a Balance That Will Protect Both People and Their Environment," *Ecological Illness Law Report*, June 1988.

401 JoAnn Gutin, "Plastics A-Go-Go," *Mother Jones*, March/April 1992.

401 Diane Brown, letter to the editor, *Chicago Tribune*, October 15, 1991.

402 Casey Bukro, "From coercion to cooperation: For industry and an environmentally aware public, prevention is better than pollution," Special Report on Ecology, *Chicago Tribune*, November 17, 1991.

402 Ellen Blum Barish, "When exercising takes your breath away," *The Good Health Magazine (Chicago Tribune)*, April 28, 1991.

402 Lou Marchi, "Non-Combustion Sources of Pollution," *Conscious Choice*, July/August 1992.

403 Casey Bukro, "A guide to helping the Earth," Special Report on Ecology, *Chicago Tribune*, November 17, 1991.

403 Ellen Freilich, "Manufacturers hopping aboard 'green' consumer bandwagon," *Chicago Tribune*, January 2, 1990.

403 Casey Bukro, "Environmental marketing ripe for shady green claims," *Chicago Tribune*, April 22, 1991.

404 Casey Bukro, "In '90s, the color of money is 'green'," *Chicago Tribune*, August 31, 1992.

405 Sheryl De Vore, "Be it resolved: to protect environment," *Pioneer Press*, December 26, 1991.

407 Juliet Schor, *The Overworked American: The Unexpected Decline of Leisure*, New York, Basic Books (Harper/Collins), 1991.

407 Smithsonian program, transcribed for *Ecolife*, March 1992.

407 Jerry Mander, "The Media and Environmental Awareness," in *The Environmental Handbook: Prepared for the First National Environmental Teach-in*, Garrett De Bell, editor, New York, Ballantine Books, 1970.

408 Karin Winegar, "The upscale learn to scale down," *Chicago Tribune*, January 3, 1991.

409 American Psychological Association, "National Health Objectives for the Year 2000," *Science Agenda*, Winter 1990.

409 Don Marquis, "the life and times of archy and mehitabel," New York, Doubleday & Co, 1935.

410 Committee on Neurotoxicology and Models for Assessing Risk, National Research Council, *Environmental Neurotoxicology*, Washington D.C., National Academy Press, 1992.

410   Wendell Berry, as quoted by Bill McKibben in "Prophet in Kentucky," *New York Review of Books*, June 14, 1990.

411   Wendell Berry, "Economy and Pleasure," *What Are People For?*, San Francisco, North Point Press, 1990, pp. 141–44.

412   "Databank: New Poll," *Common Ground*, July/August 1992.

413   Donella H. Meadows, Dennis L. Meadows, Jørgen Randers, and William W. Behrens III, *The Limits to Growth: A Report for the Club of Rome's Project on the Predicament of Mankind*, New York, Universe Books, 1972, p. 150.

Chapter 14

415   In 1968 the *New York Times* commissioned poet Archibald MacLeish to memorialize the Apollo 8 mission to the moon. MacLeish wrote the following: "To see the earth as it truly is, small and blue and beautiful in that eternal silence where it floats, is to see ourselves as riders on the earth together, brothers on the bright loveliness in the eternal cold—brothers who know now they are truly brothers."

416   Rachel Carson, *Silent Spring*, New York, Fawcett World Library, 1962, pp. 17–18.

417   Samuel S. Epstein and Shirley Briggs, "If Rachel Carson Were Writing Today: *Silent Spring* in Retrospect," *Environmental Law Reporter* 17:10180, June 1987.

417   Josh Barbanel, "PCBs may be culprit in seals' mysterious illness," *Chicago Tribune*, January 14, 1992.

418   "Statement from the Work Session on 'Chemically Induced Alterations in Sexual Development: the Wildlife/Human Connection,'" a preliminary report from the Wingspread workshop, Racine, Wisconsin, July 26–28, 1991; Theo Colborn and Coralie Clement, editors, *Chemically-Induced Alterations in Sexual and Functional Development: The Wildlife/ Human Connection, Volume XXI, Advances in Modern Environmental Toxicology*, M.A. Mehlman, series editor, Princeton, New Jersey, Princeton Scientific Publishing Co., 1992.

419   Thomas A. Mably, Robert W. Moore, Donald L. Bjerke, and Richard E. Peterson, "The Male Reproductive System Is Highly Sensitive to In Utero and Lactational TCDD Exposure," *Banbury Report 35: Biological Basis for Risk Assessment of Dioxins and Related Compounds*, Cold Spring Harbor Laboratory Press, 1991.

419   Janet Raloff, "The Gender Benders," *Science News*, January 8, 1994.

419   Janet Raloff, "That Feminine Touch: Are men suffering from prenatal or childhood exposures to 'hormonal' toxicants?," *Science News*, January 22, 1994.

419   Janet Raloff, "EcoCancers," *Science News*, July 3, 1993.

420   Jon R. Luoma, "New Effect of Pollutants: Hormone Mayhem," *New York Times*, March 24, 1992.

420 Raloff, January 8, 1994.

420 Mary O'Brien, "Scientific Evidence Grows on Endocrine Disruption by Persistent Organochlorines," *Zero Discharge News*, Spring 1992.

420 Theo Colborn, "Listening to the Lakes: Faltering Great Lakes Wildlife Populations Point the Way to Human Health Hazards," *Pesticides and You*, June 1992.

421 James Brooke, "Chernobyl Said to Affect Health of Thousands in a Soviet Region," *New York Times*, November 3, 1991.

421 Peter Montague, *RACHEL's Hazardous Waste News* #372, January 13, 1994.

422 Peter Montague, *RACHEL's Hazardous Waste News* #355, September 16, 1993.

423 W.K. Burke, "As the World Burns," *In These Times*, March 18–24, 1992.

423 "Bush shift on ozone-depleting chemicals," *Chicago Tribune*, February 12, 1992.

423 In 1984 CFCs from a plane's rain repellent invaded the plane's cockpit high over California, causing chemical injury to one of the pilots, who sued and won $2,454,000.

424 Pamela Zurer, *Chemical & Engineering News*, May 28, 1993; as cited in "*Post* and *Times* Coverage Prompt Unusual Rebukes," National Safety Council's *Environment Writer*, July 1993.

424 In the early 1980s women using 1,1,1-trichloroethane to clean telephone parts in a New Mexico electronics plant won workers' compensation for their manifested confusion, disorientation, muscle weakness, and balance and memory problems; their workbenches were "practically swimming" in the chemical, said their lawyer.

425 Stephen Jay Gould, in *Earth Ethics*, edited by Thomas Barrett, as cited in *Common Ground*, March/April 1992.

425 Casey Bukro, "In 1990s, environment may be politically explosive issue," *Chicago Tribune*, December 31, 1989; Barry Commoner, *The Closing Circle*, New York, Alfred A. Knopf, 1971, pp. 33–48.

425 Julie Hutchinson, "Doctor offers a prescription to heal the planet," *Chicago Tribune*, April 26, 1992.

425 Chris Petrakos, "How mankind can grow a new mind," *Chicago Tribune*, August 15, 1989, in a review of *New World New Mind: Moving Toward Conscious Evolution*, New York, Doubleday, 1989.

425 *Chicago Tribune*, March 6, 1994.

426 Kaye H. Kilburn, "Conserve Brains First, Else All May Be Lost," *Archives of Environmental Health*, May/June 1993.

426 Susan Cooper, introduction to article by Theo Colborn in *Pesticides and You*, June 1992.

427 David Warsh, "2 'eco' systems come together in theory, practice," *Chicago Tribune*, May 24, 1992.

427 Herman E. Daly, from "Covering the Environment," *Gannett Center Journal*, Summer 1990; as cited in the *Chicago Tribune*, October 30, 1990.

429 Barry Commoner, *Making Peace with the Planet*, New York, Pantheon, 1990, p. 196.

Afterword

433 "America's Nuclear Shame, Part 3: The Scientists," transcript of CNN special, March 13, 1994.

Index

Abrams, Robert, 227, 229, 311
Adamkus, Valdus, 351
adaptation to chemicals, 36, 280
after-shave lotion, risks from, 147
Agency for Toxic Substances and Disease Registry (ATSDR): funding to study EI/MCS, 74; on secrecy in legal cases, 336
air "fresheners," 60, 291, 386; risks from, 146; removal of, 347
alachlor, 210
alcoholism, 267
aldicarb, 248
aldrin, 332
alkylphenol novolac resin, 120, 256
allergies: as altered reactivity, 33; as IgE-mediated, 33; to corn, 265; to food, 256, 266, 380; to grains, 25, 267
Alley, Kirstie, 223
American Academy of Environmental Medicine (AAEM), 41, 359
American Chemical Society: number of new chemicals, 108; on the ozone layer, 424
Americans with Disabilities Act (ADA), 345-348; right to breathe, 346
amyotrophic lateral sclerosis (ALS), 52
animal victims of chemicals, 417-420; Florida panther, 419; immune-system damage, 417; toxic chemicals in

whales, 417; Wingspread conference, 418
antiperspirants, 123
arthritis, 36, 44, 367
Ashford, Nicholas, 33, 106, 384, 385
aspartame, 249
asthma, 52; and perfume, 293; occupational hazard, 114; side effects of drugs used for, 364; substances that can trigger, 52
autoimmune diseases, 53
Baker, Gordon, 108, 117, 329
baking out, 112
Barsky, Arthur, 50
Beasley, Joseph D., 51, 263, 372; drugs vs. nutrients, 387; on modern medicine, 358; on self-care, 386
Becker, Charles, 53
bedding, safe and unsafe, 152
Beebe, Glenn and Sharon, 176
benzene, 101, 110, 113, 121, 133, 304, 328; in carpeting, 181; in cigarette smoke, 51, 60; in drinking water, 145; in umbilical cords, 50; lawsuit concerning, 331; where found, 37
Berry, Wendell, 410
Berthold-Bond, Annie, 223, 405
betanaphthylamine, 124, 127
Bhopal, India, 70
Bierman-Lytle, Paul, 114, 137, 196

biological markers for chemical injury, 43, 329

birds, pet, killed by chemicals, 54

birth defects, 302; and toxic industrial chemicals, 128

Blumberg, Jeffrey, 270

Bower, John and Lynn, 135

Boxer, Robert W., 295

Brodeur, Paul, 212, 313

Broughton, Alan, 181, 191

Brower, David, 394, 426

butadiene, 329, 335

buying aids: researching what you buy, 153

Caldicott, Helen, 425

canaries, human, in workplaces, 103

cancer: and pesticides, studies of, 209-212; breast cancer, 211, 317; from chemicals, foods, and pesticides, 39; in children and the elderly, 210, 314; in Kanawha County, West Virginia, 75; in Mahoning Valley, Ohio, 106; lower survival rates for blacks, 110; of the bladder, workers with, 125; present and projected rates of, 39; treatment of, 379

candida, 16, 33, 49, 386

carbon tetrachloride, 60, 133

Carnow, Bertram, 105, 402

carpeting: adverse health effects from, 174-177; chemicals in, 175-176; dust in, 148, 177; in EPA headquarters, 169; in schools, 309; lawsuits concerning, 176, 179, 182; number of chemicals in, 181; testing of, by Anderson Laboratories, 181; union's petition about, 178; warning labels for, 182

Carson, Rachel, 20, 30, 146, 212, 394; publication of *Silent Spring*, 41, 416

Cartwright, Raymond, 340

chemical injury, 36, 75, 82, 106, 112, 224, 329, 359; Bill of Rights for those with, 353; recourse through lawsuits, 331-337; recourse through the ADA, 346

Chemical Injury Information Network (CIIN), 55

chemical sensitivity: difficulties of coping with, 48; incidence of, 32, 51; increase in, 74; possible mechanism of action, 382; recovering from, 49; support groups for, 49, 55-56

chlordane, 123, 209; in imported beef, 247

chlorine: compounds of, a major problem, 67; in drinking water, alternatives for, 146

chloroform: in indoor air, 60, 133; in umbilical cords, 50

chlorpyrifos, lawsuit concerning, 233, 332

Christmas decorations, risks from, 150

chronic fatigue syndrome (CFS), 33, 49

Clark, John B. and Merrill, 216, 245

clean air, none left, 75

cleaning products: safer, 155; toxic, 112, 141

Clement, Coralie, 228

clinical ecology, 41

Colborn, Theo, 66, 228, 419, 420

command and control, 69; failure of, 75-80

Commoner, Barry: five laws of ecology, 425; on buying green, 403; on safer substitutes, 428; pollution an incurable disease, 69

computers, risks from, 149

Cone, James, 122

Connor, Martin, 283

continuing-education courses on environmental medicine, 42

corporate crime, 342-345

cosmetics: absorption into the bloodstream, 282; inadequate toxicity testing of, 278; injuries caused by, 278; number of chemicals in, 278

cosmetics and the FDA, 287-288

Crohn's disease, 267

Cullen, Mark R., 51, 116, 359

cyanide, 136; in tobacco smoke, 51

Dadd, Debra Lynn, 112, 293, 316, 408

Davis, Devra Lee, 316, 372

Davis, Earon, 179, 324, 333, 381, 399

DDT: and breast cancer, 211; in Great Lakes, 64; on cotton crops, 151; persistence of, 221

depression: associated with chemicals,

382; incidence of, 385; secondary to EI/MCS, 381

detergents, scented, 282

detoxification, 16-18, 28-29

diapers, risks from, 147

diethylstilbestrol (DES), 363

dimethylformamide, 116

dioxin, 78, 153; in Agent Orange, 119, 302; in semen, 304; in the workplace, 119

disinfectants, 147, 386, 426

dose-related curve, 10, 383

double-blind study, the, 43, 381, 384, 422

drinking water: chemicals in, 145; outdoor air pollution and, 64-66

drug marketing: abuses of, 373-377; and doctors' incomes, 376; Congressional hearings on, 374; effect on doctors of, 375

drug research, 371-373; mistaken priorities, 372; sources of bias, 371

drugs and the FDA, 363-366

drugs, prescription and nonprescription: additive effects, 365; deaths from, 360; "disease shifting," 364; insufficient testing of, 362; insufficient reporting of side effects of, 363; mistakes in prescribing, 362; misuse of, 360; side effects of analgesics, 365

dry cleaning, 27, 60, 123, 133

Eaton, S. Boyd, 267, 317

economic growth, 412

economy vs. ecology, 426

Ehrlich, Paul, 425

EI/MCS: other names for, 33-37; severe cases of, 46-48

elderly, the: dangers to, from chemicals, 313-316; overuse of medications, 314; toxic cleaning products in nursing homes, 316

electromagnetic fields (emfs): in schools, 313; lawsuit concerning, 332; risks from, 143

environmental control unit, 44-45, 384

Environmental Health Association of Dallas, 55

Environmental Health Center, Dallas, 41

Environmental Health Network (EHN), 55

environmental medicine, attacks on, 379-386

environmental organizations, 395-399; industry influence on, 397; lack of attention to human health by, 395; wrong focus of, 400-406

environmental refuges, 47-49

EPA: air pollution standards, 68; and indoor air, 59-62, 81, 172; good and bad, 351-353; history of, 348-350; TEAM study, 59

EPA and carpeting: costs to taxpayers, 173; early warnings, 169; employees' petition, 178; policy dialogue, 180; workers developing EI/MCS, 167-170

epidemiology, popular, 341

Epstein, Samuel S.: cancer rates, 39; need for labeling of pesticides in food, 258; on hormones in meat, 317; on wrong pesticide safety data, 246; pesticide misuse, 220, 224; rBGH, 261; runaway chemical technology, 29, 417

ethanol-based products, risks from, 111

ethylene dibromide, 208

fabric softeners, 141, 225, 339; in diapers, 147; scented, 282

fabrics, risks from, 151

Fairechild, Diana, 234

Falck, Frank, 211

Farnsworth, Norman, on herbs, 388

FDA: see cosmetics and the FDA; drugs and the FDA; food and the FDA

Feldman, Jay, 224, 231, 246

fetuses, dangers to, from chemicals, 301-304

food: from depleted soils, 268; irradiation of, 261; over-reliance on grains, 267; sources of drug-free beef, 245; structural fats, 268; what to eat, 265-268; whom to believe, 261-265

food and the FDA: Delaney Clause, 257; *de minimus* rule, 257; Environmental Working Group study of pesticides, 257; FDA's inadequacies, 258; labeling, 258; NAS study of pesticide risk to children, 257; rBGH, 260

food, chemicals in: acquired while en route to the consumer, 255; additives, 248-253; antibiotics, hormones, and veterinary drugs, 243-245; dyes, 250; flavorings, 251; from packaging, 254; MSG, 252; pesticides, 245-248; sweeteners, 249, 265; waxes, 253

food supplements, 268-271; effectiveness of, 269; safety of, 268

formaldehyde: adverse health effects, 190; and cancer, 188; and the immune-system, 191; from insulation, 193; from mattresses, 112; from particleboard, 134, 195; from pillowcase, 26; government standards for, 200; handling problems with, 198; in carpeting, 176; list of products containing, 202; most at risk from, 197; testing for, 197; unsafe levels of, 196

4-phenylcyclohexene (4-PC), 171

fragrances: and asthma, 283; and babies, 292; aroma industry, 285-287; coping with others' use of, 295; individual differences, 289; ingredients unknown, 286; lawsuits concerning, 294; neurotoxicity of, 280; number of chemicals in, 278; secondhand scents, 290-293; toxic chemicals from, in indoor air, 281; toxic chemicals in, 281; toxicity of, 281-283

full-spectrum light, 139

furniture, risks from, 148

Gaby, Alan R., 267, 304

Galland, Leo, 263

Gibbs, Lois, 89

global warming, 422

glycol ethers: in common products, 153; in electronics industry, 118; in printing industry, 115

Godish, Thad, 156, 190, 196, 199, 200

Gould, Stephen Jay, 335, 425

Great Lakes, pollution in, 64-67

green, a murky hue, 402-406

Greider, William, 76, 124

Gulf War veterans, 118; chemical expo-

sures of, 53; environmental unit for, 45

hay fever, 52

hazardous occupations, 109; aerospace and computer industries, 117; armed forces, 118; chemical industry, 110; chlorine-based industries, 119; construction, 113; farming, 109; garment industry, 115; health care industry, 110-113; landfill and toxic waste industries, 121; office work, 99, 120; printing industry, 114

hazardous workplaces, 304; arts and crafts, 312; beauty shops, 279; dry-cleaning shops, 123; florists and nurseries, 123; laboratories, 101, 110; picture-framing shops, 328

headache clinic, 21

headaches: and food, 266; cause of, 29, 32; incidence of, 53; migraine, 19, 32, 266; number of chemicals that can cause, 53; severity of, 22

health care, U.S.: cost of, 46; dissatisfaction with, 360; insufficient testing of medical procedures, 361; need for outcomes research, 360; often inappropriate, unnecessary, ineffective, negligent, or dangerous, 360-362; role of medical schools, 378

healthy homebuilding, 134-140

healthy office buildings, 138

heating system, 140, 141

Heuser, Gunnar, 330

Hirzy, J. William, 172, 350, 351

home furnishings, safer, 140-153

Horner, Beth, 220

housing and HUD, reasonable accommodation, 337-339

Human Ecology Action League (HEAL), 55

Humber, Randy, 340

Hunter, Beatrice Trum, 244-265

illnesses with environmental component, 51-54

implants and other devices: risks from, 367-371; lack of action by the FDA, 368; lawsuits concerning silicone breast implants, 369

incineration: costs of, 79; dangers from, 77; dangers from, to workers, 122

indoor air pollution: deaths from, 62, 133; greater risks from, 60; lack of attention to, 60; lack of funding for, 61; sources of, 62; study of, in ten public buildings, 82; TEAM study, 59

Indoor Air Quality Act: of 1989, hearings on, 167, 171; of 1991, 81; of 1993, 171

industrial accidents involving chemicals, 106

infants and children, dangers to, from chemicals, 304-308

informed consent, need for, 383, 431

insect repellents, risks from, 150, 306

integrated pest management (IPM), 222, 233, 311

International Joint Commission (IJC), 66, 427

isocyanates, 78, 82, 114, 330; in Bhopal, India, 70; in carpeting, 174; in Galesburg, Illinois, 71; in Institute, West Virginia, 70

Jaffe, Russell, 214

job-related illness: court cases concerning, 116-117; incidence of, 103; lack of response to, 104; misdiagnosis and misreporting of, 108; types of, 105

Kawasaki syndrome, 177

Kennedy, Joseph, 171

Kerr, William D. Jr., 22

Kilburn, Kaye, 425

Kinney, Joseph, 171

Lamielle, Mary, 333, 345

Landrigan, Philip, 103, 104

Lautenberg, Frank R., 337

Lawson's Laws, 318

lead poisoning, 306, 310; from paint, lawsuit concerning, 332

lead, risks from, 144

learning disabilities and chemicals, 307

leather products, risks from, 153

Levin, Alan S., 35, 215, 233

Levine, Herb, 347

Lieberman, Allan, 99

Lively-Diebold, Bobbie, 171, 351

living with less, 406-410

Love Canal, New York, 50, 301, 305

malathion, 220

Marchi, Louis, 230, 402

Martin, Richard W., 53

McLellan, Robert K., 121

Mekdeci, Betty, 302

mercury poisoning, 111, 142, 307

methyl bromide, 223

methyl chloroform: see 1,1,1-trichloroethane

methyl ethyl ketone, 115, 281

methylene chloride, 112, 329; as "inert" ingredient, 213; in indoor air, 281; in paint strippers, 142

migraines, 19, 32, 266

Miller, Claudia, 33, 106

Miller, James M., 115, 121, 326

Mitchell, George, 81, 167

Molloy, Susan R., 293, 340, 345, 353

monosodium glutamate, 252

Monro, Jean, 266

Montague, Peter: chemicals in mothers' milk, 304; industry's output of chemicals, 50; "gold standard," 90; on the EPA, 350; on global warming, 422; use of toxic wastes in pesticides, 231

Moore, Helen, the nuisance factor, 354

Moses, Marion, 207-231

Mott, Lawrie, 208

MSDSs, 127, 295

Mukatis, W. Alfred, 101

multiple chemical sensitivities, recognition of, by EPA, 172

"mystery" illnesses, 53, 118, 417

Nader, Ralph, 124, 250, 287

National Academy of Sciences (NAS), incidence of chemical sensitivity, 32

National Center for Environmental Health Strategies (NCEHS), 55

National Human Adipose Tissue Survey (NHATS), 27, 73, 208

National Safe Workplace Institute, 103

natural gas, 111, 223; combustion products from stoves using, 142

negative-ion generator, 28

neurotoxicity: risks of, for children, 306; in the workplace, 107; lack of testing for, 104, 281

NIOSH: bulletins by, 124; lack of notification of endangered workers, 125; toxic chemicals in cosmetics, 279

Nutrition for Optimal Health Association (NOHA), 266

O'Brien, Mary H., 230, 239, 420

O'Connor, John, 89

occupational illness: see job-related illness

occupational risks, lack of media coverage of, 126

Occupational Safety and Health, Committees on, 123

Oetzel, Mary, 140

1,1,1-trichloroethane, 65, 115; as "inert" ingredient, 213; as ozone-depleter, 423; in indoor air, 281; toxicological profile of, 424

organic chemicals, national output of, 50

organic farming, 216

organic produce, more nutrients in, 242

organic solvents, workplace exposure to, neurotoxic effects of, 107

orrisroot, 21

OSHA, 213; ineffectiveness of, 124-125; lack of support from, 116

Ott, John, 139, 312

ozone layer depletion, 422-424

Paigen, Beverly, 301, 305

paint, toxicity of, 113

panic disorder, 53

paper products, risks from, 152

paradichlorobenzene, 60, 133, 151; in air "fresheners," 291

Parkinson's disease, 52

PCBs, 15; and breast cancer, 211; in Great Lakes, 64; in semen, 304; lawsuit concerning, 333

PELs, 125

pentachlorophenol, 138, 170, 433

perchloroethylene, 60, 123, 133; in Christmas decorations, 150

perfume: see fragrances

pesticides: and cancer, studies of, 209-212; and the "Casey" decision, 231; carbamates, 214; "circle of poison," 221, 247; commercial and government use of, 219-222; deaths from, 205, 231; doctors' lack of recogni-tion of poisoning by, 225; false advertising of, 229; farm use of, 216-219; FIFRA, 229; fraudulent testing of, 228; GAO reports about, 227; home, garden, and lawn use of, 222-227; hotline information ignored, 230; immune-system effects of, 214; in blood, 27; in body fat, 208; in drinking water, 145; in groundwater, 208; in rain, 208; in semen, 304; inadequate regulation and testing of, 227-230; increasing use of, 215; "inert" ingredients in, 230; IPM, 222; lawsuits concerning, 231-233; loss of effectiveness of, 216; neurotoxicity of, 213; organophosphates and organochlorines, 210-214; risks to migrant farm workers, 218; school use of, 222; use of B.t. for gypsy moths, 220; use of malathion for medflies, 220; use of, in mosquito abatement, 219; use of, on planes, 234; where encountered, 207

PET scans, 329

petroleum: from spills, 37; products from, 38

phenol, 299

phenol-formaldehyde resins, 118

phthalic anhydride, 330

plants, cleaning indoor air, 156

Plumlee, Lawrence, 170

pollution prevention, 67, 80, 89, 428; Greenpeace policy on, 70; in the workplace, 128

polycyclic aromatic hydrocarbons (PAHs), in carpeting dust, 148, 177

Porter, Warren P., 214, 228

pressure-treated wood, risks from, 138, 207

public health professionals, lack of attention to EI/MCS, 399

QUEEGs, 329

rain barrel effect, 34, 38

Randegger, Ed and Suzanne, 35

Randolph, Theron G., 23-27, 111, 134, 170, 299, 310, 323, 416; alcoholism as form of grain addiction, 267; and the environmental control unit, 23, 41, 384; dangers to teachers, 317;

dismissal of, 378; effect of petro-chemicals on health, discovery of, 40, 415

Rea, William J., 36, 222; and the environmental control unit, 41; and the EPA, 170; and safe homebuilding, 139; and SBS, 85; named First World Professor of Environmental Medicine, 41

recourse through individual efforts, 339-342

reproductive system: effect of chemicals on, 128, 304, 418-421; estrogen-mimicking chemicals, 419

right-to-know, 70, 125, 397

Rimland, Bernard, 268

risk assessment, 86-92

Roberts, Elyse, 224

Rogers, Sherry, 41, 46, 299, 379; on babies' environments, 305; on cosmetics, 282

Ross, Gerald, 317

rotation diet, 24-26, 266; for maintaining weight loss, 267

Roueché, Berton, 212

rubber latex: in carpeting, 183; toxicity of, 113

Ryan, Kevin, 231, 300

Samuels, Jack, 253

Sanders, Bernard, 180

Sanjour, William, 351-353

Schakowsky, Jan, 260

schools: arts and crafts, 312; dangers to children, from chemicals, 308-313; fluorescent lighting in, 312; IPM in, 311; pesticides in, 311; sick school syndrome, 310

Schwartz, George R., 252

sensitization to chemicals, 34, 71, 82, 172, 223, 383

Shapiro, Steve, 161, 351

Share, Care, and Prayer, 55

Sherman, Janette, 107, 205, 226, 228

Shields, Megan, 16

Shrier, Dona, 151

sick building syndrome: and architects, 121; causes of, 61; costs of, 62, 84; lawsuits concerning, 84, 335; prevalence of, 61, 120; recognition of, by

EPA, 82, 172; sick school syndrome, 310; symptoms of, 51

Slocum, Marna, 324

Small, Bruce, 309

smog, urban, 72

soap pads, risks from, 144

soaps, antibacterial, risks from, 112, 154, 223, 254, 316

social security disability, obtaining benefits, 324-326

specific etiology, doctrine of, 42

SPECT scans, 329

Spencer, Peter, 279

Spengler, John, 121, 190

sperm count, worldwide drop in, 53, 421

Steinman, David, 246

Stevenson, Adlai, 425

Stone, Thomas, 36

styrene, 329; in carpeting, 175; in drinking water, 145; in packaging, 254, 345; in tankers, 255; in umbilical cords, 50

sulfites, in alcohol, 253

support groups, 49, 225; list of, 55

Swift, Jerry, 263

TEAM study, 59, 172, 308

television sets and video cassette recorders, chemical fumes from, 149

TePas, Theodore, 250

third line medicine, 42

Thoreau, Henry David, 393, 408

Thrasher, Jack, 181, 191

threshold limits, need to discard, 125

tobacco smoke, secondhand, 51, 133, 308; danger to fetuses from, 304; lawsuit concerning, 333

toluene, 101, 110, 113, 116, 121, 329; in body fat, 27, 73; in carpeting, 176; in drinking water, 145; in indoor air, 281; in printing industry, 115; lawsuit concerning, 331; where found, 38

toxic chemicals: in baby products, 305; safer substitutes for, 128, 428

toxicity, lack of testing for, 105

toxicological profiles, 74, 424

Toxics Release Inventory (TRI), 71-73; chemicals reported in, 65

toxics use reduction, 81, 89, 428
toxic waste dumps, cost of cleaning up, 79
trichloroethylene, in drinking water, 145, 343
triclocarban and triclosan, toxicity of, 154, 316
trimellitic anhydride, 330
Tronêt, Lorens, 225
U.S. Congress, environmental Acts and agencies, 67-68
universal reactors, 47
urethane, in alcohol, 254
ventilation problems, 83-86; ASHRAE standards, 85
vitamins and minerals, research on, 269
Vojdani, Aristo, 330
volatile organic compounds (VOCs), 348; cancer risk from, 60; in paint, 142; study of, in indoor air, 82, 281
Werbach, Melvyn R., 42, 263

Wilkenfeld, Irene, 193, 311
Wisner, R. Michael, 16
Wolfe, Sidney, 124, 375, 383
Wolff, Mary S., 211
women, more at risk, 316-318
workers' compensation, difficulty of obtaining benefits: in Colorado, 329; in Illinois, 327; in New York State, 326; in Washington State, 329
workers, endangered, lack of notification of, 125
worldwide health damage, 421
Wyden, Ron, 278, 287, 288, 376
xylene, 110, 113, 329; as "inert" ingredient, 213, 231; in body fat, 73; in carpeting, 176; in drinking water, 145; in indoor air, 281; in printing industry, 115; where found, 38
Young, Bambi Batts, 107, 213
Ziem, Grace, 34, 368
Zuckerman, Adie, 34